Sustainable Approaches in Pharmaceutical Sciences

Sustainable Approaches in Pharmaceutical Sciences

Edited by

Kamal Shah
Professor of Pharmaceutical Chemistry
Institute of Pharmaceutical Research, GLA University,
Mathura, India

Durgesh Nandini Chauhan
Assistant Professor
Columbia College of Pharmacy, Raipur, India

Nagendra Singh Chauhan
Senior Scientific Officer Grade-2
Drugs Testing Laboratory Avam Anusandhan Kendra,
Government Ayurvedic College Campus, Raipur, India

WILEY Blackwell

This edition first published 2024

Registered Offices
John Wiley & Sons, Inc., 111 River Street, Hoboken, NJ 07030, USA
John Wiley & Sons Ltd, The Atrium, Southern Gate, Chichester, West Sussex, PO19 8SQ, UK

For details of our global editorial offices, customer services, and more information about Wiley products visit us at www.wiley.com.

Wiley also publishes its books in a variety of electronic formats and by print-on-demand. Some content that appears in standard print versions of this book may not be available in other formats.

A catalogue record for this book is available from the Library of Congress

Hardback ISBN: 9781119889847; ePub ISBN: 9781119889861; ePDF ISBN: 9781119889854;
oBook ISBN: 9781119889878

Cover Image: © Marchu Studio/Shutterstock
Cover Design: Wiley

Set in 9.5/12.5pt STIXTwoText by Integra Software Services Pvt. Ltd, Pondicherry, India
Printed and bound by CPI Group (UK) Ltd, Croydon, CR0 4YY

C9781119889847_201023

Contents

List of Contributors

Dina A. Ahmed
Analytical Chemistry Department
Faculty of Pharmacy
Cairo University
Cairo, Egypt

Imran Ali
Department of Chemistry
Jamia Millia Islamia
Jamia Nagar, New Delhi, India

Maha Mohammad AL-Rajabi
Faculty of Chemical Engineering &
Technology and Centre of Excellence for
Biomass Utilization (CoEBU)
Universiti Malaysia Perlis (UniMAP)
Arau, Perlis, Malaysia

Ashish Baldi
Pharma Innovation Lab, Department of
Pharmaceutical Sciences and Technology
Maharaja Ranjit Singh Punjab Technical
University
Bathinda, Punjab, India

Shiv Bahadur
Institute of Pharmaceutical Research
GLA University
Mathura, UP, India

Muhammad Bilal
School of Life Science and Food
Engineering
Huaiyin Institute of Technology
Huaian, China

Martina Bonelli
Department of Medicine and Aging
Sciences, Section of Legal Medicine
University of Chieti–Pescara 'G. d'Annunzio'
Chieti, Italy

Pedro Brandão
Egas Moniz Center for Interdisciplinary
Research (CiiEM) and Egas Moniz School
of Health & Science
Caparica, Portugal

Rishita J. Chauhan
Department of Pharmaceutical Chemistry
and Quality Assurance
L. M. College of Pharmacy
Ahmedabad, Gujarat, India

Durgesh Nandini Chauhan
Columbia College of Pharmacy
Raipur, India

Nagendra Singh Chauhan
Drugs Testing Laboratory Avam
Anusandhana Kendra
Raipur, CG, India

Ugo de Grazia
Fondazione IRCCS Istituto Neurologico
Carlo Besta
Laboratory of Neurological Biochemistry
and Neuropharmacology
Milan, Italy

Cristian D'Ovidio
Department of Medicine and Aging Sciences, Section of Legal Medicine
University of Chieti–Pescara 'G. d'Annunzio'
Chieti, Italy

Tejas M. Dhameliya
Department of Pharmaceutical Chemistry and Quality Assurance
L. M. College of Pharmacy
Ahmedabad, Gujarat, India

Anuradha K. Gajjar
Department of Pharmaceutical Chemistry and Quality Assurance
L. M. College of Pharmacy
Ahmedabad, Gujarat, India

Taruna Grover
Department of Chemistry
Lovely Professional University
Jalandhar-Delhi, Punjab, India
Aarti Industries Research and Technology Center
Dhirubhai Ambani Knowledge City
Navi Mumbai, Maharashtra, India

Nazim Hussain
Centre for Applied Molecular Biology (CAMB)
University of the Punjab
Lahore, Pakistan

Jegam Noel Joseph
Chemistry of Heterocycles and Natural Product Research Laboratory
Department of Chemistry, School of Advanced Sciences
Vellore Institute of Technology
Vellore, Tamil Nadu, India

Abuzar Kabir
International Forensic Research Institute, Department of Chemistry and Biochemistry
Florida International University
Miami, FL, USA

Marcello Locatelli
Department of Pharmacy
University of Chieti–Pescara 'G. d'Annunzio'
Chieti, Italy

Hayam M. Lotfy
Analytical Chemistry Department
Faculty of Pharmacy
Cairo University
Cairo, Egypt

Rajesh K. Maheshwari
Department of Pharmacy
SGSITS
Indore, Madhya Pradesh, India

Somdutt Mujwar
Chitkara College of Pharmacy
Chitkara University
Rajpura, Punjab, India

Atish S. Mundada
SNJBs SSDJ College of Pharmacy
Neminagar, Chandwad
Nashik, Maharashtra, India

Subh Naman
Pharma Innovation Lab, Department of Pharmaceutical Sciences and Technology
Maharaja Ranjit Singh Punjab Technical University
Bathinda, Punjab, India

Reem H. Obaydo
Analytical Chemistry Department
Faculty of Pharmacy
Ebla Private University (EPU)
Aleppo, Syria

Deepak D. Patil
K.K. Wagh College of Pharmacy
Nashik, Maharashtra, India

Marta Pineiro
Coimbra Chemistry Centre (CQC)–Institute of Molecular Sciences (IMS)
Department of Chemistry
University of Coimbra
Coimbra, Portugal

Radhika
Institute of Pharmaceutical Research
GLA University
Mathura, UP, India

Hassan Rafique
Centre for Applied Molecular Biology (CAMB)
University of the Punjab
Lahore, Pakistan

Selvaraj Mohana Roopan
Chemistry of Heterocycles and Natural Product Research Laboratory
Department of Chemistry, School of Advanced Sciences
Vellore Institute of Technology
Vellore, Tamil Nadu, India

Enrica Rosato
Department of Pharmacy
University of Chieti–Pescara 'G. d'Annunzio'
Chieti, Italy

Yasmin Rostom
Analytical Chemistry Department
Faculty of Pharmacy
Cairo University
Cairo, Egypt

Muhammad Usama Saeed
Centre for Applied Molecular Biology (CAMB)
University of the Punjab
Lahore, Pakistan

Sarah S. Saleh
Analytical Chemistry Department
Faculty of Pharmacy
October University for Modern Sciences and Arts (MSA)
Giza, Egypt

Victoria Samanidou
Laboratory of Analytical Chemistry, Department of Chemistry
Aristotle University of Thessaloniki
Thessaloniki, Greece

Fabio Savini
Pharmatoxicology Laboratory
Hospital 'Santo Spirito'
Pescara, Italy

Joseph Selvin
Chemistry of Heterocycles and Natural Product Research Laboratory
Department of Chemistry, School of Advanced Sciences
Vellore Institute of Technology
Vellore, Tamil Nadu, India

Kamal Shah
Institute of Pharmaceutical Research
GLA University
Mathura, UP, India

Sanyam Sharma
Pharma Innovation Lab, Department of Pharmaceutical Sciences and Technology
Maharaja Ranjit Singh Punjab Technical University
Bathinda, Punjab, India

Angela Tartaglia
Department of Pharmacy
University of Chieti–Pescara 'G. d'Annunzio'
Chieti, Italy

Teow Yeit Haan
Department of Chemical and Process Engineering and Research Centre for Sustainable Process Technology (CESPRO)
Faculty of Engineering and Built Environment
Universiti Kebangsaan Malaysia
Bangi, Selangor Darul Ehsan, Malaysia

Halil Ibrahim Ulusoy
Department of Analytical Chemistry
Faculty of Pharmacy
Cumhuriyet University
Sivas, Turkey

Maulikkumar D. Vaja
Department of Pharmaceutical Chemistry
Saraswati Institute of Pharmaceutical
Sciences
Gandhinagar, Gujarat, India

Preface

This book is aimed at an audience of advanced-level students, experts, and scientists working in the design, synthesis, analysis, and isolation of pharmaceuticals using green approaches. The field of pharmaceutical sciences will always remain in demand. As was seen in the COVID-19 pandemic, medicine plays a vital role in society. The demand for it cannot be overlooked. This book consists of all the possible facets or resources that may minimise the adverse effects associated with synthesis, isolation, or extraction, so that these possible approaches will save human and environmental health. Readers from different fields (students, researchers, industrialists, scientists) will get all the best green approaches associated with the development, design, or origination of pharmaceuticals.

The book has 11 chapters authored by scientists around the globe. Chapter 1 focuses on green technologies, the benefits associated with them, white biotechnology, and green chemistry. The impact of green approaches in the pharmaceutical industry is considered regarding the use of greener solvents, nanoparticle formulation, antimicrobial bandages, and green synthesis of drugs. This chapter will be useful for researchers, scientists, or industrialists who are working in the areas of green technologies or green chemistry.

Chapter 2 discusses green approaches to designing active pharmaceutical ingredients. This chapter narrates various ways like microwave irradiation technology, ultrasound-mediated synthesis, molecular sieving, and grinding and milling techniques. These methods are considered sustainable technologies and have become part of a valuable green protocol to produce pharmaceutically active drugs.

Chapter 3 covers the topic of microextractive methods capable of generating high recovery values for the analytes even from very complex matrices. The chapter includes techniques such as dispersive liquid–liquid microextraction, microextraction by packed sorbent, liquid–liquid extraction, solid-phase microextraction, solid-phase extraction, and fabric-phase sportive extraction. These techniques have been widely applied in many fields including bioanalysis, ecology, food, natural compounds, forensic science, and toxicology. This chapter examines recent applications of these novel procedures, highlighting the main benefits and outcomes that have been reported in the literature. Special attention is given to green approaches and the development of innovative procedures that have been optimised in agreement with green analytical chemistry principles.

Chapter 4 considers the impact of green sustainable approaches in the pharmaceutical industry. This chapter adopts the concept of minimising the utilisation of hazardous material, an approach in which scientists are effectively working to the 12 principles applicable for the betterment of the chemical strategy adopted. The numerous benefits of the exploration of green chemistry on a commercial scale are discussed along with the bioresources, chemical manufacturing, and organic transformation that affect the industrial process. The principles of green chemistry are elaborated by giving various examples compared to conventional methods at the industrial level.

Chapter 5 describes techniques of analysis that involve the selection of an appropriate solvent so as to achieve the sustainability of a chemical production process. Green methods using hydrotropy, mixed hydrotropy, and mixed solvency are simple, cost-effective, and safe. Mixed hydrotropic solubilisation also overcomes the use of a large concentration of hydrotropic agents that are required in monohydrotropy. The mixed solvency approach renders green analytical methods utilisable in ultraviolet spectrophotometric analysis, titrimetric analysis, thin-layer chromatography, high-performance liquid chromatography, and also in formulation. A systematic approach to experimentation is lacking. The different blends used in mixed solvency have not received systematic development and a rational approach. The proper justification for the use of components in a blend is missing. It is an opportunity for researchers to systematically utilise a mixed solvency approach for spectrophotometric development and formulation.

Chapter 6 discusses the role of and need for artificial intelligence (AI) in drug targeting, drug design, identification, and prediction of probable mechanisms of action. The chapter also narrates the prediction of the biological behaviour of a newer molecule to know whether it is going to possess therapeutic potency or not and also to identify the associated problem that is supposed to be obstructing its pharmaceutical impact. The chapter shows the path of the AI-based drug discovery process over the traditional wet lab-based hit-and-miss methods, which is essentially utilised in the drug discovery regime prior to moving to experimental procedures.

Chapter 7 emphasises hydrogels as a topical drug-delivery system and the role of green chemistry in developing functionalised hydrogels for drug delivery. Green chemistry plays a critical role in functionalised hydrogels in the pharmaceutical industry for the formulation of effective and safe systems for drug delivery. Recent developments in hydrogels that respond to specific trigger factors during topical drug delivery are also outlined. Finally, the adoption of green chemistry in developing functionalised hydrogels is discussed.

Chapter 8 is based on advanced approaches in green univariate spectrophotometric methods based on basic mathematical techniques, such as subtraction, division, and multiplication, for assaying the components of multicomponent mixtures in their different pharmaceutical dosage forms utilising inexpensive, affordable, and ecofriendly facilities. The pharmaceutical industry and market has shown a tremendous evolution where different new pharmaceuticals and pharmaceutical combinations have been introduced in order to increase patient compliance and obtain the required outcomes. At the same time, this evolution has raised a challenge in the field of drug analysis, where new applicable methods of analysis need to be developed and validated to ensure that the right doses will reach patients free from any undesired compounds such as impurities, adulterants, or interfering substances that may lead to undesirable side effects.

Chapter 9 provides details about the basic mechanism of cyclodextrin inclusion complex formation by grinding, discussing various challenges associated with the grinding process and different techniques of grinding, with the identification of critical material attributes, critical process parameters, and critical quality attributes through an Ishikawa fishbone diagram and criticality assessment by quality risk management based on the quality target product profile. The insights into this green chemistry quality by design approach provide a case study for creating complex molecular structures through multicomponent reactions and solvent-free synthesis on an industrial scale with consistent quality.

Chapter 10 focuses on the production of carbon nitride quantum dots from bulk graphitic carbon nitride (g-C_3N_4) and their applications. The chapter outlines the synthesis of quantum dots, with bulk g-C_3N_4 serving as a major contributor and numerous top-down subsidiary methods being employed. The photon emission efficiency of the subtypes of methods that have been performed can be seen clearly in their quantum yields. Even though the technique has proven to be extremely useful, there are still a number of application fields that need to be explored where there is scope for improvement.

Chapter 11 discusses mechanochemical approaches that have several advantages for active pharmaceutical ingredient (API) synthesis, from access to unexplored reactivity to high compliance with sustainability parameters and green chemistry principles. The wide variety of apparatus, the number of variables to optimise, and safety concerns regarding scale-up procedures remain some of the most relevant challenges in years to come in the field of mechanochemistry. The still fairly unexplored field of continuous manufacturing under mechanochemical conditions might open the door to new, safer, and cleaner API synthesis protocols, easily applied in the industrial setting. The chapter will inspire scientists, medical professionals, or industrialists to work on green technology or synthesis in the pharmaceutical sciences.

Last, but not least, we would like to express our earnest gratitude to all the authors who have taken time from their busy schedules to be part of this endeavour and offered impeccable chapters that added both magnitude and significance to this book. We welcome suggestions and criticisms from our readers. Special thanks are due to our families for their sustenance and inspiration. We express our acknowledgement to the publishing and production team, especially Bhavya Boopathi and her team, for their substantial, skilful, and motivating management.

Kamal Shah
Durgesh Nandini Chauhan
Nagendra Singh Chauhan

1

Green and Sustainable Approaches in Pharmaceutical Sciences

Shiv Bahadur[1], Radhika[1], Durgesh Nandini Chauhan[2], Nagendra Singh Chauhan[3] and Kamal Shah[1]

[1] *Institute of Pharmaceutical Research, GLA University, Mathura, UP, India*
[2] *Columbia Institute of Pharmacy, Raipur, CG, India*
[3] *Drugs Testing Laboratory Avam Anusandhana Kendra, Raipur, CG, India*

CONTENTS

1.1 Introduction

The pharmaceutical industry contributes around $1.27 trillion to the global economy, making it one of the world's largest contributors. At the same time, these businesses emit around 1.9 million metric tonnes of carbon dioxide each year. Environmental protection is a constant goal for the regulatory agencies that oversee various sectors across the world, including pharmaceuticals. Sadly, however, firms' in-house systems are not as good as they should be. Several creative concepts for environmental protection have been developed, but most of them have failed because of a lack of engagement with the world's largest pharmaceutical companies [1, 2].

New environmentally friendly, safe, and effective pharmaceuticals are the goal of all pharmaceutical firms. In order to achieve this goal, the industry must switch from synthetic to eco-friendly materials. Companies in a number of sectors have begun to use green chemistry techniques in an attempt to replace their old-fashioned ways of manufacturing [3]. Ecologically friendly green chemistry's primary goals are to maximise energy efficiency, reduce waste, and employ renewable energy sources for power generation.

Sustainable Approaches in Pharmaceutical Sciences, First Edition. Edited by Kamal Shah, Durgesh Nandini Chauhan, and Nagendra Singh Chauhan.

Green chemistry may help limit the amount of waste products that are generated throughout the process of synthesis, such as solvents, contaminants, and exhausted reagents. Pharmaceutical corporations have broad influence in this area and could make significant contributions. As a result, it is important to investigate various green chemical methods and discover the gaps in their use [4].

In the pharmaceutical industry, green chemistry techniques are in great demand and have been developed in recent decades within a new approach that addresses issues such as pollution, limited environmental resources, and renewable sources of materials. The pharmaceutical industry is under increasing pressure to improve both its production efficiency and the implications of its products as environmental degradation and better testing procedures are becoming more widely known. Employing green chemistry practices does not necessarily equate to cost-effectiveness, however. Incorporating the concepts of green chemistry may be seen as an extra challenge, and the commercialisation of green technology is being thwarted by a lack of capital investment [5].

In order to implement green processes, various modifications must be made to the lengthy global supply chain. In addition to intellectual property and fail-fast requirements, challenges such as safety and the occupational health management of those participating in the process must be considered. Although green chemistry lessens the sector's dependency on fossil fuels, there is still a dearth of real government subsidies for alternative energy resources and setting up pharmaceutical enterprises. New restrictions on environmental contamination of water sources, both from industrial waste and from the residues of medications and medicines discharged in water bodies as municipal liquid waste, are another issue facing pharmaceutical companies. Even at very low levels, research has shown that drugs and their metabolites damage lakes, rivers, and coastal areas. Fish and other benthic creatures are particularly vulnerable to the effects of large quantities of drugs. Pharmaceutical companies are generally aware of these issues and take them seriously, but the rules in place do not always benefit the industry [3].

The difficulty of obtaining readily available green feedstock materials has been cited as a fundamental obstacle to the widespread use of green synthesis. If such materials cannot be sourced, it is probably because they do not exist at the right degree of detail or simplicity. They may not be in a format that is easy to use or tailored to a particular industry.

A broad range of solutions are needed to deal with the issues that arise in the use of green and sustainable chemistry. As an example, green chemistry training that emphasises the fundamentals of process excellence in design, biocatalysis, and the selection of solvents and reagents is highly recommended. While reducing carbon emissions should be a priority, it is equally important to employ renewable energy resources wisely, manage water use efficiently, and reduce trash output [6]. However, although the scientific community has largely embraced the idea of green chemistry, the technological progress of green chemistry has yet to be achieved via education and awareness. Traditional chemical industries must undergo a major shift to become more sustainable. There must be collaboration between education, politics, and economics, as well as a multidisciplinary commitment to equality and metrics [2, 7].

Research institutions and universities have been working for years towards greener chemistry, which is now being used in numerous industries. There is still a lot of work to be done, not just in terms of research but also in terms of how we think about chemistry and synthesis and what it can do for our well-being and advancement in technology and society. There will come a point in the future when pharmaceutical chemists will no longer need to be taught about green chemistry since it will be included in the natural sequence of operations. Green chemistry is now gaining significance on a world scale. Not only does it help the environment, it also results in high-quality goods with few hazardous residues. If the current situation of the pharmaceutical sector and the difficulties it faces, such as environmental issues, high costs, and other challenges, are examined, it is clear that green chemistry offers a novel approach for improving living standards while reducing environmental problems [6]. Reductions in the use of harmful chemicals and solvents and the substitution of those materials with more environmentally friendly, renewable alternatives may lower emissions and save water. The pharmaceutical business and medicine production might be transformed in the future by green chemistry. It benefits the ecology and the economy at the same time. As a consequence, the conventional pharmaceutical industry will be transformed into one that is more environmentally friendly and sustainable [2, 7].

Even so, green chemistry ideas and practices have been effectively adopted by pharmaceutical companies in a number of countries [8]. Some of the successful end goods and technologies that have gained prominence in recent years are described in the rest of this chapter.

1.2 Green Solvents

Green solvents can be employed as an alternative to traditional solvents. In their green chemistry principles, Anastas and colleagues advocated the use of 'safer solvents and auxiliaries'. Combustible organic solvents are used in various synthesis processes; nevertheless, these conventional solvents are damaging to the environment and poisonous. Thus, green solvents are currently replacing conventional solvents in numerous industries [9, 10]. There is a wide variety of solvents, and the choice of a suitable solvent for a particular reaction can be crucial to the success of a reaction technique. When choosing a solvent for a reaction, the qualities that should be considered are chemical compatibility with reagents and products; solubility of reagents; and procedure temperature [2, 7].

Sertraline hydrochloride, a greener solvent, was produced using chemical reagents such as toluene, hexane, tetrahydrofuran (THF), and metal salts such as titanium tetrachloride ($TiCl_4$). When these solvents were substituted with water and the palladium on carbon (Pd/C) catalyst was removed, it provided a more selective and environmentally friendly method.

1.2.1 Water as a Solvent

The ever-increasing demand for a more sustainable approach in synthesis operations has led to a growing interest in using water as a solvent. The use of water as a solvent in chemical synthesis is one of the best ways to minimise the release of dangerous compounds into the environment, according to green chemistry. When using water as a solvent, reactions are frequently conducted under mild experimental conditions and consequently the catalysts are frequently reused, which reduces the overall price of the product [6].

1.2.2 Ionic Liquids

In the context of green solvents we can discuss ionic liquids, which, at least for a time, are considered not only as designer solvents but also as green solvents, primarily because they require negligible vapour pressure and do not contribute to the problem of volatile organic compounds [11]. Green technology involves the synthesis of biodiesel and bioethanol from transesterification of vegetable oil. During biodiesel production, a vast amount of the by-product glycerol is produced and discarded. This glycerol has tremendous potential for applications in the pharmaceuticals, food, and explosives sectors [12].

1.3 Nanoparticle Formulations

Nanoparticles are particles that range in size from 1 nm to 100 nm. The improved characteristics of nanoparticles are a result of their vast surface area. Historically, physical and chemical processes were used to create nanoparticles. The increased demand for nanoparticles resulted in their mass fabrication. Therefore, a commercial approach for synthesising metal nanoparticles was established. However, the actual technology utilised to create nanoparticles is environmentally harmful and poisonous, involving the use of hazardous solvents and large amounts of energy. Due to the existence of by-products, the colloidal solution is also contaminated by the classical synthesis technique.

To address this issue, green nanoparticle production was developed. Not only are these nanoparticles environmentally friendly, they are also cost-effective and may be employed for large-scale production [13, 14]. Synthesising nanoparticles using methods that are clean, non-toxic, and environmentally benign adheres to green chemistry principles such as prevention, less dangerous chemical synthesis, developing safer compounds, and real-time pollution prevention [15].

Nanotechnology in the field of pharmaceuticals is at the developmental stage [16]. Green nanoparticles are more biocompatible than their chemical counterparts. The three key advantages of employing green nanoparticles are as follows (Figures 1.1 and 1.2):

- They are environmentally friendly.
- They are non-toxic.
- Many microorganisms like yeast, fungi, bacteria, plants, etc. can be used for the synthesis of nanoparticles.

1.4 Antimicrobial Bandages

A bandage is a piece of material used to cover a wound or a wounded body part. It offers support to the wound and surrounding tissue. This adheres to the first and twelfth principles of green chemistry (see Chapter 2). Wound-healing dressings can be made by green nanoparticle synthesis, in which bandages are impregnated with nanoparticles [17]. For instance, silver nanoparticles were generated by impregnating a bandage with the weed species *Tridax procumbens*, which has demonstrated antibacterial action against Gram-positive and Gram-negative bacteria. Nanoparticles have also been produced using *Prosopis farcta*

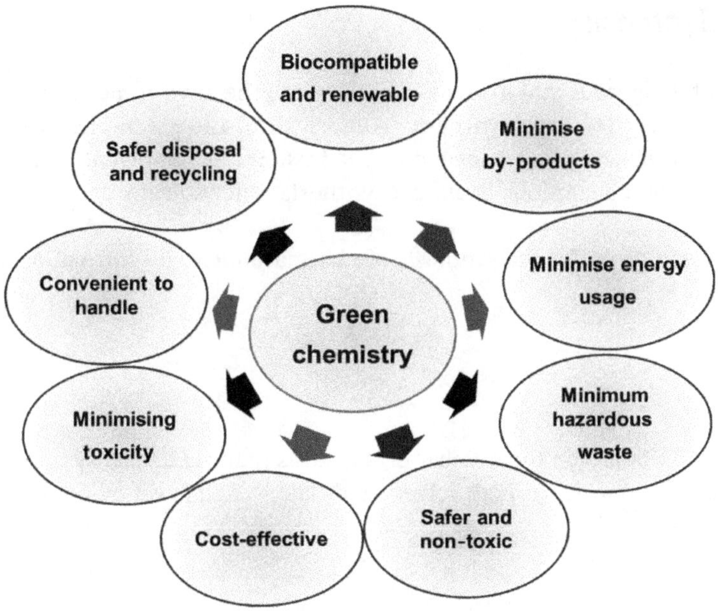

Figure 1.1 Potential advantages of green chemistry.

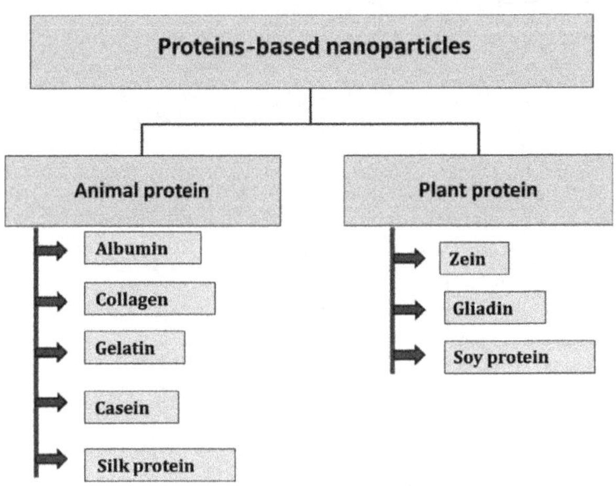

Figure 1.2 Protein-based nanoparticles.

and occasionally a time-saving, environmentally safe, and inexpensive synthesis of silver (Ag) and philosopher's wool (zinc oxide, ZnO). On cultures of *Acinetobacter baumannii* and *Bacteroides* genus *aeruginosa*, the minimal inhibitory concentrations (MIC) of these Ag and ZnO nanoparticles as well as their mixture were determined. Cotton wound bandages were impregnated with nanoparticles of Ag and ZnO and mixed Ag/ZnO nanoparticles in the vicinity of the calculated MIC and their antimicrobial activity was evaluated in vitro; all nanoparticle types demonstrated a high medication activity for the bandages [18].

1.5 Green Drug Synthesis

To prevent the release of dangerous and toxic by-products into the environment, green techniques have been created for drug synthesis. Almost all of the green chemistry principles have been used in the same endeavour, for instance it is preventive and involves atomic economy, less hazardous chemical synthesis, safer solvents, catalysis, and so on [19].

Some examples have been given for the synthesis of pharmaceuticals by conventional and green methods.

1.5.1 Ibuprofen

See Figures 1.3 and 1.4.

During green synthesis of ibuprofen the number of steps was reduced. Green synthesis of ibuprofen utilises hydrogen fluoride as both solvent and catalyst and fewer by-products are formed during the reaction.

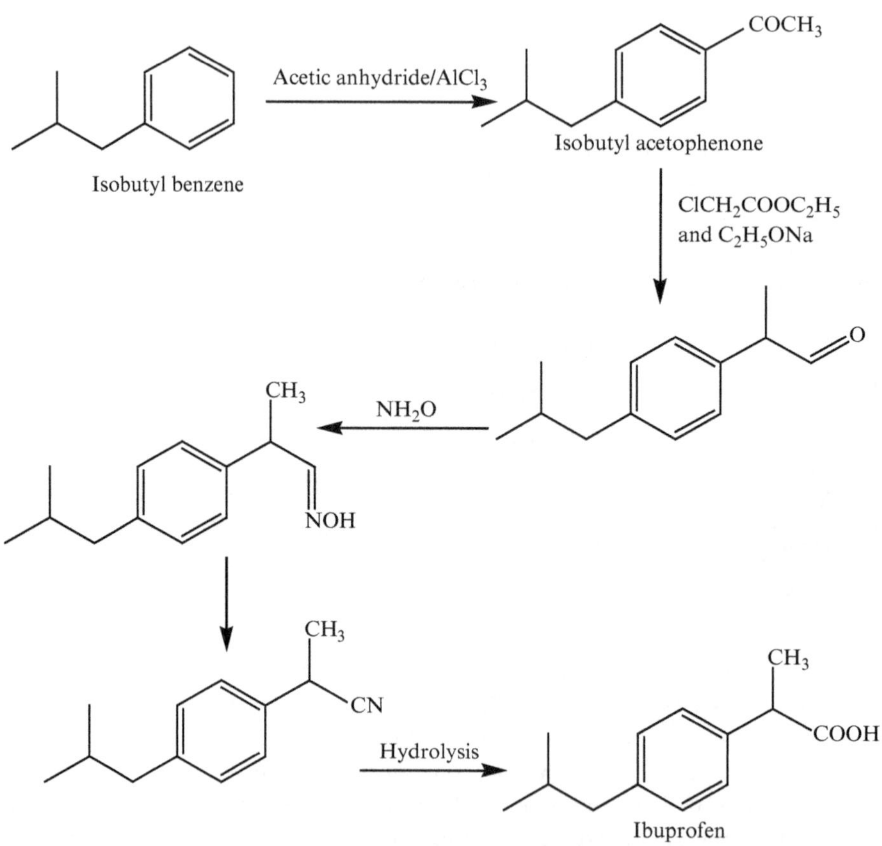

Figure 1.3 Conventional synthesis of ibuprofen.

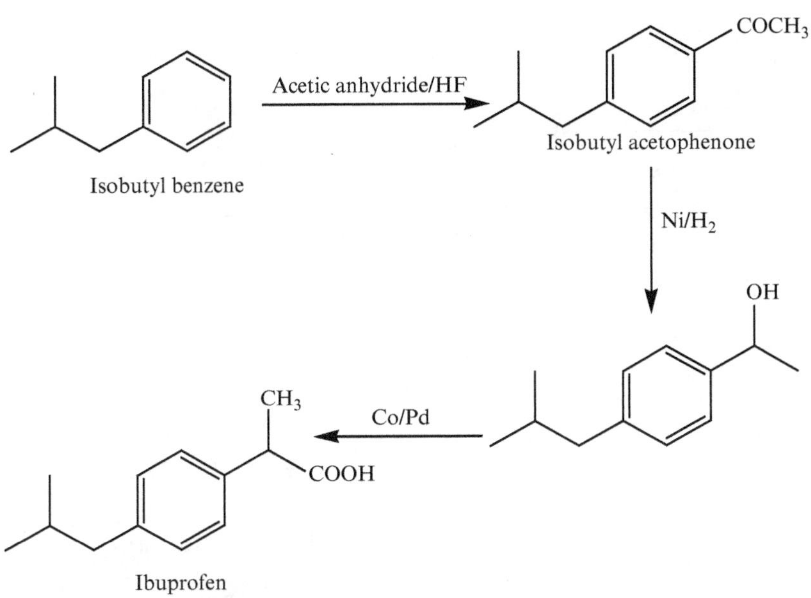

Figure 1.4 Green synthesis of ibuprofen.

1.5.2 Sildenafil

See Figures 1.5 and 1.6.

The advantages of green synthesis of sildenafil are:

- The proposed green method reduces waste production.
- It enhances the yield.
- There is less consumption of solvent: the 22 l of solvent previously used for production of 1 kg sildenafil is now reduced to 7 l.

1.5.3 Paroxetine

See Figures 1.7 and 1.8.

1.5.3 Quinapril hydrochloride

See Figure 1.9.

The green synthesis has increased the yield from 58% to 90%. The method utilises fewer solvents and minimises the use of acetic acid, acetone, and toluene.

1.6 Green Nanotechnology

The major objective of nanotechnology includes the development of structures and devices of the required shape and size at a nanometer scale. Nanotechnology includes any biomedical devices whose structural features are less than 100 nm in size. These types of materials are known as nanoparticle aggregates, nanostructures, and nanocomposites.

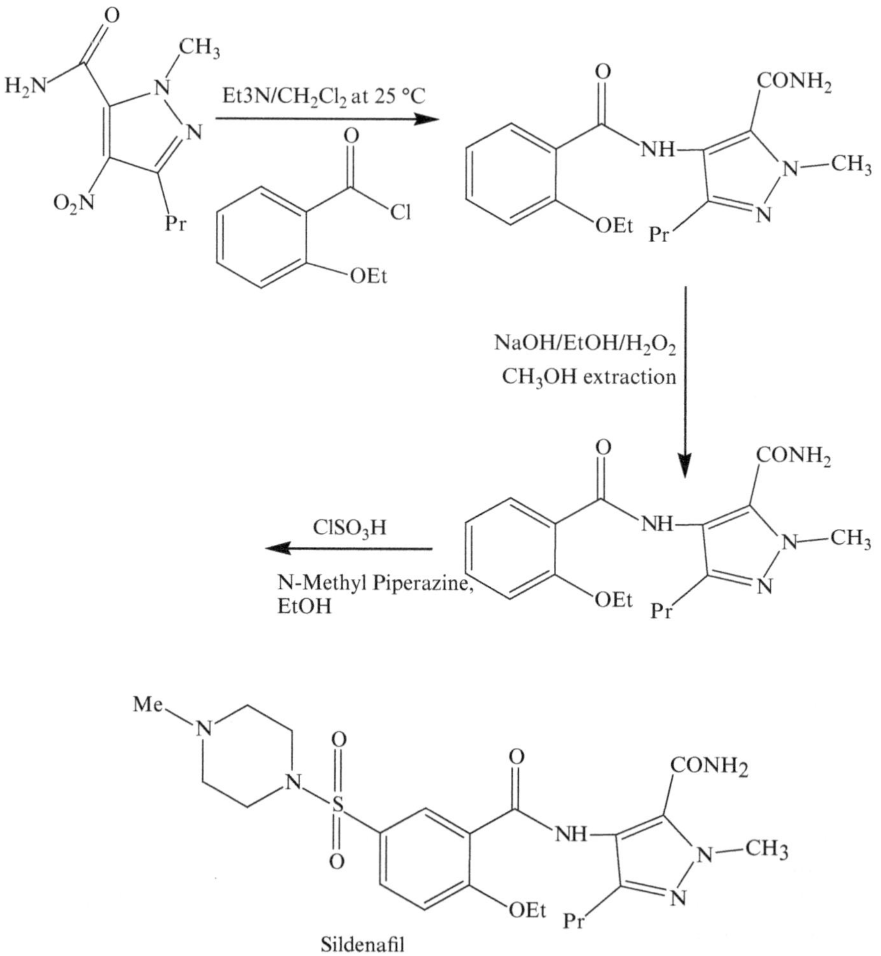

Figure 1.5 Conventional synthesis of sildenafil.

Nanomaterials have major features depending on size that are due to their optical and electrical properties, shape, and surface activity.

In the last few decades several nanomaterials have been invented that have multifunctional and intelligent properties and can be used in the pharmaceutical sciences, especially in the diagnosis and treatment of cancer [10, 20]. Other products that have been developed include electrodes in batteries, carbon nanotubes, and those used in cosmetic and food sciences. While synthetic nanomaterials have several benefits, they may have various hazardous effects on the environment. Hence, their applications have been limited due to the various side effects [21].

Currently many scientists are working in the search for safe and effective natural nanomaterials through green synthesis routes, most commonly known as green nanotechnology. Green nanotechnology-based products could be more environmentally friendly and may replace synthetic nanomaterials [22]. The different by-products formed in synthetic

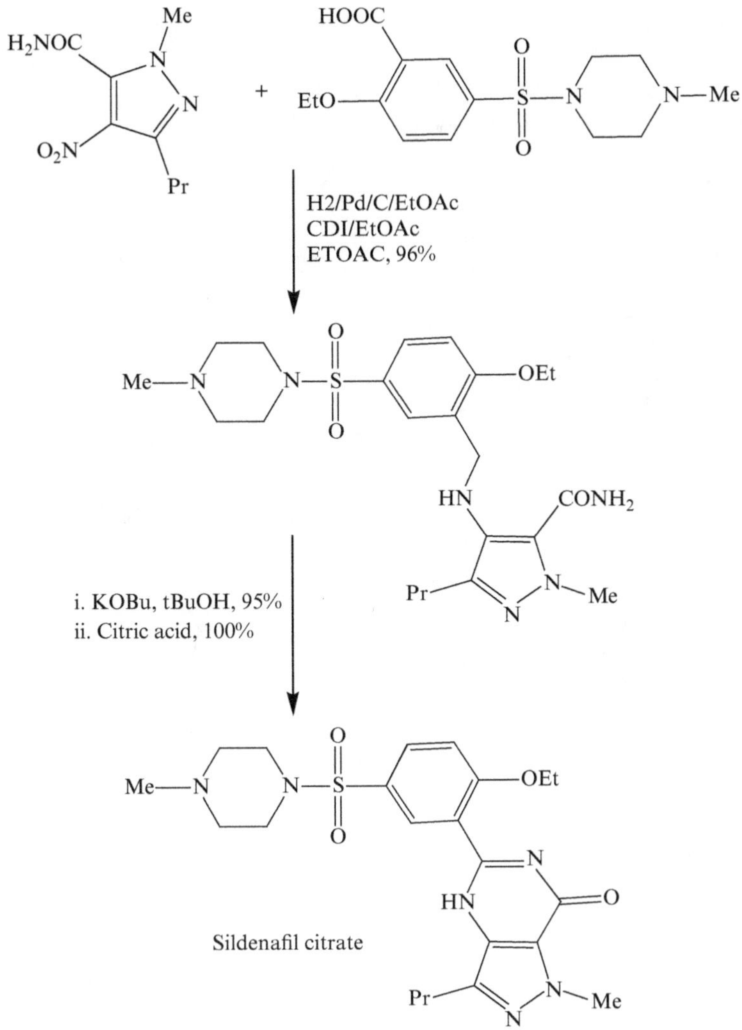

Figure 1.6 Green synthesis of sildenafil.

nanomaterials can be minimised through green nanotechnology and several limitations can be overcome. Now eco-nanotoxicological research has been widely considered in different areas of nanotechnology-based products. There are several advantages of green nanotechnology over synthetic technology, such as its cost-effectiveness and minimal environmental hazards. This technology can enhance sustainability by reducing various risk factors for toxicity and the safety of human beings. The use of green resources for the production of nanotechnology-based products could solve several environmental issues. For instance, green nanotechnology approaches based on magnetite nanoparticles (NPs) are used for the removal of toxicity from chlorinated organic solvents to eliminate arsenic from water [23].

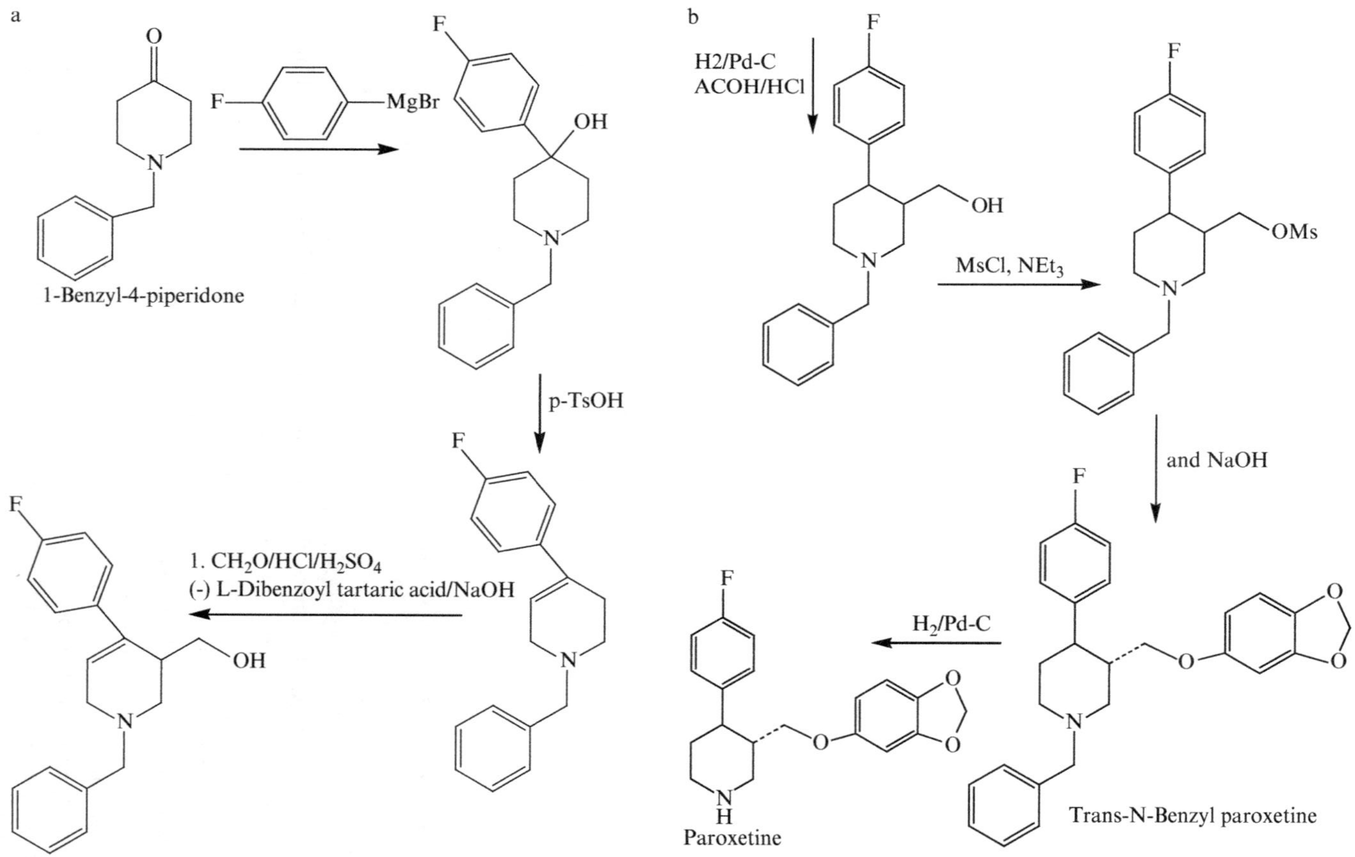

Figure 1.7 (a, b) Conventional synthesis of paroxetine.

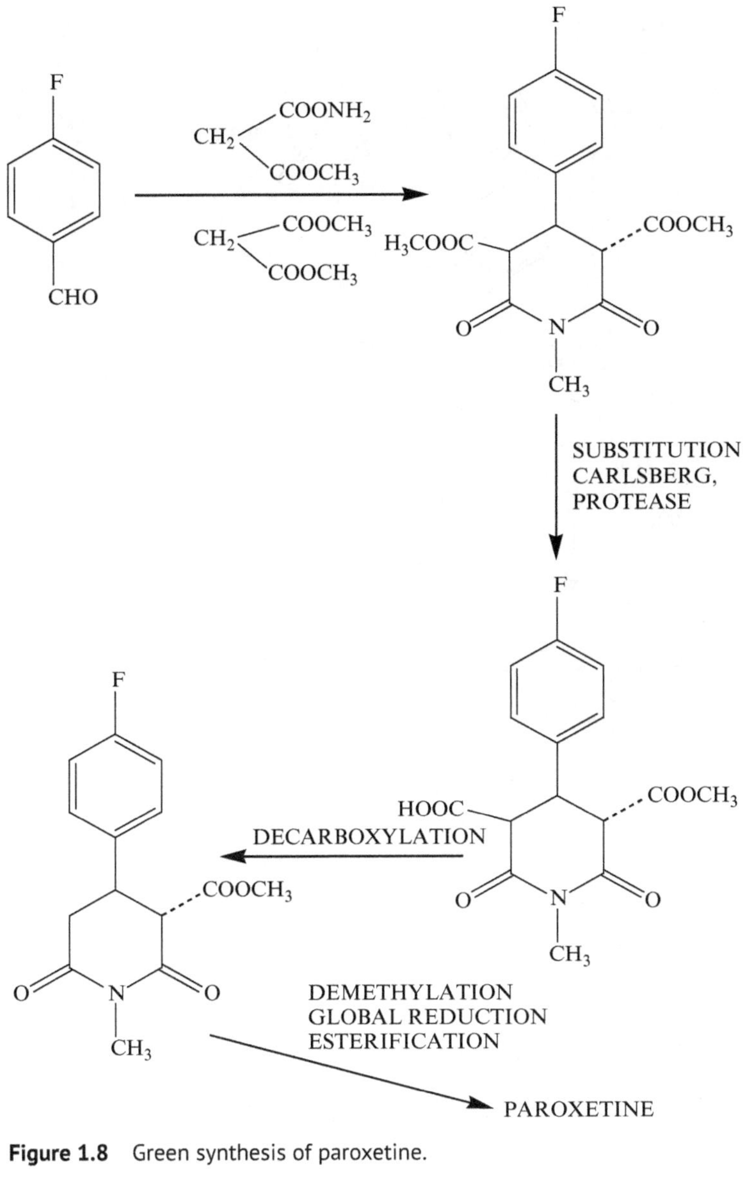

Figure 1.8 Green synthesis of paroxetine.

Green nanotechnology-based sensors for coliform bacteria as pollutants may enhance the detection ability compared to existing methods. Furthermore, these approaches will be helpful in reducing greenhouse gases, weight, and the use of fossil fuels. Nanomembranes may also be produced through green nanotechnology that are used for the separation of individual components from a complex mixture more effectively than via nanocatalysts [10]. Green nanotechnology methods can also use water instead of synthetic solvents, which may reduce the toxicity of several products [24].

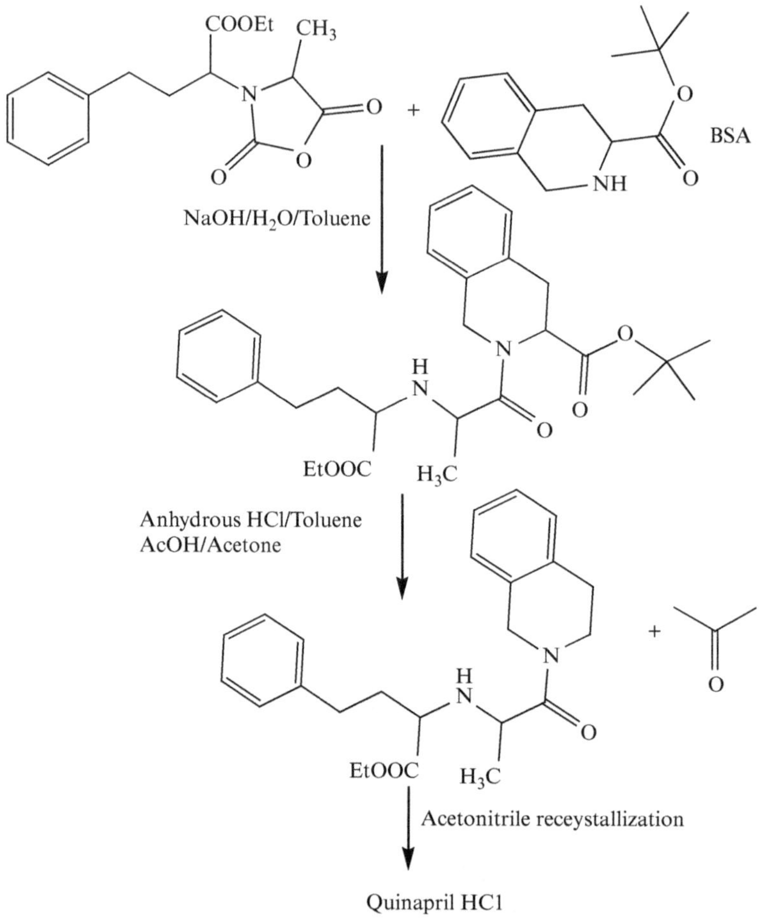

Figure 1.9 Green synthesis of quinapril hydrochloride.

1.7 Benefits of Green Technologies

Green science-based approaches are a major area of research throughout the world and more than 1000 scientific papers have been published on green technologies-based products. Green technologies decrease the release of hazardous waste materials into the environment. Green science includes various research areas such as green solvents, alternative energy sciences, molecular designs, bio-based transformations, and catalyst designs to minimise various hazardous substances. The release of hazardous waste substances such as methyl isobutyl ketone, hydrochloric acid, and trichloroethylene may be minimised through green nanotechnology [25]. Furthermore, these green techniques have an important role in novel production methods for fuel cells, solar cells, and solar batteries for storing energy. Green methods minimise the environmental hazards in next-generation catalysts for the production of chemicals and promote the sustainable development of new technology. Nanotechnology is playing a key role in several industrial sectors for new developments towards sustainability. Green nanotechnology enhances the synthesis of environmentally friendly nanomaterials and nanoproducts in which no toxic ingredients are used [2].

Green nanotechnology has been applied in different areas of science and technology such as nanosensor membranes, nanoscale membranes, and nanocatalysts. This green technology produces eco-friendly materials that can be used for various purposes like water purification, cleaning of environmental pollutants, and hazardous waste sites. Further, these nanomaterials weigh less and thus are easier to transport. Nanotechnology helps in the development of fuel cells and light-emitting diodes, self-cleaning nanoscale surface coatings and batteries with enhanced life. All these environmentally friendly innovations are energy efficient, address recycling, safety, and health concerns, and involve renewable resources. Hence, these green nanotechnologies may be helpful in the production of materials as well as products that have several advantages over synthetic materials, such as improved safety and less toxicity along with being environmentally friendly. Industrial pollutants could be controlled to a significant extent, since green nanomaterials can be helpful in the monitoring and prevention of different kinds of industrial pollutants [10, 26].

Furthermore, hazardous and toxic materials may be used to improve the ecosystem of the environment as part of the green nanotechnology-related remediation process. Energy generation and energy saving can be achieved through thermal discs and solar panels that use the sun as a heat source for the production of electrical energy in an environmentally friendly way. Sustainable and green chemical products including detergents, cleaning agents, and insecticides may be produced through environmentally safe and green reagents, such as orange coconut oil, peppermint, and glycerin, avoiding the use of any toxic or hazardous materials [27].

Currently most products are produced with materials that are not eco-friendly such as plastics, which are not biodegradable and can be toxic. Green technology uses sustainable and recyclable materials while developing products. Hence, green materials could be good for health as well as environmentally friendly.

1.8 White Biotechnology and Green Chemistry

At the start of the twentieth century, the relationship between industrial microbiology and technical chemistry proved beneficial to both fields. It is worth noting that during World War I, an anaerobic fermentation of glycerol and butanol was used as a feedstock for explosions and synthetic rubber. Biotechnological processes, on the other hand, had poor productivity and effluent issues that necessitated the development of more effective and 'cleaner' chemical technologies. Many novel ideas on the use of biofuel for bulk chemical synthesis were proposed as a result of the 1970s oil crisis. Anaerobic fermentation and dehydration processes provide the most commonly utilised petrochemicals [10]. To describe nations with a surplus of agricultural goods but few oil reserves, such as the United States, the term 'biorefinery' is employed. Chemicals, fuels, electricity, goods, and materials are produced in the 'clusters of bio-based industries' or the biorefinery.

The European chemical industry coined the term 'white biotechnology' to characterise the use of biotechnological ideas in chemistry. In contemporary biotechnology, white biotechnology serves industry by making use of living cells like moulds, yeasts, or bacteria as well as enzymes in order to generate products and services. White biotechnology is a potential component of green chemistry as described by Anastas and Warner in 1998 [28], which brings together chemistry, biology, and contemporary technology. In the design, production, and use of chemical products, green chemistry uses a set of principles that decrease or eliminate the usage or synthesis of hazardous compounds. In turn, white biotechnology procedures tend to focus on environmental considerations. Despite the fact that these features are seldom discussed in depth, they should always be present and active in current technology.

Some of the environmental implications of biotechnology and green chemistry include the use of renewable feedstock; novel high-performance microorganisms; online monitoring of substrates and products in bioreactors; optimisation of biotechnological processes by consideration of the complete process, including generation of feedstock, fermentation, and separation of the result; and sustainable socioeconomic and regional development [29].

1.9 Conclusion

Green chemistry is a subdiscipline of chemistry that puts an emphasis on durability, and is hence also known as sustainable chemistry. Sustainability in green chemistry is achieved by the employment of either a natural chemical moiety or a chemical synthesis technique that causes minimum harm to the environment. The significance of green chemistry and its industrial applications have been discussed in this chapter.

References

1 Vijay Kumar, P.P.N., Pammi, S.V.N., Kollu, P. et al. (2014). Green synthesis and characterization of silver nanoparticles using Boerhaavia diffusa plant extract and their anti bacterial activity. *Industrial Crops and Products* 52: 562–566.

2 Mishra, M., Sharma, M., Dubey, R. et al. (2021). Green synthesis interventions of pharmaceutical industries for sustainable development. *Current Research in Green and Sustainable Chemistry* 4: 100174.

3 de Oliveira Souza, H., dos Santos Costa, R., Quadra, G.R., and dos Santos Fernandez, M.A. (2021). Pharmaceutical pollution and sustainable development goals: going the right way? *Sustainable Chemistry and Pharmacy* 21: 100428.

4 Bruce, S. (2008). Cosmeceuticals for the attenuation of extrinsic and intrinsic dermal aging. *Journal of Drugs in Dermatology* 7 (2 Suppl.): s17–s22.

5 Mestres, R. (2005). Green chemistry—views and strategies. *Environmental Science and Pollution Research International* 12 (3): 128–132.

6 Khataei, M.M., Epi, S.B.H., Lood, R. et al. (2022). A review of green solvent extraction techniques and their use in antibiotic residue analysis. *Journal of Pharmaceutical and Biomedical Analysis* 209: 114487.

7 Singh, R.M., Pramanik, R., and Hazra, S. (2021). Role of green chemistry in pharmaceutical industry: a review. *Journal of University of Shanghai for Science and Technology* 23: 291–299.

8 De Marco, B.A., Rechelo, B.S., Tótoli, E.G. et al. (2019). Evolution of green chemistry and its multidimensional impacts: a review. *Saudi Pharmaceutical Journal* 27 (1): 1–8.

9 Huguet-Casquero, A., Gainza, E., and Pedraz, J.L. (2021). Towards green nanoscience: from extraction to nanoformulation. *Biotechnology Advances* 46: 107657.

10 Anastas, P.T., and Kirchhoff, M.M. (2002). Origins, current status, and future challenges of green chemistry. *Accounts of Chemical Research* 35 (9): 686–694.

11 Karić, N., Vukčević, M., Ristić, M. et al. (2021). A green approach to starch modification by solvent-free method with betaine hydrochloride. *International Journal of Biological Macromolecules* 193: 1962–1971.

12 Takla, S.S., Shawky, E., Hammoda, H.M., and Darwish, F.A. (2018). Green techniques in comparison to conventional ones in the extraction of Amaryllidaceae alkaloids: best solvents selection and parameters optimization. *Journal of Chromatography A* 1567: 99–110.

13 Brandt, F.S., Cazzaniga, A., and Hann, M. (2011). Cosmeceuticals: current trends and market analysis. *Seminars in Cutaneous Medicine and Surgery* 30 (3): 141–143.

14 Kaul, S., Gulati, N., Verma, D. et al. (2018). Role of nanotechnology in cosmeceuticals: a review of recent advances. *Journal of Pharmaceutical (Cairo)* 27: 3420204.

15 Assali, M., and Zaid, A.N. (2022). Features, applications, and sustainability of lipid nanoparticles in cosmeceuticals. *Saudi Pharmaceutical Journal* 30 (1): 53–65.

16 Constable, D.J.C. (2021). Green and sustainable chemistry – the case for a systems-based, interdisciplinary approach. *iScience* 24 (12): 103489.

17 Pleissner, D., and Kümmerer, K. (2020). Green chemistry and its contribution to industrial biotechnology. *Advances in Biochemical Engineering/Biotechnology* 173: 281–298.

18 Vázquez, L., Bañares, C., Torres, C.F., and Reglero, G. (2020). Green technologies for the production of modified lipids. *Annual Review of Food Science and Technology* 11: 319–337.

19 Wrooman, A., Krötzsch, E., Carvajal, Z.Y.G., and Hernández-Gutiérrez, R. (2021). Green metallic nanoparticles for cancer therapy: evaluation models and cancer applications. *Pharmaceutics* 13 (10): 1719.

20 Guo, K.W. (2011). Green nanotechnology of trends in future energy. *Recent Patents on Nanotechnology* 5: 76–88.

21 Iavicoli, I., Leso, V., Ricciardi, W. et al. (2014). Opportunities and challenges of nanotechnology in the green economy. *Environmental Health* 13: 78.

22 Nath, D., and Banerjee, P. (2013). Green nanotechnology – a new hope for medical biology. *Environmental Toxicology and Pharmacology* 36 (3): 997–1014.

23 Ahmad, S., Munir, S., Zeb, N. et al. (2019). Green nanotechnology: a review on green synthesis of silver nanoparticles – an ecofriendly approach. *International Journal of Nanomedicine* 14: 5087–5107.

24 Cascione, M., Rizzello, L., Manno, D. et al. (2022). Green silver nanoparticles promote inflammation shutdown in human leukemic monocytes. *Materials (Basel)* 15 (3): 775.

25 Domingo-Echaburu, S., Dávalos, L.M., Orive, G., and Lertxundi, U. (2021). Drug pollution & sustainable development goals. *Science of the Total Environment* 800: 149412.

26 Sahoo, T., Panda, J., Sahu, J. et al. (2020). Green solvent: green shadow on chemical synthesis. *Current Organic Synthesis* 17 (6): 426–439.

27 Jahangirian, H., Lemraski, E.G., Webster, T.J. et al. (2017). A review of drug delivery systems based on nanotechnology and green chemistry: green nanomedicine. *International Journal of Nanomedicine* 12: 2957–2978.

28 Anastas, P.T., and Warner, J.C. (1998). *Green Chemistry: Theory and Practice*. Oxford: Oxford University Press.

29 Stottmeister, U., Aurich, A., Wilde, H. et al. (2005). White biotechnology for green chemistry: fermentative 2-oxocarboxylic acids as novel building blocks for subsequent chemical syntheses. *Journal of Industrial Microbiology & Biotechnology* 32 (11–12): 651–664.

2

Green Approaches in Conventional Drug Synthesis

Hassan Rafique[1], Nazim Hussain[1], Muhammad Usama Saeed[1] and Muhammad Bilal[2]

[1] *Centre for Applied Molecular Biology (CAMB), University of the Punjab, Lahore, Pakistan*
[2] *School of Life Science and Food Engineering, Huaiyin Institute of Technology, Huaian, China*

CONTENTS

2.1 Introduction

The outcomes of environmental changes and the necessity to decrease carbon footprints are the key concerns of today. Nevertheless, the devotion to reducing carbon emissions has already been in place in the public sector for a long time. The familiarity with anthropogenic and natural sources of environmental pollutants has appeared as a requirement that moves ahead of state boundaries to achieve a global aspect. Hence, several studies have pointed to the application of novel technologies in a variety of sustainable environmental programmes [1, 2]. These are green approaches that may reveal distinct environmentally friendly methods for sustainable administration and cleaning of the environment. Sustainable development has turned out to be a motto for both developing and developed countries.

The green synthesis approach can be defined as 'an emerging area in the field of bio-nanotechnology that offers environmental and economic benefits as a substitute for physical and chemical methods'. In this approach, non-toxic reagents that are biosafe and ecofriendly are employed [3]. Green synthesis highlights techniques that follow a consistent and ecofriendly pathway with moderate reactions, using non-toxic precursors, and generating fewer wastes to safeguard a sustainable environment. As a result of this green approach, the design and

Sustainable Approaches in Pharmaceutical Sciences, First Edition. Edited by Kamal Shah, Durgesh Nandini Chauhan, and Nagendra Singh Chauhan.

production of new goods/drugs that are biodegradable, reusable, and safe are now taking place [4]. For instance, green synthesis uses microorganisms that are known as 'bio-nanofactories' because they are environmentally effective, cost-effective, fast, affordable, and exceptionally structured with a capacity for metal uptake while retaining security levels [5].

Even though we are living in the modern world of technology, the conventional use of chemotherapy such as antibiotics for bacterial infection is causing the problem of antibiotic resistance in persistent bacterial strains. Along with this comes the issue of non-targeted delivery effects of conventional chemicals and resistant drugs of the same family in a single bacterial strain. The repercussions are changes in drug dosages and intolerable toxicity of therapeutic agents [6]. The solution to this is greener synthesis in the field of nanoparticles, which exemplifies the progress over other approaches because it is modest, cost-efficient, and comparatively reproducible, and often results in more durable products. As has been mentioned, microorganisms can also be utilised to produce nanoparticles [7], but the synthesis is time-consuming and only a restricted number of shapes and sizes are suitable for the method compared to routes involving plant-based materials. Plants yield stable nanoparticles compared to other methods and it is undemanding to scale up. Bio-fabricated nanoparticles are being researched for their use in anticancerous, antimicrobial activities and in drug-delivery systems as well. Therefore, currently numerous scientists are diverting from synthetic methods to green approaches, because in green synthesis energy is not needed and there is lower requirement for high temperatures and pressures, or for toxic chemicals, and the contamination risk is also lower [8].

2.2 Green Chemistry Perspective

The scientific question confronting the chemical sector while planning the future for Earth is: What are going to be the nature and production methods of the chemicals desirable for a sustainable civilisation? Chemistry has an extensive record of designing beneficial products and procedures with remarkable performance; nevertheless, this scientific progress has frequently been understood by considering a limited definition of function, where unfavourable outcomes are not justified. Likewise, the resultant chemical products are frequently planned for their intended use while depending on conditional controls to limit exposures to risks that have not been assessed, possibly owing to the significant lack of models, as demonstrated by the array of unintended unfriendly consequences [9]. Into this comes the concept of green chemistry, which is also acknowledged as sustainable chemistry. It is characterised as a methodology for chemistry that endeavours to decrease pollution. This basis also tries to enhance the output yield of chemical products by adjustment of the chemicals being devised, produced, and consumed. In 1991, the US Environmental Protection Agency (EPA) initiated a research programme called 'Alternative Synthetic Pathways for Pollution Prevention' under the umbrella of Pollution Prevention Act 1990, which indicated a revolutionary departure from existing EPA initiatives in highlighting the elimination/reduction of the generation of toxic substances, as opposed to handling hazardous substances after they have been generated and circulated in the ecosystem. This idea was then extended to initiation of the production of safer chemicals and substances with greener methods. In 1996, 'green chemistry' was officially accepted as a term [10].

With the opening of green approaches and green chemistry, it is vital to acknowledge that the utility of such methods is a 'double-edged sword'. Terms like 'environmentally friendly', 'green', and 'sustainable' have become hackneyed and lost their genuine meaning due to their unrestricted use in the mass media, commercials, and scientific discourse. In fact, there is a tangible scepticism among consumers related to 'green' goods, and sometimes these are perceived as a simple marketing trick. Thus, it is important that scepticism about the extensive misuse of the related terminology does not become an obstacle to green chemistry. The ethical outcomes of the objectives of green chemistry have resulted in ample consultation. Even though these debates are productive, we must be careful not to miss the decisive vision of green chemistry to create an infrastructure to permit the development of new methods that reduce the generation of hazardous products [11–14]. Regrettably, misrepresentations are perhaps the major obstacle to the adoption of a green approach in academia as well as at an industrial level.

Two common misunderstandings regarding green chemistry are:

- It is a myth and is generated by industry as a promotional tool to market and make profits from possibly toxic products.
- It is an ecological movement whose concerns force costly yet poor-performance products onto customers.

Though these opinions are far from reality, nevertheless for green chemistry to accomplish its objectives of pollution regulation and the dream of a sustainable environment, it must be commercially successful. For a product to be profitable, it must have exceptional performance at a reduced cost. It is obvious that customers will not consume or purchase substandard goods just because they are 'green' or have a 'green' label. Therefore, in order to have a genuine influence on social use, green technology has to be sustainable from both perspectives, cost as well as performance [15–18].

Paul Anastas (one of the pioneers of green chemistry) argued that the production of pollutants can be inhibited or reduced through improving the methodologies for producing chemicals. To explain in detail, the following 12 principles of green chemistry were devised in 1998 by Anastas and John Warner [19]:

1) Lower or absolutely prevent the production of derivatives.
2) Make use of renewable feedstocks.
3) Encourage the development of real-time analysis of chemical products before harmful substances can form.
4) Use safer auxiliaries and solvents in chemical processes.
5) Avoid waste generation wherever possible.
6) Promote the 'atom economy'.
7) Employ appropriate catalysts.
8) Plan the production of less toxic and safer products.
9) Synthesise chemical by-products that are less hazardous.
10) Plan energy-efficient chemical manufacturing processes.
11) Create chemicals that break down into non-toxic products after their consumption.
12) Promote essentially safer chemistry to avoid accidents from taking place.

The atom economy, initially proposed by Barry Trost (an American chemist) in 1973, was developed as a key concept among researchers of green chemistry. It was devised to surmount the shortcomings of the conventional 'yield' concept that was used for determining the productivity of chemical reactions. In the past, chemists conventionally considered just the amount of primary chemical product they aimed to produce, to calculate the yield; that is, the target molecule and not the by-products, which might include materials that are not environmentally friendly. On the other hand, the atom economy considers all reactants and products, and therefore offers a more dependable statistic on whether the reaction yields unwanted by-products or not.

2.3 Green Approaches in Drug Synthesis

Every day thousands of people in the developing world die due to curable infections, in spite of considerable improvements in the treatment of those diseases [20]. This is because of the unavailability of drugs due to high cost. So we must consider both the cost of the product and its environmental impact when designing a sustainable 'green' product. Even though the barrier to treatment of these infections is not only economic, budgets do restrict access to medications in developing countries [20–22].

To formulate techniques to reduce the expense of anti-retroviral agents or other pharmaceutical agents, it is important to recognise the inherent correlation between the cost of the product and the retail price. For a standard drug that is well marketed at a dose of 100 mg, the cost can be broken down into three categories, with their percentage contributions to the market price [23–25]:

- Active pharmaceutical ingredient (API): 65–75%.
- Preparation and packaging cost: 10–20%.
- Profit: 5–15%.

This cost fragmentation provides a variety of options for intervention. Thus, it can help to bring down the cost and can be split into two interconnected groups:

- Cost reduction of the API.
- Finding the optimum dose of the API with the optimum effect.

In the development stage of a novel drug, often the simplest composition that efficiently provides an effective dose in blood plasma is preferred for production to save cost, time, and complexity in the development process. In human subjects, the quantity of a given drug present in blood plasma after intravenous injection is known as its percentage bioavailability. In contrast, the quantity of drug present in blood plasma after the introduction of a specific dose form is known as the relative bioavailability of that drug-delivery system. Numerous drugs show comparatively low bioavailability after oral dosing, and in developing countries essential medicines are delivered orally. In oral dosage, the rest of the drug is excreted out of the body either as a metabolite or a parent without interacting with the target to provide a definite therapeutic effect. Additionally, the excretion of key APIs has an environmental impact. According to De Jeorder et al., reducing the cost of a drug can be achieved through the following practices [26]:

- Improving drug composition, which can help in reduction of the dose.
- Setting a green dose (reducing side effects with optimum tolerability).
- Reducing the cost through the application of green chemistry.

Therefore, finding the optimum dose of a drug that is convenient, safe, and still enhances the bioavailability of the drug can be regarded as an improvement in dosing along with having a green influence too [26]. The next sections will discuss the green approaches that are being employed in drug synthesis.

2.3.1 Microwave-Assisted Synthesis

There is a concept that microwaves have the ability to penetrate into any kind of substance, thus they can be transformed into heat in that substance. In turn, the extent to which materials can be heated depends on their dielectric properties. Thus, with materials that have higher dielectric loss it is easier to attain a resonant state in a field of microwaves, therefore the absorption of microwaves will be efficient. Many mechanisms from the technique of microwave irradiation can be regulated, such as drug polymer interaction and the dissolution properties of substances with the help of proper heating mechanisms. Through this technique numerous benefits can be accomplished, such as higher-quality products and improved energy effectiveness with decent time requirements [27].

The quest to use microwave irradiation for the synthesis of organic products has been flourishing for many years. It requires fundamental knowledge of the theory of dielectric heating and the availability of materials and methods for the particular synthesis. Its wide use in reducing reaction times has led to its approval in several fields of organic chemistry; this characteristic is of great significance in high-speed pharmaceutical manufacturing and it has become the mainstream heating source in company laboratories. This technique offers new clues for drying and heating in the field of drug synthesis [28]. Revolutionising chemical synthesis, the technique can help in producing small molecules within a fraction of the time of conventional methods. It ensures swifter reactions and saves fossil fuels or other sources of energy that can be used for heat production, because in this technique microwaves work as a source of heat. The main gain of this method is uniform heating of materials, as depicted in Figure 2.1. Conduction and dipolar polarisation are the basic mechanisms involved in this technique. The ability of microwaves to generate uniform heat can enhance the interaction between the drug and the polymer, therefore can enable substantial structural adjustments. Microwave irradiation will continue to play a key role in drug discovery processes [29, 30]. In this regard, the present state of the art is full of examples of recent applications in drug synthesis.

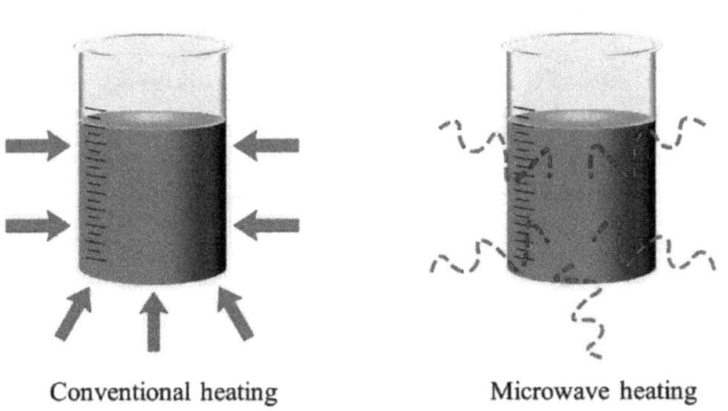

Figure 2.1 Comparison visualisation of conventional and microwave heating.

Many reports have been published on attempts at green synthesis and the therapeutic efficiencies of drugs produced through microwave-assisted synthesis. For instance, novel ionic liquids, with moieties of imidazolium and pyridazinium, were synthesised by microwave irradiation; they showed promising antimicrobial activities and were expected to have the same bioactivity as the parent drug [31]. Further, microwave-assisted synthesis can be used in improving the solubility of drug moieties in order to enhance a drug's oral bioavailability. To do so, production of nanocomposites has been considered a better choice. Keeping this in mind, bio-nanocomposites (BNCs) of an insoluble drug called glipizide were produced by a microwave-assisted mechanism for better solubility and demonstrated enhanced bioavailability [32, 33]. A more recent study reported on the microwave-assisted synthesis of new derivatives of thiazolyl coumarin and explored their antitumor potential through various methods [34].

A microwave-assisted technique is also used for improving drug-delivery systems; that is, to load gold nanoparticles on a hydroxyapatite surface coated with collagen through microwave irradiation for optimised drug (doxorubicin) loading and releasing purposes in biomedical applications [35]. It is acknowledged that nitrogen-containing heterocycles are of great interest for researchers as they are bioactive compounds found in nature. Therefore, researchers have applied microwave-assisted organic synthesis (MAOS) in order to develop complex N-heterocyclic structures. This method has been found to be applicable in the synthesis of various compounds such as herbicides, vitamins, and antibacterial, antifungal, and anticancerous agents. The synthesis of N-heterocycles including the indoles, pyridines, pyrroles, pyrrolidines, 1,2,3,-triazoles, pyrazoles, and imidazoles, which are of great importance in medicinal uses, has been reported in different publications [36].

2.3.2 Ultrasound-Mediated Synthesis

In conventional drug synthesis a lot of waste is generated due to the use of large amounts of chemicals or solvents and processes that may or may not be toxic, hazardous, and energy consuming along with posing a threat to environmental sustainability. Thus, in recent decades many medical industries have moved to greener approaches for drug discovery, manufacturing, and delivery [37]. We have discussed microwave-assisted synthesis as a green approach to drug development; another green approach to drug synthesis is an energy-efficient activation technique called ultrasound-mediated synthesis, also known as 'sonochemistry'. It involves the application of ultrasound to promote a chemical reaction. In recent years it has been employed in organic synthesis and drug discovery, as it dramatically reduces the time to reaction. It offers low cost, enhanced purity, and excellent yields compared to conventional methods.

For instance, it is reported that synthesis of heterocyclic compounds can be accelerated with the application of sonochemistry [38]. This technique has been used for catalyst-free synthesis of various compounds. Two examples are mentioned here for illustration. The first is the ultrasound-mediated catalyst-free synthesis of rhodanine derivatives in water. For this, researchers developed a one-pot catalyst-free protocol. In the reaction the ultrasound probe was of 20 KHz frequency with 3–5 minutes' duration [39]. Similarly, an enzyme inhibitor called dihydropyrano[2,3-c]pyrazol is considered very appealing for its biological properties [40]. The beneficial effect of ultrasound treatment on the catalyst-free synthesis of dihydropyrano[2,3-c]pyrazol has been reported where the ultrasound probe was of 40 KHz frequency [41]. Therefore, it can be said that ultrasound-mediated synthesis of pharmaceutical products can help in reducing the number of reagents such as catalysts or other solvents that are required for the conventional synthesis of the same products. Using ultrasound in a synergistic way, drug synthesis can take place in different conditions such as in water, bio-sourced solvents, ionic liquids, and solventless condition [42].

2.3.3 Molecular Sieving

Put simply, sieving is the process of separation based on the size and shape of the components of any mixture. Take this process to the molecular level (micro to nano scale), it is called 'molecular sieving'. The ability to make extraordinary nanofilters that can separate molecules based on the desired shape, scale, and surface type does help in engineering better products. There are different techniques for molecular sieving including continuous-flow molecular sieving, electrostatic sieving, hydrodynamic sieving, ogston sieving, and many others [43]. The molecular sieving approach is of high significance in medicinal industries as it helps to manufacture products that are really difficult to produce through conventional methods. Hindered alkyl ether, for example, has value in various applications of medicinal chemistry, but is really difficult to synthesise through conventional reactions. Xiang et al. reported the synthesis of hindered alkyl ether through electrogenerated carbocations and documented higher yields, lower labour, and subsequent decrease in the number of steps required in the conventional method [44].

We can also shed light on the green aspect of molecular sieving in the pharmaceutical production of antibiotics. It is widely known that wastewater from pharmaceutical companies that manufacture antibiotics has a great impact on the ecological environment. Therefore, it is necessary to treat that wastewater before releasing it into ecological water bodies, as it may contain antibiotic residues such as tetracycline. Here is where the application of molecular sieving in the form of nanosheets or nanofilters can filter the pharmaceutical wastewater or can be used to recover the valuable organic molecules [45]. In a research article, Zhi Song and his colleagues demonstrated the efficiency of ZIF-8/GO – a composite film – in the removal of tetracycline from pharmaceutical wastewater with a 99% removal rate [46].

Molecular sieving, particularly nanofiltration, can be of great importance in the drug discovery and development process due to its capabilities of molecular transportation and separation. Take, for instance, silica or mesoporous membranes, which can serve as a template for synthesis and support for nanocatalysts and nanomaterials, as well as surface modifiers for optical and electrochemical sensing. It has been demonstrated that the permeability and selectivity of silica nanochannel membranes can be tuned and improved by different modification methodologies [47]. Due to these abilities of mesoporous/nanomaterial structures, controlled drug delivery can be achieved. With the advent of silica-based nanomaterials, like MCM-48 or SBA-15, systematic drug-delivery systems are now possible [48]. Hence, it is highly recommended that we should adopt the new techniques and apply them for the betterment of the environment.

2.3.4 Milling Approach

For any drug to be effective, factors such as the drug's solubility, its dissolution characteristics, and its membrane permeability are of great significance and these parameters define the efficiency of its bioavailability. Regardless of the route of administration, drug dissolution (the transfer of solid drug into the liquid phase, the surrounding physiological fluid) is a critical factor for therapeutic effectiveness. Drug solubility is the quantity of drug that transfers into solution as soon as an equilibrium is established between the drug solute and the undissolved drug in order to develop a saturated solution at a particular temperature. Furthermore, the extent to which a drug gets dissolved and becomes available at the targeted site of action is known as drug bioavailability.

To overcome the challenge of poor water solubility of a drug, various techniques are in place such as the use of complexing agents or cosolvents. Apart from these, the technique of milling is also employed to enhance drug solubility through mechanical energy. Comminution, size reduction, grinding, and milling are terms frequently used interchangeably. Milling is regarded as a 'top-down' approach, in which fine particles are produced by applying mechanical energy to physically break down the coarse particles. The instruments that can be used for this purpose may include cutter mills, pestles and mortars, roller mills, and runner mills. Advances in technology now enable us to produce ultrafine particles [49]. As this approach allows solvent-free or solventless processes, it is considered a green approach and has wide applications in industrial and research sectors [50]. An antifungal drug called griseofulvin signifies one example of many drugs where milling enhances solubility and absorption.

The mechanism by which milled products improve solubility and dissolution is that milling helps in reducing the size of particles and also alters the size distribution. The size properties can be measured by light-scattering techniques like laser diffraction. Due to the reduced size comparing to their non-milled counterparts, milled particles acquire a greater specific area. Furthermore, they also have higher surface energy, and this increases the dissolution rate of the milled drug along with the thinner diffusion boundaries. On the other hand, milling also alters the shape of particles and thus improves the surface roughness. There are different techniques of milling to produce nanoparticles, namely wet milling, media milling, higher-pressure homogenisation, and cryogenic milling [49].

Of the many milling methods, liquid-assisted grinding (LAG) is worth mentioning here. A review was published by Ying et al. on the synthesis of APIs and other drug-like fragments through the use of LAG. They documented the possible synthesis of sulfonylureas, chiral amines, peptides, hydantoins, fenbufen, metallo-drugs, procainamide and paracetamol, levopraziquantel, indole derivatives, sulfonyl guanidines, quinazolinones, pyranochromenones, quinoxalines, n-demethylation of alkaloids, and benzo-fused heteroaromatic compounds. The process of synthesis using LAG is called mechano-synthesis and this study comes under the umbrella of mechanochemistry, which is a significant representative of green chemistry. Through the adoption of such green chemistry approaches, drugs and drug-like fragments can be produced with high efficiency while having less impact on the environment [50].

2.4 Bio-fabricated Nanoparticles

Bio-fabricated nanoparticles (BFNPs) are nanoparticles (particles with size in nanometers) which are derived or synthesised from living organisms such as plants or microorganisms or from their extracted materials. As has been mentioned, nanoparticles have wide applications in numerous fields such as agriculture, industry, and medicines. We do not discuss the drawbacks of the conventional chemical synthesis of nanoparticles, but rather in this section cover the impact of the green approach to synthesising nanoparticles.

Using the green approach advances the nanoparticles' characteristics and impedes various sources of toxicity. This environmentally friendly approach does not require supplementary reagents and the process often involves a minimum number of steps. Additionally, with the help of the green approach the blood compatibility and stability of nanoparticles can be enhanced. For example, silver nanoparticles (AgNPs) fabricated through an extract of *Zingiber officinale* were revealed to be more stable than their chemically synthetic variant, which lost their surface charge and subsequently aggregated in some physiological conditions; in contrast, BFNPs were stable at 20–50 °C for up to 30 days. Therefore, by using the green approach for the synthesis of nanoparticles we can enhance their surface properties and enhance them with natural biocompatible constituents.

There are several methods for synthesising BFNPs, which include [51]:

- Photosynthesis of metallic nanoparticles (MNPs).
- Biosynthesis of MNPs through microbes.
- Biomolecule-mediated synthesis of MNPs.
- Intracellular synthesis of MNPs.
- Green synthesis of organic nanoparticles.

BFNPs have diverse applications in different fields, particularly in medicine. BFNPs are being researched and employed in drug-delivery systems, anticancer activities, antimicrobial activities, and for diagnostic purposes. For an overview, the anticancer activities of BFNPs are outlined in Table 2.1.

Table 2.1 Summary of anticancer potential of bio-fabricated nanoparticles (BFNPs).

BFNPs	Bio-template	Significance	Cancer	Reference
Fatty acid-capped AgNPs (LIV-AgNPs)	Polyherbal Liv52 drug extract (papaya leaf extract)	Dose-dependent cytotoxic effect	Colon cancer	[52]
AgNPs	*Justicia adhatoda*	Anticancer activity at 100 μg/ml concentration	Cervical cancer	[53]
Platinum NPs	*Psidium guajava*	Effective cytotoxicity	Breast cancer	[54]
CuONPs	*Ocimum americanum*	Dose-dependent cytotoxic effect	Lung adenocarcinoma	[55]
AuNPs	*Ganoderma lucidum*	Cytotoxicity	Colon cancer	[56]
AuNPs	Isolated porphyran from marine red algae	pH-dependent release reduces the toxicity of doxorubicin	Glioma	[57]
AgNPs	*Melia azedarach*	Superior cytotoxicity	Dalton's ascites lymphoma (DAL)	[58]

(Continued)

Table 2.1 (Continued)

BFNPs	Bio-template	Significance	Cancer	Reference
AuNPs	Bacteria strain of *Delftia* sp.	pH-responsive drug release and elevated cytotoxicity	Lung cancer	[59]
AgNPs	Plant *Piper longum*	Effective cytotoxic and antioxidant properties	Breast cancer	[60]
AgNPs	Plant gum ghatti and gum olibanum	Cytotoxicity enhanced by decreasing NP size	Cervical cancer	[61]
AgNPs	*Tritirachium oryzae* W5H	Cytotoxic effect	Breast and prostate cancer	[62]

AgNP, silver nanoparticle; AuNP, gold nanoparticle; CuONP, copper oxide nanoparticle; NP, nanoparticle.

2.5 Green Approaches in Malaria Treatment

Malaria is a parasitic disease that is spread through protozoal vectors that are common in underdeveloped and developing countries. The malarial parasite *Plasmodium* affects humans and is the reason for millions of deaths worldwide every year [63]. Although this disease is pandemic, it is severe in tropical and subtropical regions. Plants are an important conventional source of medicines for malaria. Artemisinin and quinine are the two main drugs for malarial treatment that are derived from plants [6]. The use of these drugs is now facing the problem of resistance by the parasite, and nanobiotechnology, a greener approach, appears to be an efficient tool to combat this issue.

Nanoparticles designed and manufactured through an environmentally friendly approach play a strategic role in the field of medicine and show potential against *Anopheles* larvae, a vector of the malarial parasite. Substantial bio-efficacy against the larvae has been demonstrated by nanoparticles extracted from plants. Excellent antiplasmodial activity of bio-fabricated nanoparticles is also reported by studies of their use against *Plasmodium berghei* and *Plasmodium falciparum*. Different nanoparticles such as silver (Ag), gold (Au), selenium (Se), titanium (Ti), zinc oxide (ZnO), and many more are being employed for this purpose [6, 64].

Another approach to prevent malarial infection is 'vector control', which is discussed in the next section. With an approach to develop green methods for drug synthesis and ecofriendly therapeutical agents, it is not irrelevant to say that 'preventive measures' for the infection are also considered a green approach.

2.6 Green Approaches in Dengue Treatment

Dengue, a viral disease, spreads through a vector that is an *Aedes* sp. mosquito. Dengue fever is caused by four DENV serotypes. It represents an important health problem for the general public and is endemic in more than 120 countries [65]; around 390 million infections are caused by dengue each year in tropical and subtropical areas. In 2015 a vaccine for dengue was licensed but it did not prove to be a general solution due to certain factors. In this regard, vector control is still the best approach for the containment of the virus.

Further, vector control through environmental intervention symbolises a green approach as there is a low risk of toxicity and contamination of the environment [66]. Here the term 'ecofriendly vector' applies, which is the release of modified species of the same arthropod vector but lacking the ability to harbour the virus in the environment, thus reducing the spread of infection. In another green approach nanoparticles extracted and fabricated from plants are being used as pesticides for the control of mosquitos [67]. For instance, AgNPs fabricated through a seed extract of *Moringa oleifera* are reported to be an effective tool against *Aedes aegypti*, a major vector of dengue serotype DENV-2 [68]. In recent research, the anti-dengue effect of leaf extract from *Carica papaya* was examined through in vitro and in silico studies. The results highlighted that DENV-2 viral inhibition was >90% by botanically synthesised AgNPs from extracts of *C. papaya* [69].

2.7 Green Synthesis of Different Drugs

This section considers some of the drugs or pharmaceutical derivatives that are reported to be being synthesised in a green approach.

2.7.1 Quinoline-Based Imidazole Derivatives

Naturally occurring quinoline-based therapeutics, alkaloids, and synthetic analogues are significant regarding their biological activities. Some quinoline derivatives have different pharmaceutical properties, for instance primaquine is an important agent in antimalarial activity and dibucaine is a valuable anaesthetic. Many derivates of quinoline have been developed for treatments of different diseases such as HIV, malaria, antibacterial infections, and tumours. Desai and his colleagues reported the successful synthesis of quinoline derivatives through the microwave-assisted heating of reactants in a solvent-free reaction. They also observed the high yield and rate of reaction carried out by microwave irradiation compared to conventional methods for heterocyclic compounds like quinoline-based derivatives [70].

2.7.2 Benzimidazoles

Another important class of bioactive heterocyclic compounds that have significant applications in therapeutics are moieties of benzimidazoles. Due to their broad range of pharmaceutical activity, benzimidazole moieties are being used as antibacterial, antiviral, antiulcer, antifungal, and anti-inflammatory agents. There are different synthetic methodologies for benzimidazoles [71], but a review on green approaches has been conducted by Asif. He demonstrated the available greener methodologies for the synthesis of benzimidazoles such as using microwave irradiation, a green catalyst, a solvent-free reaction, and a green solvent [72].

2.7.3 Chalcone Derivatives

Bacterial infections are a major clinical issue in the developing countries of Asia, Africa, and South America. Drugs used against these Gram-positive and Gram-negative pathogens include norfloxacin, amoxicillin, and ciprofloxacin, but there are some side effects of using these drugs such as hypertension, dizziness, and nausea, not to forget the bacterial resistance. Therefore, the approach of using antibacterial agents is gaining much attention and is of high significance. In this regard, chalcone derivatives have been reported to have antibacterial, antiviral, antifungal, anticancer, and insecticidal properties. Chalcone-based heterocyclic compounds have significantly enhanced antibacterial and antiviral activities. Khan has reported on the synthesis of novel chalcones under microwave irradiation [73], which has also been discussed by Furthermore, many schemes have been shown by Shntaif [74].

2.8 Conclusion

Green synthesis, whether in medicine or other fields such as food and industry, is receiving a great deal of attention and effort as the need for environmental sustainability is being acknowledged around the whole world. Regarding the synthesis of pharmaceutically active compounds, there are several green approaches that can be useful for improving product quality and yield as well as for the environment. A green approach can help in saving the fossil fuels that are used in conventional methods as the source of heat, for instance the microwave-assisted approach as discussed in this chapter is an efficient heating process. Similarly, ultrasound-assisted synthesis can help in reducing the use of solvents. Furthermore, we can obtain molecules of the desired size and shape via molecular sieving, which also assists in reducing waste production through the entire process. For increasing the efficiency of a drug or pharmaceutical agent, such as its solubility and dissolution, milling is of great significance. These approaches are considered green due to their lower impact on the environment and increased efficiency of production with less complex methodologies. Production of BFNPs also comes under green synthesis and many reports have been published regarding their applications and efficiency in drug synthesis and drug-delivery systems.

Although there are many efforts to improve environmental sustainability, there is a call for a detailed search for green methods that can be applied to replace conventional methods to huge effect, so that the environment can be left safer and more sustainable for future generations. To summarise:

- Green synthesis highlights techniques that adhere to a consistent and ecofriendly pathway with moderate reactions to safeguard a sustainable environment.
- Green chemistry, also called sustainable chemistry, is defined as an endeavour in chemistry to reduce pollution. It attempts to enhance the yield output of chemical products by adjusting how chemicals are devised, produced, and used.
- Four green approaches are briefly covered in this chapter.
- Microwaves work as a source of heat for the reaction to occur. The main gain of this method is uniform heating.

- Ultrasound-assisted synthesis, also termed sonochemistry, involves the application of ultrasound to promote a chemical reaction.
- Molecular sieving has the ability to make use of nanofilters that can separate molecules based on their desired shape, scale, and surface type, and helps in engineering better products.
- To overcome the challenge of poor water solubility of drugs, an approach called milling is also being employed for the purpose of enhancement of drug solubility through mechanical energy.
- Bio-fabricated nanoparticles are synthesised from living organisms such as plants or microorganisms or from their extracted materials.

References

1 Agrawal, P.K., Shrivastava, R., and Verma, J. (2019). Bioremediation approaches for degradation and detoxification of polycyclic aromatic hydrocarbons. In: *Emerging and Eco-friendly Approaches for Waste Management* (eds. R.N. Bharagava, and P. Chowdhary), 99–119. Singapore: Springer.

2 Mishra, S., Chowdhary, P., and Bharagava, R.N. (2019). Conventional methods for the removal of industrial pollutants, their merits and demerits. In: *Emerging and Eco-friendly Approaches for Waste Management* (eds. R.N. Bharagava, and P. Chowdhary), 1–31. Singapore: Springer.

3 Mtibe, A., Mokhothu, T.H., John, M.J. et al. (2018). Fabrication and characterization of various engineered nanomaterials. In: *Handbook of Nanomaterials for Industrial Applications* (ed. C.M. Hussain, 151–171. Amsterdam: Elsevier.

4 Venkatachalam, C.D., Sengottian, M., and Ravichandran, S.R. (2021). Green synthesis of nanoparticles—metals and their oxides. In: *Nanomaterials* (eds. R.P. Kumar, and B. Bharathiraja), 79–96. Amsterdam: Elsevier.

5 Soumya, M., Rajeshkumar, S., and Venkat Kumar, S. (2017). A review on biogenic synthesis of gold nanoparticles, characterization, and its applications. *Resource-Efficient Technologies* 3 (4): 516–527. https://doi.org/10.1016/j.reffit.2017.08.002.

6 Leili, M., Kaushik, P., Muhammad, B. et al. (2021). Green nanoparticles to treat patients with Malaria disease: an overview. *Journal of Molecular Structure* 1229: 129857. https://doi.org/10.1016/j.molstruc.2020.129857.

7 Tsekhmistrenko, S., Bityutskyy, V., Tsekhmistrenko, O. et al. (2020). Bacterial synthesis of nanoparticles: a green approach. *Biosystems Diversity* 28 (1): 9–17.

8 Chella Purushothaman, D., and Arun, K.T. (2018). Green synthesis of nanomaterials. In: *Micro and Nano Technologies: Synthesis of Inorganic Materials* (eds. S.M. Bhagyaraj, O.S. Oluwafemi, N. Kalarikkal, and S. Thomas), 169–184. Cambridge: Woodhead Publishing. https://doi.org/10.1016/B978-0-08-101975-7.00007-5.

9 Zimmerman, J.B., Anastas, P.T., Erythropel, H.C., and Leitner, W. (2020). Designing for a green chemistry future. *Science* 367 (6476): 397–400.

10 Jeon, J. (2018). Green chemistry. *Encyclopedia Britannica*. https://www.britannica.com/science/green-chemistry.

11 Jiménez-González, C., and Constable, D.J. (2011). *Green Chemistry and Engineering: A Practical Design Approach*. Chichester: Wiley.
12 Matlack, A. (2010). *Introduction to Green Chemistry*. Boca Raton, FL: CRC Press.
13 Perosa, A., and Zecchini, F. (2007). *Methods and Reagents for Green Chemistry: An Introduction*. Chichester: Wiley.
14 Sheldon, R.A. (2008). Green and sustainable chemistry: challenges and perspectives. *Green Chemistry* 10: 359–360.
15 Bell, M.M., and Ashwood, L.L. (2015). *An Invitation to Environmental Sociology*. Berkeley, CA: Sage.
16 Brundtland, G.H. (1987). *Report of the World Commission on Environment and Development: 'Our Common Future'*. New York: UN.
17 Redclift, M. (2005). Sustainable development (1987–2005): an oxymoron comes of age. *Sustainable Development* 13 (4): 212–227.
18 Taylor, M. (2011). *Public Policy in the Community*. London: Macmillan International Higher Education.
19 Anastas, P.T., and Warner, J.C. (1998). Principles of green chemistry. In: *Green Chemistry: Theory and Practice*, 29. Oxford: Oxford University Press.
20 Van Boeckel, T.P., Gandra, S., Ashok, A. et al. (2014). Global antibiotic consumption 2000 to 2010: an analysis of national pharmaceutical sales data. *Lancet Infectious Diseases* 14 (8): 742–750. https://doi.org/10.1016/S1473-3099(14)70780-7.
21 Abdullahi, A.A. (2011). Trends and challenges of traditional medicine in Africa. *African Journal of Traditional, Complementary and Alternative Medicines* 8 (5 Suppl): 115–123. http://doi.org/10.4314/ajtcam.v8i5S.5.
22 Samb, B., Desai, N., Nishtar, S. et al. (2010). Prevention and management of chronic disease: a litmus test for health-systems strengthening in low-income and middle-income countries. *Lancet* 376 (9754): 1785–1797.
23 Falco, A., Barrajón-Catalán, E., Menéndez-Gutiérrez, M., Falco, A. et al. (2013). Melittin-loaded immunoliposomes against viral surface proteins, a new approach to antiviral therapy. *Antiviral Research* 97 (2): 218–221. https://doi.org/10.1016/j.antiviral.2012.12.004.
24 Pinheiro, E.D.S., Antunes, O.A.C, and Fortunak, J.M.D. (2008). A survey of the syntheses of active pharmaceutical ingredients for antiretroviral drug combinations critical to access in emerging nations. *Antiviral Research* 79 (3): 143–165. https://doi.org/10.1016/j.antiviral.2008.05.001.
25 Mas, V., Falco, A., Brocal, I. et al. (2006). Identification of selective inhibitors of VHSV from biased combinatorial libraries of N,N′-disubstituted 2,5-piperazinediones. *Antiviral Research* 72 (2): 107–115. https://doi.org/10.1016/j.antiviral.2006.04.005.
26 De Joarder, D., Sarkar, R., and Mukhopadhyay, C. (2020). Sustainable green technologies for synthesis of potential drugs targeted toward tropical diseases. In: *Green Approaches in Medicinal Chemistry for Sustainable Drug Design* (ed. B.M. Banik), 75–93. Amsterdam: Elsevier.
27 Zhang, X.B., Shi, N.Q., Yang, Z.Q., and Wang, X.L. (2014). [Application of microwave irradiation technology to the field of pharmaceutics]. *Yao Xue Xue Bao* 49 (3): 303–309.
28 Santagada, V., Frecentese, F., Perissutti, E. et al. (2009). Microwave assisted synthesis: a new technology in drug discovery. *Mini-Reviews in Medicinal Chemistry* 9 (3): 340–358. http://doi.org/10.2174/138955751090903034 0.

29 Sadler, S., Moeller, A.R., and Jones, G.B. (2012). Microwave and continuous flow technologies in drug discovery. *Expert Opinion on Drug Discovery* 7 (12): 1107–1128. http://doi.org/10.1517/17460441.2012.727393.

30 Yadav, A.R., and Mohite, S.K. (2020). A brief review: microwave chemistry and its applications. *Research Journal of Pharmaceutical Dosage Forms Technology* 12 (3): 191–197. http://doi.org/10.5958/0975-4377.2020.00033.6.

31 Aljuhani, A., El-Sayed, W.S., Sahu, P.K. et al. (2018). Microwave-assisted synthesis of novel imidazolium, pyridinium and pyridazinium-based ionic liquids and/or salts and prediction of physico-chemical properties for their toxicity and antibacterial activity. *Journal of Molecular Liquids* 249: 747–753. https://doi.org/10.1016/j.molliq.2017.11.108.

32 Divya, G., Deepika, J., Dolly, R., and Akash, K. (2018). Microwave synthesized nanocomposites for enhancing oral bioavailability of drugs. In: *Applications of Nanocomposite Materials in Drug Delivery* (eds. Asiri, A.M. Inamuddin, and A. Mohammad), 619–632. Woohead Publishing. https://doi.org/10.1016/B978-0-12-813741-3.00027-3.

33 Rajashree, N., Abhisek, S., and Nayak, P.L. (2011). Preparation and characterization of chitosan–polylactide composites blended with Cloisite 30B for control release of the anticancer drug paclitaxel. *Carbohydrate Polymers* 83 (2): 988–994. https://doi.org/10.1016/j.carbpol.2010.09.009.

34 Gabr, M.T., El-Gohary, N.S., El-Bendary, E.R. et al. (2017). Microwave-assisted synthesis and antitumor evaluation of a new series of thiazolylcoumarin derivatives. *EXCLI Journal* 16: 1114–1131. http://doi.org/10.17179/excli2017-208.

35 Mondal, S., Hoang, G., Manivasagan, P. et al. (2019). Rapid microwave-assisted synthesis of gold loaded hydroxyapatite collagen nano-bio materials for drug delivery and tissue engineering application. *Ceramics International* 45 (3): 2977–2988. https://doi.org/10.1016/j.ceramint.2018.10.016.

36 Henary, M., Kananda, C., Rotolo, L. et al. (2020). Benefits and applications of microwave-assisted synthesis of nitrogen containing heterocycles in medicinal chemistry. *RSC Advances* 10 (24): 14170–14197. http://doi.org/10.1039/D0RA01378A.

37 Tucker, J.L., and Faul, M.M. (2016). Industrial research: drug companies must adopt green chemistry. *Nature* 534 (7605): 27–29. http://doi.org/10.1038/534027a.

38 Mohammadi Ziarani, G., Kheilkordi, Z., and Gholamzadeh, P. (2020). Ultrasound-assisted synthesis of heterocyclic compounds. *Molecular Diversity* 24 (3): 771–820. http://doi.org/10.1007/s11030-019-09964-1.

39 Rostamnia, S., and Lamei, K. (2011). A rapid, catalyst-free, three-component synthesis of rhodanines in water using ultrasound. *Synthesis* 2011 (19): 3080–3082. http://doi.org/10.1055/s-0030-1260158.

40 Tatu, P., Prosanta, S., Tapio, J.N. et al. (2017). Design, synthesis, and biological evaluation of 2,4-dihydropyrano 2,3-c pyrazole derivatives as autotaxin inhibitors. *European Journal of Pharmaceutical Sciences* 107: 97–111. https://doi.org/10.1016/j.ejps.2017.07.002.

41 Yi, Z., Hui, W., Yu, H. et al. (2011). A novel and environment-friendly method for preparing dihydropyrano 2,3-c pyrazoles in water under ultrasound irradiation. *Ultrasonics Sonochemistry* 18 (3): 708–712. https://doi.org/10.1016/j.ultsonch.2010.11.012.

42 Draye, M., Chatel, G., and Duwald, R. (2020). Ultrasound for drug synthesis: a green approach. *Pharmaceuticals* 13 (2): 23.

43 Han, J., Fu, J., and Schoch, R.B. (2008). Molecular sieving using nanofilters: past, present and future. *Lab on a Chip* 8 (1): 23–33.

44 Xiang, J., Shang, M., Kawamata, Y. et al. (2019). Hindered dialkyl ether synthesis with electrogenerated carbocations. *Nature* 573 (7774): 398–402. http://doi.org/10.1038/s41586-019-1539-y.

45 Kandambeth, S., Biswal, B.P., Chaudhari, H.D. et al. (2017). Selective molecular sieving in self-standing porous covalent-organic-framework membranes. *Advanced Materials* 29 (2): 1603945. https://doi.org/10.1002/adma.201603945.

46 Song, Z., Ma, Y.-L., Li, C.-E. et al. (2019). Molecular sieving film prepared by vacuum filtration for the efficient removal of tetracycline antibiotics from pharmaceutical wastewater. *Advances in Materials Science and Engineering* 2019: 3532576. http://doi.org/10.1155/2019/3532576.

47 Zhou, P., Yao, L., Chen, K., and Su, B. (2020). Silica nanochannel membranes for electrochemical analysis and molecular sieving: a comprehensive review. *Critical Reviews in Analytical Chemistry* 50 (5): 424–444.

48 Vallet-Regí, M., Balas, F., and Arcos, D. (2007). Mesoporous materials for drug delivery. *Angewandte Chemie* 46 (40): 7548–7558. https://doi.org/10.1002/anie.200604488.

49 Loh, Z.H., Samanta, A.K., and Heng, P.W.S. (2015). Overview of milling techniques for improving the solubility of poorly water-soluble drugs. *Asian Journal of Pharmaceutical Sciences* 10 (4): 255–274. https://doi.org/10.1016/j.ajps.2014.12.006.

50 Ying, P., Yu, J., and Su, W. (2021). Liquid-assisted grinding mechanochemistry in the synthesis of pharmaceuticals. *Advanced Synthesis Catalysis* 363 (5): 1246–1271. https://doi.org/10.1002/adsc.202001245.

51 Kumar, S., Lather, V., and Pandita, D. (2015). Green synthesis of therapeutic nanoparticles: an expanding horizon. *Nanomedicine* 10 (15): 2451–2471. https://doi.org/10.2217/nnm.15.112.

52 Ansari, M.A., Asiri, S.M.M., Alzohairy, M.A. et al. (2021). Biofabricated fatty acids-capped silver nanoparticles as potential antibacterial, antifungal, antibiofilm and anticancer agents. *Pharmaceuticals* 14 (2): 139. http://doi.org/10.3390/ph14020139.

53 Mathiyazhagan, N., Devarajan, N., Sabariswaran, S. et al. (2021). Biofabrication and characterization of AgNPs synthesized by Justicia adhatoda and efficiency on multi-drug resistant microbes and anticancer activity. *Inorganic Chemistry Communications* 134: 109071. https://doi.org/10.1016/j.inoche.2021.109071.

54 Manzoor, S., Bashir, D.J., Imtiyaz, K. et al. (2021). Biofabricated platinum nanoparticles: therapeutic evaluation as a potential nanodrug against breast cancer cells and drug-resistant bacteria. *RSC Advances* 11 (40): 24900–24916. http://doi.org/10.1039/D1RA03133C.

55 Manikandan, D.B., Arumugam, M., Veeran, S. et al. (2021). Biofabrication of ecofriendly copper oxide nanoparticles using Ocimum americanum aqueous leaf extract: analysis of in vitro antibacterial, anticancer, and photocatalytic activities. *Environmental Science and Pollution Research* 28 (26): 33927–33941. http://doi.org/10.1007/s11356-020-12108-w.

56 Elumalai, D., Suman, T.Y., Hemavathi, M. et al. (2021). Biofabrication of gold nanoparticles using Ganoderma lucidum and their cytotoxicity against human colon cancer cell line (HT-29). *Bulletin of Materials Science* 44 (2): 132. http://doi.org/10.1007/s12034-021-02435-0.

57 Venkatpurwar, V., Shiras, A., and Pokharkar, V. (2011). Porphyran capped gold nanoparticles as a novel carrier for delivery of anticancer drug: in vitro cytotoxicity study.

International Journal of Pharmaceutics 409 (1–2): 314–320. https://doi.org/10.1016/j.ijpharm.2011.02.054.

58 Sukirtha, R., Priyanka, K.M., Antony, J.J. et al. (2012). Cytotoxic effect of Green synthesized silver nanoparticles using Melia azedarach against in vitro HeLa cell lines and lymphoma mice model. *Process Biochemistry* 47 (2): 273–279. https://doi.org/10.1016/j.procbio.2011.11.003.

59 Kumar, C.G., Poornachandra, Y., and Mamidyala, S.K. (2014). Green synthesis of bacterial gold nanoparticles conjugated to resveratrol as delivery vehicles. *Colloids and Surfaces B: Biointerfaces* 123: 311–317. https://doi.org/10.1016/j.colsurfb.2014.09.032.

60 Reddy, N.J., Vali, D.N., Rani, M., and Rani, S.S. (2014). Evaluation of antioxidant, antibacterial and cytotoxic effects of green synthesized silver nanoparticles by Piper longum fruit. *Materials Science and Engineering: C, Materials for Biological Applications* 34: 115–122. https://doi.org/10.1016/j.msec.2013.08.039.

61 Kora, A.J., and Sashidhar, R.B. (2015). Antibacterial activity of biogenic silver nanoparticles synthesized with gum ghatti and gum olibanum: a comparative study. *Journal of Antibiotics (Tokyo)* 68 (2): 88–97. http://doi.org/10.1038/ja.2014.114.

62 Al-Tawarah, N.M., Qaralleh, H., Khlaifat, A.M. et al. (2020). Anticancer and antibacterial properties of verthemia iphionides essential oil/silver nanoparticles. *Biomedical and Pharmacology Journal* 13 (3): 1175–1185. https://dx.doi.org/10.13005/bpj/1985.

63 Rahman, K., Khan, S.U., Fahad, S. et al. (2019). Nano-biotechnology: a new approach to treat and prevent malaria. *International Journal of Nanomedicine* 14: 1401–1410. http://doi.org/10.2147/IJN.S190692.

64 Hamed, B., Zahra, A., Mohammad Taghi, R. et al. (2019). Nanobiotechnology as an emerging approach to combat malaria: a systematic review. *Nanomedicine: Nanotechnology, Biology and Medicine* 18: 221–233. https://doi.org/10.1016/j.nano.2019.02.017.

65 Rozera, R., Verma, S., Kumar, R. et al. (2019). Herbal remedies, vaccines and drugs for dengue fever: emerging prevention and treatment strategies. *Asian Pacific Journal of Tropical Medicine* 12 (4): 147–152. http://doi.org/10.4103/1995-7645.257113.

66 Buhler, C., Winkler, V., Runge-Ranzinger, S. et al. (2019). Environmental methods for dengue vector control – a systematic review and meta-analysis. *PLOS Neglected Tropical Diseases* 13 (7): e0007420. http://doi.org/10.1371/journal.pntd.0007420.

67 Benelli, G., Maggi, F., Pavela, R. et al. (2018). Mosquito control with green nanopesticides: towards the One Health approach? A review of non-target effects. *Environmental Science and Pollution Research* 25 (11): 10184–10206. https://doi.org/10.1007/s11356-017-9752-4.

68 Sujitha, V., Murugan, K., Paulpandi, M. et al. (2015). Green-synthesized silver nanoparticles as a novel control tool against dengue virus (DEN-2) and its primary vector Aedes aegypti. *Parasitology Research* 114 (9): 3315–3325. https://doi.org/10.1007/s00436-015-4556-2.

69 Bere, A.W., Mulati, O., Kimotho, J., and Ng'ong'a, F. (2021). Carica papaya leaf extract silver synthesized nanoparticles inhibit dengue type 2 viral replication in vitro. *Pharmaceuticals* 14 (8): 718. https://doi.org/10.3390/ph14080718.

70 Desai, N.C., Maheta, A.S., Rajpara, K.M. et al. (2014). Green synthesis of novel quinoline based imidazole derivatives and evaluation of their antimicrobial activity. *Journal of Saudi Chemical Society* 18 (6): 963–971. https://doi.org/10.1016/j.jscs.2011.11.021.

71 Kathirvelan, D., Yuvaraj, P., Babu, K. et al. (2013). A green synthesis of benzimidazoles. *Indian Journal of Chemistry* 52B: 1152–1156. http://nopr.niscair.res.in/handle/123456789/20511.

72 Asif, M. (2019). Green synthesis of benzimidazole derivatives: an overview on green chemistry and its applications. *Chemical Methodologies* 3 (6): 620–631. https://dx.doi.org/10.33945/SAMI/CHEMM.2019.6.1.

73 Salman, A.K., and Abdullah, M.A. (2017). Green synthesis, characterization and biological evaluation of novel chalcones as anti bacterial agents. *Arabian Journal of Chemistry* 10: S2890–S2895. https://doi.org/10.1016/j.arabjc.2013.11.018.

74 Shntaif, A.H. (2016). Green synthesis of chalcones under microwave irradiation. *International Journal of ChemTech Research* 9 (02): 36–39.

3

Modern Green Extraction Techniques

Marcello Locatelli[1], Enrica Rosato[1], Cristian D'Ovidio[2], Martina Bonelli[2], Halil Ibrahim Ulusoy[3], Abuzar Kabir[4], Imran Ali[5], Fabio Savini[6], Ugo de Grazia[7], Victoria Samanidou[8] and Angela Tartaglia[1]

[1] *Department of Pharmacy, University of Chieti–Pescara 'G. d'Annunzio', Chieti, Italy*
[2] *Department of Medicine and Aging Sciences, Section of Legal Medicine, University of Chieti–Pescara 'G. d'Annunzio', Chieti, Italy*
[3] *Department of Analytical Chemistry, Faculty of Pharmacy, Cumhuriyet University, Sivas, Turkey*
[4] *International Forensic Research Institute, Department of Chemistry and Biochemistry, Florida International University, Miami, FL, USA*
[5] *Department of Chemistry, Jamia Millia Islamia, Jamia Nagar, New Delhi, India*
[6] *Pharmatoxicology Laboratory – Hospital 'Santo Spirito', Pescara, Italy*
[7] *Fondazione IRCCS Istituto Neurologico Carlo Besta, Laboratory of Neurological Biochemistry and Neuropharmacology, Milan, Italy*
[8] *Laboratory of Analytical Chemistry, Department of Chemistry, Aristotle University of Thessaloniki, Thessaloniki, Greece*

CONTENTS

3.1 Introduction

Sample pre-treatment is one of the extremely critical and error-prone steps of the entire analytical procedure. Analysis selectivity and sensitivity could be improved through proper clean-up and pre-concentration of the sample. Sample preparation presents as a key aim the concentration and isolation of target analytes and is therefore an inevitable step for the success of analytical processes, especially when complex sample matrices are involved [1]. Several efforts have been made to simplify this crucial and often underestimated preliminary analytical phase as much as possible. Most of the analyses are carried out on complex sample matrices, which are not suitable for direct injection into analytical instruments. Therefore, sample preparation is necessary because matrix components could interfere with target analytes and may reduce the performance of the analytical instrument. For

Sustainable Approaches in Pharmaceutical Sciences, First Edition. Edited by Kamal Shah, Durgesh Nandini Chauhan, and Nagendra Singh Chauhan.

these reasons, all modern techniques aim to obtain a suitable sample for analysis by isolating and concentrating the analytes of interest.

Since the early days of introducing and developing sample preparation techniques, numerous procedures and technologies have been devised over the years, beginning with traditional and conventional ones, such as liquid-liquid extraction (LLE) and solid phase extraction (SPE). However, despite their wide applicability in different fields, some limitations have emerged such as high volumes of organic solvents, long application times, and additional steps often required. In this scenario, microextraction techniques have emerged in the last two decades to try to cross established boundaries [2].

Nowadays, sustainable development is a cornerstone of any new area and this concept has also been extended to the chemical field, and in particular to analytical chemistry. As a result, principles that aim to consider environmental health and safety during the development of new analytical procedures were introduced [3]. The 'green chemistry' model was presented in 1998 [4], and subsequently the concept of green analytical chemistry (GAC) emerged in 2000. The principles of GAC have helped analytical chemists to make laboratory activities more environmentally friendly through the reduction of toxic chemicals and solvents in analytical processes, minimisation of energy consumption, minimisation of wastes, and improvement of operator safety [5, 6]. These critical issues for GAC principles included in analytical procedures are schematised in Figure 3.1.

For all analyses, except those that use direct techniques, the sample should be treated in the first step. In this context it is possible to use different approaches, such as non-invasive methods or applying statistical analyses for sample selection in order to get as much information from as few samples as possible and interpret results without error. Once the samples have been obtained for analysis, the preparation step is fundamental. This phase, in addition to leading to a sample suitable for instrumental analysis (most complex matrices are not suitable for direct analysis), must be ecocompatible. The analytical challenge is therefore focused on making sample preparation techniques as green as possible, through the mechanisation, contraction, and simplification of extraction procedures.

This chapter will discuss procedures for sample preparation, handling, and extraction according to the values of ecocompatibility outlined in GAC, with particular attention to the use of greener solvents and to the application of simple and miniaturised microextraction procedures that require minimal amounts of solvents and reagents.

3.2 Ecofriendly Sample Preparation Techniques

The optimal approach to minimise the use of solvents and reagents would be direct analysis, avoiding the preliminary phase. However, direct procedures are only suitable for analysing clean and non-interferential matrices. In general, most analyses involve complex matrices, rich in compounds and interferences. These samples are therefore not suitable for immediate injection but require preliminary steps that make them suitable for subsequent instrumental analysis.

3.2.1 Solid Phase Extraction

SPE was one of the earliest techniques developed for the isolation and extraction of target analytes. This technique generally uses SPE cartridges that contain the packed solid porous

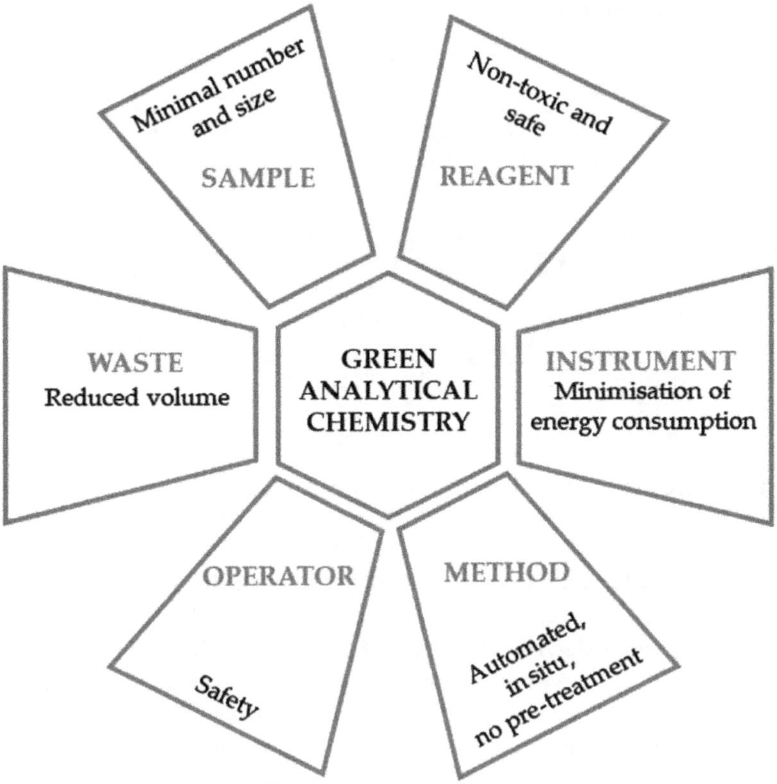

Figure 3.1 Important components of sample preparation procedure with regard to green analytical chemistry.

material for the absorption mechanism. The general procedure is based on the interaction between the absorbing solid phase and the solution containing the analytes, which, passing through the SPE bed, are retained or not by the packaged phase. The separation relies on the differential affinity between the packaging materials contained within the cartridge (Figure 3.2).

SPE is recognised as more advantageous and greener than LLE, as it employs reduced volumes of solvent and generates little waste. In addition, the whole process can be automated. Although SPE is one of the most popular techniques, some disadvantages have been found such as the non-uniformity of the bed, the restricted selectivity of certain conventional absorbents, and the clogging of the cartridge that could occur with very complex matrices [6].

Thanks to the many advantages of this technique, interest around it has grown and several studies have been published in recent years. These latest studies emphasise GAC and how to make sample pre-treatment through SPE more environmentally friendly.

Trenholm and co-workers have described an online SPE–LC–MS/MS (solid phase extraction–liquid chromatography–tandem mass spectrometry) instrument configuration for the direct analysis and evaluation of pharmaceutical markers in water [7]. The extraction was performed using Symbiosis™ Pharma (Spark Holland, Emmen, The Netherlands), an automated workstation, coupled to an LC system in the XLC mode operated through Analyst®

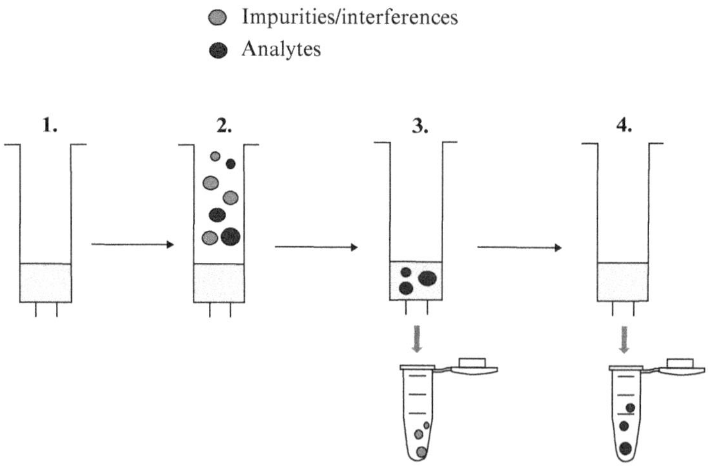

Figure 3.2 Schematic representation of solid phase extraction procedure.

1.4.2 (Applied Biosystems, Foster City, CA, USA). Waters Oasis HLB Prospekt cartridges (Milford, MA, USA) were used. The retained analytes were then eluted directly to the LC column using 200 μL methanol (MeOH). This online SPE has considerably reduced the amount of solvents (solvent usage is 54-fold lower for this method compared to the offline one), with a 98% reduction in the amount of environmental pollution. The obtained data have proven also that the most sustainable laboratory methods represent an alternative approach capable of maintaining high levels of sensitivity, selectivity, and robustness.

Laise C. da Silva et al. have described an online SPE method for the extraction of compounds from apple pomace [8]. The Extract-US system (FAPESP 2013/04304–4, patent pending) was used for the extraction process. Because of the environmental impact of MeOH, ethanol (EtOH) has been assessed as a replacement solvent. EtOH was used as both an initiation and an extraction solvent. The data were then matched with those obtained using MeOH and the differences in recovery observed were not statistically significant, suggesting that lower-toxicity solvents can be used in the extraction method.

Shirani and collaborators have described a green method for cobalt (Co), nickel (Ni), and chromium (Cr III) in nutrition and environmental samples using needle hub in-syringe solid phase extraction (NH-IS-SPE) based on a novel functionalised bio-polyamide [9]. For the first time, a functionalised bio-polyamide with high adsorption efficiency was launched. The developed method is therefore environmentally friendly thanks to the use of bio-polyamide. The optimised extraction showed numerous improvements such as reduced time, excellent linearity, and a higher enrichment factor compared to similar methods.

Nanomaterials (NMs) are now largely replacing conventional adsorbent materials in solid extraction technologies. NMs present a significant surface area that enhances the adsorption and interaction capacity of target analytes; in addition, they present high thermal, mechanical, and electronic stability. The most commonly described nano-based adsorbents are magnetic nanoparticles (MgNPs), carbon nanomaterials (CNMs), and silica nanoparticles (SiNPs) [10].

Shi and collaborators have reported a new method for the analysis of pesticide remains in fruit juice using graphene-based pipette tip SPE [11]. The graphene material synthesised was characterised by different techniques. Graphene was then packed in a cartridge. The reported work observed reduced consumption of absorbent material and solvents, as well as reduced extraction and analysis time, maintaining exceptional analytical performance with good linearity, low detection limit, recovery, and adequate accuracy.

Magnetic solid phase extraction (MSPE) is another green procedure, which has achieved wide applicability due to its environmental compatibility, fast separation process, and great adsorption efficiency. This technique is based on magnetic interaction between magnetic material dispersed in the solution and target analytes. After the absorption process, separating the magnetic material from the solution can be accomplished by using a magnet. Subsequently, the desorption solution is analysed after desorption (Figure 3.3). This technique makes the pre-treatment procedure significantly simpler, avoiding filtration or other physical procedures to separate the phases [12]. The magnetic nanoparticles consist primarily of iron (Fe) and related oxides (Fe_3O_4 or γ-Fe_2O_3) and some Co, Ni, and their oxides.

Several articles have evaluated the application of MSPE in various fields. Selected applications of MSPE in different areas are listed in Table 3.1. MSPE has emerged as a preparation procedure for the evaluation of numerous compounds with different advantages, including the increase in analysis performance as well as the eventual automation of the procedure.

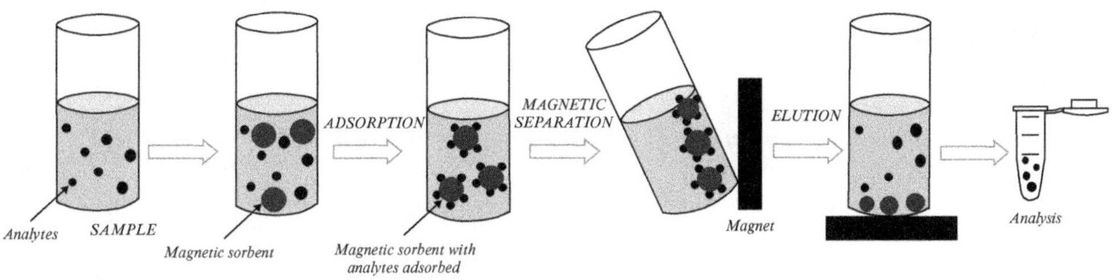

Figure 3.3 Schematic illustration of magnetic solid phase extraction procedure.

Table 3.1 Modern applications of magnetic solid phase extraction in the analysis of various samples.

Analytes	**Matrix**	**Instrumentation**	**Magnetic material**	**Recovery (%)**	**References**
Fluoroquinolones	Tap water	UPLC–UV	Fe_3O_4@ Cys@ MIL125–NH_2	83.8–109.4	[13]
Bifenox Dichlobenil Diclofop methyl	Wheat flour	HPLC–DAD	HCSs@ Fe3O4–MWCNTs–COOH	88.8–96.6	[14]
Pyrethroid	Organic and conventional vegetables	HPLC–UV	PSt/MNPs	91.6–116.2	[15]

(Continued)

Table 3.1 (Continued)

Analytes	Matrix	Instrumentation	Magnetic material	Recovery (%)	References
Sulfonamides	Meat samples	HPLC–DAD	Fe_3O_4@ JUC–48	76.1–102.6	[16]
Sulfonamides	Milk	HPLC–DAD	HCP/Fe_3O_4	84.0–105.0	[17]
Atrazine Propazine Prometryn	Milk and rice	HPLC–DAD	AC–OFX MNPs	81.0–109.0	[18]
Triazine herbicides	Rice	HPLC–UV	Fe_3O_4@ SiO_2–GO/ MIL–101(Cr)	83.9–103.5	[19]
Plant growth regulators	Cucumbers, tomatoes, sprouts, asparagus, lettuce	UHPLC–QTrap–MS/MS	Fe_3O_4@SiO_2/ GO/β–CD	77.7–108.3	[20]
Pesticides	Tea	GC–MS	Fe_3O_4@f–BN	84.5–122	[21]
Organophosphorus pesticides	Fruit juices	GC–FID	poly(*p*PDA–co–Th)@ Fe_3O_4	88.1–99.2	[22]
Benzoylurea insecticides	Cucumbers, tomatoes	HPLC	MP–POPs	81.8–103.5	[23]
Copper (II)	Tea, mushrooms	AAS	Fe_3O_4@C	98.3–101.0	[24]
Chromium (III) Cobalt (II) Cadmium (II) Zinc (II) Lead (II)	Aubergines, tomatoes, onion, garlic	ICP–MS	Carbon-coated Fe_3O_4	97.0–100.0	[25]
Cadmium (II) Lead (II) Copper (II)	Beans	GFAAS	MNP@ ATED	82.2–118.0	[26]
Cobalt (II) Tin (II)	Tea, juice, energy drinks	ICP–OES	Fe_2O_3@ Boletus edulis	>95%	[27]
Antimony (V)	Tap water, well water, mineral water, soft drinks, orange drinks, and beers	ET–AAS	Maghemite	95.8–104.0	[28]
Cadmium (II)	Edible oils	GFAAS	Fe_3O_4@ Al_2O_3	96.0–105.0	[29]

Table 3.1 (Continued)

Analytes	Matrix	Instrumentation	Magnetic material	Recovery (%)	References
Mercury (II)	Water and fish samples	HPLC–ICP–MS	Fe_3O_4@ SiO_2@γ-MPTS	80.7–111.0	[30]
Cobalt (II) Mercury (II)	Water and food samples	ICP–OES	γ–Fe_2O_3	80.1–96.4	[31]
Lead (II)	Fish and molluscs	FAAS	Fe_3O_4@ GO@ polyimide	95.0–106.0	[32]
Lead (II)	Vegetables and water	FAAS	Fe_3O_4/N–CQDs	97.6–99.8	[33]
Endocrine-disrupting phenols	Tea	HPLC–FLD	Fe_3O_4@COF	81.3–118.0	[34]
Alkyl phenols	Baby foods	GC–MS	$CoFe_2O_4$/ oleic acid	89.9–118.2	[35]
Alkyl phenols	Fruit juices	HPLC–DAD/ ESI–IT–MS/MS	$CoFe_2O_4$/ oleic acid	91.0–119.0	[36]

AAS, atomic absorption spectroscopy; ET-AAS, electrothermal atomic absorption spectroscopy; FAAS, flame atomic absorption spectrometry; GC-FID, gas chromatography flame ionisation detector; GC-MS, gas chromatography mass spectrometry; GFAAS, graphite furnace atomic absorption spectrometry; HPLC-DAD, high-performance liquid chromatography diode array detector; HPLC-FLD, high-performance liquid chromatography fluorescence detector; HPLC-ICP-MS, high-performance liquid chromatography–inductively coupled plasma mass spectrometry; ICP-MS, inductively coupled plasma mass spectrometry; ICP-OES, Inductively coupled plasma–optical emission spectrometry; UHPLC-QTrap MS/MS: ultrahigh-pressure liquid chromatography quadrupole ion trap tandem mass spectrometry; UPLC-UV, ultraperformance liquid chromatography ultraviolet detection.

3.2.2 Solid Phase Microextraction

Realising green analytical methodologies has been one of the primary purposes of the analytical chemistry community. The presentation of miniaturised techniques has made great strides in achieving this goal. Microextraction is a non-exhaustive technique in which the volume of the extraction step is very small. One example is solid phase microextraction (SPME) [37].

SPME represents one of the most prevalent green sample preparation techniques, proposed for the first time by Pawliszyn and Arthur [38]. It uses a coated extraction phase on a solid support. This coated thin layer (7–250 μm) acts as an extraction phase: the analytes present in the sample diffuse from the sample and are adsorbed onto the coating or its porous active surface until equilibrium is reached. The extraction phase can be performed by immersing the fibre (direct immersion solid phase microextraction, DI-SPME) or sampling the analytes from the headspace (HS–SPME). On completion of the extraction, the fibre is placed inside the injector of the analytical instrument (e.g. in gas chromatography, GC), or within the desorption solvent for LC analysis or capillary electrophoresis (CE) (Figure 3.4).

SPME has numerous advantages, including ease of operation, low cost, the possibility of automation, direct coupling between the fibre and the analysis system, and a significant decrease in the use of organic solvents from the analytical protocol [39]. SPME is considered a green extraction procedure because it unites extraction and sample injection into a single phase.

Souza-Silva et al. have reported a process using direct immersion solid phase microextraction–gas chromatography–time-of-flight mass spectrometry (DI-SPME-GC-ToF-MS) for fungicide determination in fruits [40]. In particular, a new concept of an SPME sorbent, which permits extraction by immediate absorption in complex matrices, has been employed in grape and strawberry pulp. In the SPME technique, it is necessary to pre-treat the sample to protect the fibre coating, which may deteriorate easily especially when complex and untreated matrices are directly analysed. Consequently, it is essential to find new coatings to expand the performance of this technique. Souza-Silva et al. have reported an outer coating layer of polydimethylsiloxane/divinylbenzene (PDMS/DVB), which efficiently protects the fibre. Furthermore, the opportunity to carry out SPME by direct immersion in complex matrices without performing sample pre-treatment (centrifugation, filtration, dilution, etc.) has been demonstrated. In particular, it has been shown that the smooth external morphology of the coating (PDMS/DVB/PDMS) considerably reduces the encrustations and allows the device to be rinsed when necessary. This automated method has shown

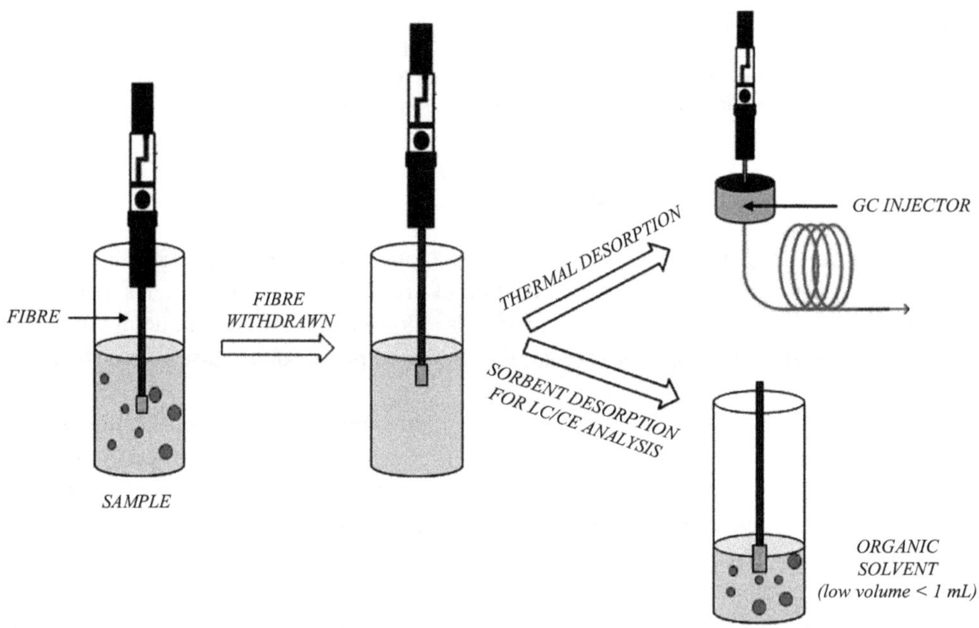

Figure 3.4 Schematic representation of solid phase microextraction. CE, capillary electrophoresis; GC, gas chromatography; LC, liquid chromatography.

promising analytical performance (precision, accuracy) using a simple, fast, and automated (minimising human mistakes) preparation protocol. Furthermore, the performance of the reported procedure was compared with QuEChERS Official Method 2007.01. As can be observed in Table 3.2, the QuEChERS method uses more solvents and chemicals, and consist of more steps that cannot be easily automated. Regarding the analytical performance, the described SPME method reached lower limits of quantification (LOQ) for both grape and strawberry analysis. Comparing the instrumental results obtained, the new SPME method allows for better clean-up, as has been observed from the chromatograms produced.

Piri-Moghadam et al. have described a procedure for the analysis of 23 targeted insecticides by thin film (TF) SPME–GC–MS [41]. The method used two types of SPME devices: PDMS/DVB and PDMS/DVB-carbon mesh-supported membranes. The extraction process with two different membranes was carried out using 30 mL of sample and after this thermal desorption was performed before the GC/MS analysis. The eco-sustainability of the method was estimated by comparison with the US EPA 8720 method, based on LLE. The new reported method significantly reduced the organic solvent volumes (only 60 μL of acetonitrile against 50 mL of dichloromethane for LLE) and only 30 mL of sample against 800 mL for LLE. In addition, numerous advantages were achieved, including increased sensitivity and reduced sample and waste volumes.

Zhang and co-workers discussed DI-SPME for the analysis of pesticides, polycyclic aromatic hydrocarbons (PAHs), and polychlorinated biphenyls (PCBs) in edible seaweeds [42]. The PDMS/DVB/DMS matrix-compatible coating of SPME fibre allowed the simultaneous quantification of 41 analytes. Due to its good accuracy and sensitivity, as well as its ecological profile, the suggested method may be judged valuable for pesticide, PCB, and PAH analysis in algae. Compared to previous studies, which mainly used LLE, this SPME procedure incorporates sampling, handling, extraction, and concentration in a single automatable step with low solvent consumption, leading to an ecological approach. In addition, by using the matrix-compatible reported coating and by carefully optimising the extraction conditions, greater sensitivity was achieved, offering a particularly appropriate approach for the evaluation of numerous analytes in the algae.

Table 3.2 Comparison between QuEChERS official method 2007.01 and the direct immersion solid phase microextraction (DI-SPME) method.

	QuEChERS Official Method	**DI-SPME Method**
Sample	15 g	9 g
Solvents	15 mL AcN	5 μL
Other compounds	$MgSO_4$ $NaCH_3COO$	–
Automation	No	Yes
Analysis	Injection of 1 μL into GC–MS	Direct injection of SPME fibre

AcN, acetonitrile; GC–MS, gas chromatography–mass spectrometry.

Pacheco-Fernandez and collaborators have described an ecological SPME fibre coating based on the metal-organic framework (MOF) CIM–80(Al) for the analysis of different samples [43]. Given the tuneable physicochemical characteristics of MOFs, numerous MOF–based sorbent coatings have been newly created. MOFs are spongy fabrics created from metal clusters and organic binders that can be easily functionalised. In this work a new stationary phase SPME was developed based on the arrest of MOF CIM-80(Al) on nitinol filaments. The new coating was then tested using HS–SPME and DI-SPME (the sample was not pre-treated in any way). The coating showed high thermal (up to 320 °C) and chemical stability even after soaking in matrices. In addition, a preliminary screening study demonstrated that CIM-80(Al) has a higher extraction efficiency than other commercial coatings.

Also in bioanalysis, the need for more ecological techniques has led to the replacement of traditional techniques with alternatives that provide minimum handling of the sample accompanied by high performance and efficiency. For example, SPME has been applied for blood analysis thanks to the introduction of biocompatible coatings, offering advantages in terms of greenness of sample preparation. Gionfriddo and co-workers have reported a new SPME coating based on polytetrafluoroethylene amorphous fluoroplastics (PTFE AF 2400) for the extraction of numerous compounds [44]. The new SPME tool was evaluated for coupling with GC and LC. The performance of the coating was evaluated using different banned doping substances, considering the rising interest in the monitoring of these compounds. The method demonstrated LOQ below the minimum required performance limits (MRPLs) set by the World Anti-Doping Agency (WADA). The new SPME offers many advantages, as it allows in vivo sampling thanks to the miniaturisation of the device. The method allows energy savings (in accordance with GAC principles), linked to the elimination of transport of biological solutions and tissues in frozen conditions necessary to preserve the integrity of the sample. Table 3.3 summarises other examples of SPME applications that consider the environmental impact of extraction.

Table 3.3 Examples of solid phase microextraction (SPME) applied in various matrices.

Analytes	Matrix	Method	Recovery (%)	References
Epoxiconazole Fluroxypyr Metribuzin Oxyfluorfen	Soil samples	HS–SPME–GC/MS	84–112	[45]
Copper Lead Chromium	Water, food	SPME–DPV	>86.4	[46]
Amaranth Ponceau 4R Allura red Carmoisine Erythrosine	Juice samples	In tube SPME–HPLC–UV	80.2–120.5	[47]

Table 3.3 (Contniued)

Analytes	Matrix	Method	Recovery (%)	References
Amphetamine-type Stimulants and synthetic cathinones	Urine	SPME–GC/MS	–	[48]
Anthracene Acenaphthene Fluoranthene Fluorene Naphthalene Pyrene Phenanthrene	Aqueous samples	In tube SPME–GC–FID	78.7–103.5	[49]
Hexachlorobenzene Chlorothalonil Fipronil Chlorfenapyr	Garlic samples	SPME–GC/MS	84.0–108.2	[50]
Epichlorohydrin Bisphenol A	Water samples	SPME–HPLC–UV	97.17–99.46	[51]
Naphthalene Acenaphthylene Acenaphthene Fluorene Phenanthrene Anthracene Fluoranthene Pyrene	Soil samples	Cooling-assisted SPME	25.1–114.5	[52]
Benzoic acid Sorbic acid Propionic acid	Food samples	HS–SPME–GC–FID	83.0–109.0	[53]
Volatile organic compounds	Air samples	SPME–GC–MS	35–88	[54]

DPV, differential pulse voltammetry; FID, flame ionised detector; GC, gas chromatography; HPLC, high-performance liquid chromatography; HS, headspace; MS, mass spectrometry; UV, ultraviolet.

3.2.3 Microextraction by Packet Sorbent

Microextraction by packed sorbent (MEPS) was recently launched as a quick and easy sample preparation technique. MEPS represents a miniature extraction technique that has shown excellent performance with minimal or no solvent consumption [55]. The miniaturisation of extraction devices represents the trend of extraction techniques as well as being one of the 12 principles of GAC (see Chapter 2). This technique is precisely the result of the miniaturisation of classical SPE and the reusable sorbent material (approximately 2–4 mg) is packaged inside a microsyringe (Figure 3.5) [56]. Very interesting advantages have been observed, including low solvent utilisation, modest sample volume (10–250 μL),

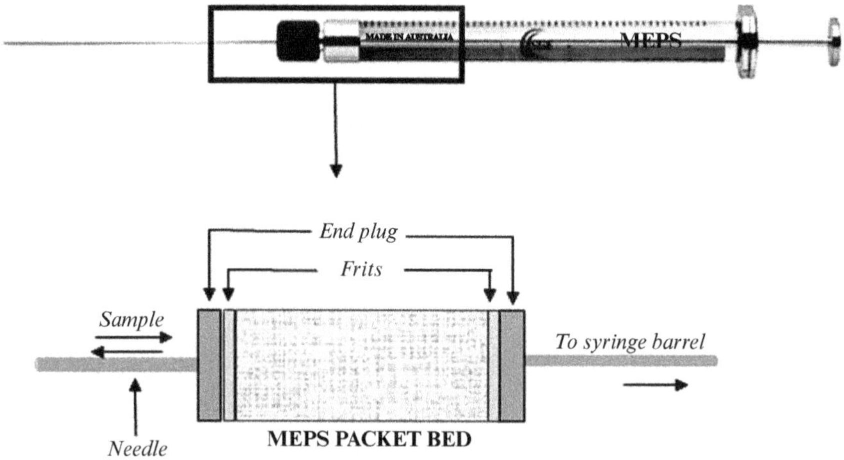

Figure 3.5 Microextraction by packed sorbent (MEPS) sorbent in syringe. Source: MDPI.

and the possibility of its being coupled with a chromatographic system [57]. Usually, washing and elution steps use no more than 20–50 μL of organic solvents. Nowadays, different packing materials are available, including C2, C8, C18, polystyrene–divinylbenzene (PS–DVB), ion exchange, and porous graphitic carbon.

Greater attention has been paid to the employment of green sorbents in MEPS too. For example, algal biomass has received increasing attention as a novel adsorbent material. Rasolzadeh and co-workers have described the use of *Chlorella vulgaris* microalgae as innovative packing for the extraction of nitrofurantoin (NFT) in urine [58]. *C. vulgaris* was inoculated in 500 mL of self-cleaned fresh modified medium at pH 7.2–7.4 and at 25 °C/18 °C ± 0.5 °C (light/dark conditions). The cells were sampled during the logarithmic growth phase and transferred to tanks and centrifuged at 1500 rpm for 15 minutes; later the pellet was rinsed twice with deionised water and then dried for about five days. The microsyringe was packed with 4 mg of sorbent (dry biomass of *C. vulgaris*) and was mounted on the alternative device for online coupling. It was observed that the packaged bio-absorbent could be used several times after washing. This original use of dried algae cells as a green absorbent material was efficiently applied to the absorption of NFT from urine samples. The proposed method was quick, ecological, and quite selective. Furthermore, algae could replace more expensive materials such as nanoporous absorbents, representing an ecological and economic alternative.

The application of this technique has increased in recent years thanks to its easy combination with chromatographic methods and good recovery (80–100%). However, the adsorption capacity of commercial adsorbents could lead to low recovery and inadequate overall sensitivity of the method. In this scenario, conductive polymers such as polyaniline, polypyrrole, and polythiophene (PTh) have been widely applied as promising sorbent materials. PTh is one of the most examined and used polymers: it is highly porous and flexible and has excellent thermal, mechanical, and chemical stability. Florez and collaborators have reported on the use of PTh as a highly suitable absorbent for MEPS for the determination of different hormones from bovine milk samples [59]. In their study, 4 mg of PTh was loaded in the MEPS syringe (Figure 3.6). Before extraction, the sorbent material was conditioned with ultrapure water (250 μL). An aliquot of bovine milk (250 μL) was spiked with 120 ng/mL of steroid standard solution; 100 μL of ultrapure water was used as washing solvent and 700 μL of MeOH : HCOOH (formic acid) (5 : 1 v/v) as eluent solvent. Later, the eluent was evaporated and the dried sample was re-dispersed in MeOH (100 μL) before the HPLC–DAD (diode array detection) analysis.

High efficiency (85–90%) was observed, confirming the versatility of PTh as extraction material. In Table 3.4 other MEPS application have been summarised.

3.2.4 Fabric Phase Sorptive Extraction

The number of microextraction techniques with high compatibility in analytical instrumentation, which minimise the use of hazardous solvents and reagents and require very small sample volumes, is continually increasing. In 2014, fabric phase sorptive extraction (FPSE) was introduced as a pioneering procedure that uses a flexible device of distinct fabrics as a substratum for designing hybrid absorptive layers. The FPSE membrane can be promptly inserted into the sample for the extraction process, avoiding tedious pre-treatment steps. Once the target analytes have been extracted, the membrane is placed in a small quantity of organic solvent (usually 150–200 μL) for the desorption process. FPSE has unified the typical extraction principles of SPME (equilibrium extraction) and SPE (exhaustive extraction) into a single technology. Moreover, FPSE proposes a wide range of absorbent chemicals, including polar, medium-polar, non-polar sorbents, cation exchangers, and anion exchangers.

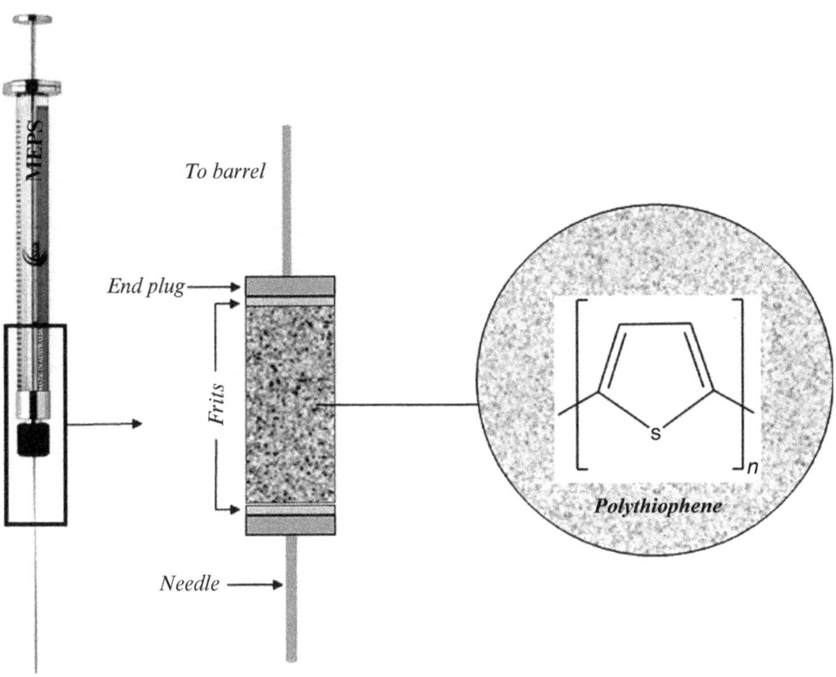

Figure 3.6 Polythiophene as adsorbent material in a microextraction by packed sorbent syringe. Source: MDPI.

Table 3.4 Some recent microextraction by packed sorbent (MEPS) applications in different fields using low volume of sample and elution solvents.

Analytes	Matrix	Sample volume	Elution solvent volume	References
Bifonazole Butoconazole Clotrimazole Econazole Itraconazole Ketoconazole Miconazole Posaconazole Ravuconazole Terconazole Tioconazole Voriconazole	Plasma and urine samples	0.15 mL for plasma, 0.2 mL for urine	150 μL MeOH	[60]
Methadone 2-Ethylidine-1,5-dimethyl-3,3-diphenyl-1-pyrrolidine (EDDP)	Hair samples	0.15 mL	100 μL 2.36% ammonium hydroxide in MeOH	[61]
Clonazolam Deschloroetizolam Nifoxipam Flubromazolam Meclonazepam Zolpidem Zaleplon Zopiclone	Plasma samples	0.10 mL	100 μL DCM-IPA-NH_4OH (78: 20 : 2 v/v/v)	[62]
Methylparaben Ethylparaben *n*-Propylparaben *n*-Butylparaben	Cosmetic samples	0.05 mL	50 μL MeOH	[63]
Endocrine-disrupting chemicals	Urine samples	0.10 mL	100 μL 80% MeOH in H_2O	[64]
Methylone	Oral fluids	0.10 mL	100 μL 2-propanol	[65]
Pyriproxyfen Deltamethrin Etofenprox	Apple juice	0.10 mL	150 μL AcN	[66]
Polybrominated diphenyl ethers	Egg samples	0.10 mL	100 μL isooctane	[67]
Polycyclic aromatic hydrocarbons	Snow samples	0.05 mL	10 μL ethyl acetate	[68]
Omeprazole (OME) enantiomers	Oral fluids and plasma samples	0.10 mL	250 μL ethanol	[69]

Table 3.4 (Continued)

Analytes	Matrix	Sample volume	Elution solvent volume	References
Cocaine and metabolites	Hair samples	0.15 mL	100 μL 2% ammonium hydroxide in MeOH	[70]
Δ9-tetrahydrocannabinol (THC) and metabolites	Urine samples	0.30 mL	100 μL 90% AcN	[71]

AcN, acetonitrile; DCM, dichloromethane; H_2O, water; IPA, isopropanol ammonium hydroxide; MeOH, methanol; NH_4OH, ammonium hydroxide.

This procedure has been employed for different compounds and in numerous matrices (food, cosmetic, biological, etc.). For example, this technique was successfully applied for the determination of hormones in environmental and biological samples [72, 73]; benzodiazepines (bromazepam, diazepam, lorazepam, and alprazolam) in blood serum [74]; azole antimicrobial drugs in biological fluids [75]; aromatase inhibitors in whole blood, plasma, and urine [76]; endocrine-disrupting chemicals (EDCs) in various biological fluids [77–81]; antidepressant drugs in urine [82] and other biological fluids [83]; antibiotic residues [84, 85] in food and biological samples; non-steroidal anti-inflammatory drugs (NSAIDs) in saliva samples [86]; β-blocker drugs from human serum and urine [87]; and phenolic compounds in human saliva samples [88].

Locatelli and co-workers [89] presented an advanced application of FPSE as an in vivo sampler for the evaluation of exhaled breath aerosol (EBA). In this work, an array of six membranes (fabric phase sorptive membrane, FPSM) possessing different characteristics (non-polar, medium-polar, and polar) was built. The FPSM array was then inserted inside the facemask and 15 volunteers were involved for the sampling. Once removed, a mixture of MeOH and AcN (150 μL) was used for the elution of extracted compounds. The samples were then analysed using LC tandem mass spectrometry through rapid screening that permitted the rapid qualitative analysis of more than 700 compounds. This study undoubtedly represents a potential implementation of biomonitoring of different compounds and its applicability could also be extended to other fields. Moreover, particular attention was paid to the sustainable profile of the method, also evaluated through the green analytical procedure index (GAPI) [90]. The GAPI allows, following the indicated parameters, critical evaluation of the specific components of the analytical procedure (solvents, energy consumption, volumes of discharge, etc.); everything is shown in a pictogram that gives a visual idea of how green the proposed apparatus or practice is. The evaluation carried out in this study showed a fairly good green profile.

FPSE represents a novel sample preparation technique that offers numerous benefits such as ease of application, superior performance, and broad applicability due to the availability of numerous adsorbents. This technique certainly reflects the principles of GAC, such as the reduced consumption of organic solvents, the possibility of analysing a complex matrix without pre-treatment steps, sample volume reduction, and the opportunity to carry out less invasive sampling. All these advantages are accompanied by excellent analytical parameters, as demonstrated by the good performance in terms of accuracy and precision in the validated methods.

3.3 Solvent-Based Microextraction Procedures

3.3.1 Liquid Phase Microextraction

LLE is a technique that involves the partitioning of analytes from an aqueous phase to a water-immiscible solvent based on solubility. It was definitely one of the first separation techniques developed and is among the most generally used. Recently, the diffusion of SPE techniques and the subsequent miniaturisation have certainly made LLE less widespread. The time requirement, the low extraction efficiency, the high chemical and solvent consumption, and the high cost are some of its disadvantages. Miniaturisation has been a key element to overcome some of these limitations, and as a result liquid phase microextraction (LPME) was launched in the 1990s [91]. LPME uses a few microlitres of a water-immiscible solvent extraction phase and an aqueous sample phase, which contains the selected analytes [92]. Dispersive liquid-liquid microextraction (DLLME), which immediately attracted scientist attention, involves the rapid addition of a dual system of solvents (extraction solvent and dispersant solvent) that leads to the formation of a turbid mixture in which the extraction solvent is spread within a type of small droplets. Extraction equilibrium is reached quickly, thanks to the wide contact area between the droplets and the sample, and the analytes are extracted. The mixture is thus centrifuged to collect the organic solvent in the lower or upper part (depending on the density of the extraction solvent) and the transferred phase is collected for instrumental analysis. Another improvement in DLLME was the application of ionic liquids (ILs) as alternative solvents. This technique, named IL-DLLME, avoiding the use of toxic solvents, is considered environmentally sustainable. ILs are considered further in the next section.

3.3.2 Ionic Liquids and Deep Eutectic Solvents

The search for more sustainable solvents and reagents has become the new challenge of the entire analytical procedure. In this context, new solvents have been proposed that contribute to greening analytical practices.

ILs are composed entirely of ions and include numerous compounds with particular characteristics such as minimal volatility, miscibility with both water and organic solvents, elevated thermal stability, and the absence of inflammability. They are identified as 'design solvents' as it is possible to vary the physical and chemical properties to replace the components and make them more suitable to meet the requirements [93]. ILs are considered eco-friendly solvents because they do not discharge toxic vapours into the surrounding environment. In contrast, the process of synthesising ILs often involves steps that limit their green characteristics; therefore, this designation is rather controversial. Research in this area is gradually moving towards further recyclable and fewer lethal preparations and advanced techniques, such as microwave irradiation and eco-assisted reactions, which have significantly expanded the environmental impact of IL synthesis in addition to leading to higher reaction yields. ILs have been successfully applied in different fields of analytical chemistry, like chromatography, CE, mass spectrometry, and extraction and (micro)extraction techniques, as a substitute for conventional reagents. In Table 3.5 some recent applications and techniques that involve the use of ILs are reported.

Table 3.5 Recent applications of ionic liquids (ILs) and deep eutectic solvents (DESs) in sample preparation techniques.

Analytes	Matrix	IL/DES	Extraction technique	Instrumental analysis	References
Resmethrin Bifenthrin Fenpropathrin Cyhalothrin	Water samples	1-Vinyl-3-butylimidazolium bis(trifluoromethylsulfonyl)-imide	MSPE	GC–MS	[96]
Ampicillin Benzylpenicillin Amoxicillin Oxacillin Cloxacillin	Milk samples	[DABCO–C_3OH]Cl or 1-(3-Hydroxypropyl)–1,4-diazabicyclo[2.2.2]octan-1-ium chloride	MSPE	UPLC–MS/MS	[97]
Docosahexaenoic Eicosapentaenoic Arachidonic acid	Breast milk	[SiO_2-MIM-BF_4] or SiO_2-1-Methylimidazolium tetrafluoroborate	SPE	ELSD–HPLC	[98]
Pioglitazone	Drug samples	1-Hexyl-3-methyl-imidazolium-hexafluorophosphate	DLLME	HPLC–UV	[99]
Fipronil Metalaxyl Paclobutrazol Myclobutanil Napropamide Thiacloprid Penconazole	Food samples	Proline/propylene glycol (1 : 3)	MSPE	HPLC–UV	[100]
Diflubenzuron Triflumuron Hexaflumuron Flufenoxuron Chlorfluazuron	Tea and fruit juices	Trihexyl tetradecyl phosphonium chloride/tetradecyl alcohol	UA–DLLME	HPLC–UV	[101]
Oxytetracycline Doxycycline Tetracycline	Water samples	Choline chloride : ethylene glycol/thymol : octanoic acid	DLLME	HPLC–UV	[102]

(Continued)

Table 3.5 (Continued)

Analytes	Matrix	IL/DES	Extraction technique	Instrumental analysis	References
Salicylic acid Oxaprozin Diclofenac Ibuprofen	Environmental water and milk samples	Guanidinium chloride and thymol	UA–DLLME	HPLC–UV	[103]
Pesticides	Tomato samples	Choline chloride/ethylene glycol (1.25 mL) and choline chloride/n-butyric acid (58 μL)	SBSE	GC–MS	[104]
Phthalate esters	Soft drinks	Thymol/octanoic acid	VA–DLLME	UHPLC–MS/MS	[105]
Phthalic acid esters	Tap and mineral water	Menthol/acetic acid	DLLME	LC–UV	[106]
Terpenes	Spices	Tetrabutylammonium bromide/dodecanol	HS–SDME	GC–MS	[107]
Organophosphorus	Water samples	Benzyltriphenylphosphonim bromide/1-undecanol	AA–LPME	GC–MS	[108]
Pb (II) Cd (II)	Vegetables	Citric acid/sucrose	HI–DES–ME	FAAS	[109]
Ketoprofen Diclofenac	Liver	Menthol/formic acid	EA–DLLME	LC–MS/MS	[110]

AA–LPME, atomic absorption liquid phase microextraction; Cd, cadmium; DLLME, dispersive liquid-liquid microextraction; EA–DLLME, effervescent-assisted dispersive liquid-liquid microextraction; ELSD–HPLC, evaporative light scattering detection–high-performance liquid chromatography; FAAS, flame atomic absorption spectrometry; GC–MS, gas chromatography mass spectrometry; HI–DES–ME, heat-induced deep eutectic solvent microextraction; HPLC–UV, high-performance liquid chromatography ultraviolet detection; HS–SDME, headspace single-drop microextraction; LC–MS/MS, liquid chromatography tandem mass spectrometry; LC–UV, liquid chromatography ultraviolet detection; MSPE, magnetic solid phase extraction; Pb, lead; SBSE, stir bar sorptive extraction; SPE, solid phase extraction; UA–DLLME, ultrasound-assisted dispersive liquid-liquid microextraction; UHPLC–MS/MS, ultra-high performance liquid chromatography–tandem mass spectrometry; UPLC–MS/MS, ultra-performance liquid chromatography–tandem mass spectrometry; VA–DLLME, vortex-assisted liquid-liquid microextraction.

Deep eutectic solvents (DESs) were introduced originally in 2001 as a change from the traditionally used organic solvents [94]. DESs could be considered a category of ILs, as they share many characteristics and properties (low vapour pressure, non-flammability, non-reactivity to water), but they cannot be considered true ILs as they are not totally composed of ions. DESs are systems formed by a eutectic mixture of Lewis or Bransted acids and bases that may contain a diffusion of anionic and/or cationic species. They are usually obtained by complexing a quaternary ammonium salt with a metal salt or chemical bond donor [95]. In addition, the preparatory phase is considered more environmentally friendly than that of ILs, and they are also easily biodegradable and recyclable, which makes them valid solvents for use in sustainable analytical procedures. DESs are often divided into four categories: DES types I, II, and IV are composed primarily of a metal salt (metal chloride hydrate) and organic salts or other neutral compounds. DES type III consists primarily of an organic salt as acceptor and hydrogen donor. Similar to DES are natural deep eutectic solvents (NADES), which are formulated using natural elements generated by cellular metabolism (urea, amino acids, sugars, choline, etc.). Several articles on analytical processes based on LLE and SPE applying DES have been published and the most recent are summarised in Table 3.5.

3.4 Conclusion

The determination/quantification of compounds in complex matrices inevitably involves a preparation phase whose primary objective is the isolation and concentration of analytes. This preliminary phase also aims to obtain a clean sample appropriate for subsequent instrumental analysis. Over the years, these preparation techniques have increasingly been oriented towards simplification, automation, and the reduction of waste. Over time, several ecofriendly methodologies have been introduced in the preparation step, including microextraction techniques that use new and greener adsorbent materials or the use of alternative green solvents. Sustainable development has now become the focus of every area, and this concept, extended to analytical chemistry with the introduction of the principles of GAC, is continually growing. In the near future, new extraction techniques are expected to be increasingly ecofriendly, leading to laboratory procedures that have as little impact on the environment as possible.

References

1 Dugheri, S., Marrubini, G., Mucci, N. et al. (2021). A review of micro-solid-phase extraction techniques and devices applied in sample pretreatment coupled with chromatographic analysis. *Acta Chromatographica* 33: 99–111. https://doi.org/10.1556/1326.2020.00790.

2 D'Ovidio, C., Bonelli, M., Rosato, E. et al. (2022). Novel applications of microextraction techniques focused on biological and forensic analyses. *Separations* 9: 1–33. https://doi.org/10.3390/separations9010018.

3 Jiménez-Skrzypek, G., Ortega-Zamora, C., González-Sálam, J., and Hernández-Borges, J. (2021). Miniaturized green sample preparation approaches for pharmaceutical analysis. *Journal of Pharmaceutical and Biomedical Analysis* 207: 114405. https://doi.org/10.1016/j.jpba.2021.114405.

4 Anastas, P.T., and Warner, J.C. (1998). *Green Chemistry: Theory and Practice*. Oxford: Oxford University Press.

5 Gałuszka, A., Migaszewski, Z., and Namiesnik, J. (2013). The 12 principles of green analytical chemistry and the significance mnemonic of green analytical practices. *Trends in Analytical Chemistry* 50: 78–84. https://doi.org/10.1016/j.trac.2013.04.010.

6 Aly, A.A., and Górecki, T. (2020). Green approaches to sample preparation based on extraction techniques. *Molecules* 25: 1719. https://doi.org/10.3390/molecules25071719.

7 Trenholm, R.A., Vanderford, B.J., and Snyder, S.A. (2009). On-line solid phase extraction LC–MS/MS analysis of pharmaceutical indicators in water: a green alternative to conventional methods. *Talanta* 79: 1425–1432. https://doi.org/10.1016/j.talanta.2009.06.006.

8 da Silva, L.C., Souza, M.C., Sumere, B.R. et al. (2020). Simultaneous extraction and separation of bioactive compounds from apple pomace using pressurized liquids coupled on-line with solid-phase extraction. *Food Chemistry* 318: 126450. https://doi.org/10.1016/j.foodchem.2020.126450.

9 Shirani, M., Salari, F., Habibollahi, S., and Akbari, A. (2020). Needle hub in-syringe solid phase extraction based a novel functionalized biopolyamide for simultaneous green separation/preconcentration and determination of cobalt, nickel, and chromium (III) in food and environmental samples with micro sampling flame atomic absorption spectrometry. *Microchemical Journal* 152: 104340. https://doi.org/10.1016/j.microc.2019.104340.

10 Khan, W.A., Arain, M.B., and Soylak, M. (2020). Nanomaterials-based solid phase extraction and solid phase microextraction for heavy metals food toxicity. *Food and Chemical Toxicology* 145: 111704. https://doi.org/10.1016/j.fct.2020.111704.

11 Shi, Z., Li, Q., Xu, D. et al. (2016). Graphene-based pipette tip solid-phase extraction with ultra-high performance liquid chromatography and tandem mass spectrometry for the analysis of carbamate pesticide residues in fruit juice. *Journal of Separation Science* 39: 4391–4397. https://doi.org/10.1002/jssc.201600498.

12 Jiang, H.L., Li, N., Cui, L. et al. (2019). Recent application of magnetic solid phase extraction for food safety analysis. *Trends in Analytical Chemistry* 120: 115632. https://doi.org/10.1016/j.trac.2019.115632.

13 Lian, L.L., Zhang, X.Y., Hao, J. et al. (2018). Magnetic solid-phase extraction of fluoroquinolones from water samples using titanium-based metal-organic framework functionalized magnetic microspheres. *Journal of Chromatography A* 1579: 1–8. https://doi.org/10.1016/j.chroma.2018.10.019.

14 Li, W.K., Zhang, H.X., and Shi, Y.P. (2018). Simultaneous determination of bifenox, dichlobenil and diclofop methyl by hollow carbon nanospheres enhanced magnetic carboxylic multi-walled carbon nanotubes. *Analytica Chimica Acta* 1011: 40–49. https://doi.org/10.1016/j.aca.2018.01.030.

15 Yu, X., and Yang, H.S. (2017). Pyrethroid residue determination in organic and conventional vegetables using liquid-solid extraction coupled with magnetic solid phase extraction based on polystyrene-coated magnetic nanoparticles. *Food Chemistry* 217: 303–310. https://doi.org/10.1016/j.foodchem.2016.08.115.

16 Xia, L., Liu, L.J., Lv, X.X. et al. (2017). Towards the determination of sulfonamides in meat samples: a magnetic and mesoporous metal-organic framework as an efficient sorbent for magnetic solid phase extraction combined with high-performance liquid chromatography. *Journal of Chromatography A* 1500: 24–31. https://doi.org/10.1016/j.chroma.2017.04.004.

17 Tolmacheva, V.V., Apyari, V.V., Furletov, A.A. et al. (2016). Facile synthesis of magnetic hypercrosslinked polystyrene and its application in the magnetic solid-phase extraction of sulfonamides from water and milk samples before their HPLC determination. *Talanta* 152: 203–210. https://doi.org/10.1016/j.talanta.2016.02.010.

18 Mohd, N.I., Gopal, K., Raoov, M. et al. (2019). Evaluation of a magnetic activated charcoal modified with non-ionic silicone surfactant as a new magnetic solid phase extraction sorbent with triazine herbicides as model compounds in selected milk and rice samples. *Talanta* 196: 217–225. https://doi.org/10.1016/j.talanta.2018.12.043.

19 Liang, L., Wang, X.H., Sung, Y. et al. (2018). Magnetic solid-phase extraction of triazine herbicides from rices using metal-organic framework MIL-101(Cr) functionalized magnetic particles. *Talanta* 179: 512–519. https://doi.org/10.1016/j.talanta.2017.11.017.

20 Chen, J.Y., Cao, S.R., Zhu, M. et al. (2018). Fabrication of a high selectivity magnetic solid phase extraction adsorbent based on β-cyclodextrin and application for recognition of plant growth regulators. *Journal of Chromatography A* 1547: 1–13. https://doi.org/10.1016/j.chroma.2018.03.004.

21 Pang, Y.C., Zang, X.H., Wang, M.T. et al. (2018). Fibrous boron nitride nanocomposite for magnetic solid phase extraction of ten pesticides prior to the quantitation by gas chromatography. *Microchimica Acta* 185: 561–568. https://doi.org/10.1007/s00604-018-3103-0.

22 Targhoo, A., Amiri, A., and Baghayeri, M. (2018). Magnetic nanoparticles coated with poly(p-phenylenediamine-co-thiophene) as a sorbent for preconcentration of organophosphorus pesticides. *Microchimica Acta* 185: 15–23. https://doi.org/10.1007/s00604-017-2560-1.

23 Wang, J.T., Jiao, C.N., Li, M.H. et al. (2018). Porphyrin based porous organic polymer modified with Fe3O4 nanoparticles as an efficient adsorbent for the enrichment of benzoylurea insecticides. *Microchimica Acta* 185: 36–44. https://doi.org/10.1007/s00604-017-2542-3.

24 Azam, S., and Amjad, M. (2015). Magnetic Fe3O4@C nanoparticles modified with 1-(2-thiazolylazo)-2-naphthol as a novel solid-phase extraction sorbent for preconcentration of copper (II). *Microchimica Acta* 182: 257–264. https://doi.org/10.1007/s00604-014-1327-1.

25 Habila, M.A., Alothman, Z.A., El-Toni, A.M. et al. (2017). Carbon-coated Fe3O4 nanoparticles with surface amido groups for magnetic solid phase extraction of Cr(III), Co(II), Cd(II), Zn(II) and Pb(II) prior to their quantitation by ICP-MS. *Microchimica Acta* 184: 2645–2651. https://doi.org/10.1007/s00604-017-2283-3.

26 Huang, Y.F., Peng, J.H., and Huang, X.J. (2019). Allylthiourea functionalized magnetic adsorbent for the extraction of cadmium, copper and lead ions prior to their determination by atomic absorption spectrometry. *Microchimica Acta* 186: 51–59. https://doi.org/10.1007/s00604-018-3101-2.

27 Özdemir, S., Yalcin, M.S., Kilinc, E., and Soylak, M. (2018). Boletus edulis loaded with γ-Fe2O3 nanoparticles as a magnetic sorbent for preconcentration of Co(II) and Sn(II) prior to their determination by ICP-OES. *Microchimica Acta* 185: 73–79. https://doi.org/10.1007/s00604-017-2605-5.

28 Narimani-Sabegh, S., and Noroozian, E. (2019). Magnetic solid-phase extraction and determination of ultra-trace amounts of antimony in aqueous solutions using maghemite nanoparticles. *Food Chemistry* 287: 382–389. https://doi.org/10.1016/j.foodchem.2019.02.112.

29 Barreto, I.S., Andrade, S.I.E., Cunha, F.A.S. et al. (2018). A robotic magnetic nanoparticle solid phase extraction system coupled to flow-bath analyzer and GFAAS for determination of trace cadmium in edible oils without external pretreatment. *Talanta* 178: 384–391. https://doi.org/10.1016/j.talanta.2017.09.063.

30 Zhu, S.Q., Chen, B.B., He, M. et al. (2017). Speciation of mercury in water and fish samples by HPLC-ICP-MS after magnetic solid phase extraction. *Talanta* 171: 213–219. https://doi.org/10.1016/j.talanta.2017.04.068.

31 Özdemir, S., Mohamedsaid, S.A., Kılınç, E., and Soylak, M. (2019). Magnetic solid phase extractions of Co(II) and Hg(II) by using magnetized C. micaceus from water and food samples. *Food Chemistry* 271: 232–238. https://doi.org/10.1016/j.foodchem.2018.07.067.

32 Mehdinia, A., Ramezain, M., and Jabbari, A. (2017). Preconcentration and determination of lead ions in fish and mollusk tissues by nanocomposite of Fe3O4@graphene oxide@ polyimide as a solid phase extraction sorbent. *Food Chemistry* 237: 1112–1117. https://doi.org/10.1016/j.foodchem.2017.06.051.

33 Mashkani, M., Mehdinia, A., Jabbari, A. et al. (2018). Preconcentration and extraction of lead ions in vegetable and water samples by N-doped carbon quantum dot conjugated with Fe3O4 as a green and facial adsorbent. *Food Chemistry* 239: 1019–1026. https://doi.org/10.1016/j.foodchem.2017.07.042.

34 Deng, Z.H., Wang, X., Wang, X.L. et al. (2019). A core-shell structured magnetic covalent organic framework (type Fe3O4@COF) as a sorbent for solid-phase extraction of endocrine-disrupting phenols prior to their quantitation by HPLC. *Microchimica Acta* 186: 108–117. https://doi.org/10.1007/s00604-018-3198-3.

35 Pastor-Belda, M., Vinas, P., Campillo, N., and Hernandez-Cordoba, M. (2017). Magnetic solid phase extraction with CoFe2O4/oleic acid nanoparticles coupled to gas chromatography-mass spectrometry for the determination of alkylphenols in baby foods. *Food Chemistry* 221: 76–81. https://doi.org/10.1016/j.foodchem.2016.10.035.

36 Vinas, P., Pastor-Belda, M., Torres, A. et al. (2016). Use of oleic acid nanoparticles for the magnetic solid-phase microextraction of alkyphenols in fruit juices using liquid chromatography-tandem mass spectrometry. *Talanta* 151: 217–233. https://doi.org/10.1016/j.talanta.2016.01.039.

37 Billiard, K.M., Dershem, A.R., and Gionfriddo, E. (2020). Implementing green analytical methodologies using solid-phase microextraction: a review. *Molecules* 25: 5297–5310. https://doi.org/10.3390/molecules25225297.

38 Arthur, C.L., and Pawliszyn, J. (1990). Solid phase microextraction with thermal desorption using fused silica optical fibers. *Analytical Chemistry* 62: 2145–2214. https://doi.org/10.1021/ac00218a019.

39 Spietelun, A., Marcinkowski, L., de la Guardia, M., and Namiesnik, J. (2013). Recent developments and future trends in solid phase microextraction techniques towards green analytical chemistry. *Journal of Chromatography A* 1321: 1–13. http://dx.doi.org/10.1016/j.chroma.2013.10.030.

40 Souza-Silva, E.A., Lopez-Avila, V., and Pawliszyn, J. (2013). Fast and robust direct immersion solid phase microextraction coupled with gas chromatography–time-of-flight mass spectrometry method employing a matrix compatible fiber for determination of triazole fungicides in fruits. *Journal of Chromatography A* 1313: 139–146. http://dx.doi.org/10.1016/j.chroma.2013.07.071.

41 Piri-Moghadam, H., Gionfriddo, E., Rodriguez-Lafuente, A. et al. (2017). Inter-laboratory validation of a thin film microextraction technique for determination of pesticides in surface water samples. *Analytica Chimica Acta* 964: 74–84. https://doi.org/10.1016/j.aca.2017.02.014.

42 Zhang, L., Gionfriddo, E., Acquaro, V., Jr., and Pawliszyn, J. (2018). Direct immersion solid-phase microextraction analysis of multi-class contaminants in edible seaweeds by gas chromatography-mass spectrometry. *Analytica Chimica Acta* 1031: 83–97. https://doi.org/10.1016/j.aca.2018.05.066.

43 Pacheco-Fernandez, I., Rentero, M., Ayala, J.H. et al. (2020). Green solid-phase microextraction fiber coating based on the metalorganic framework CIM-80(Al): analytical performance evaluation in direct immersion and headspace using gas chromatography and mass spectrometry for the analysis of water, urine and brewed coffee. *Analytica Chimica Acta* 1133: 137–149. https://doi.org/10.1016/j.aca.2020.08.009.

44 Gionfriddo, E., Boyacı, E., and Pawliszyn, J. (2017). New generation of solid-phase microextraction coatings for complementary separation approaches: a step toward comprehensive metabolomics and multiresidue analyses in complex matrices. *Analytical Chemistry* 89: 4046–4054. https://doi.org/10.1021/acs.analchem.6b04690.

45 Orazbayeva, D., Koziel, J.A., Trujillo-Rodríguez, M.J. et al. (2020). Polymeric ionic liquid sorbent coatings in headspace solid-phase microextraction: a green sample preparation technique for the determination of pesticides in soil. *Microchemical Journal* 157: 104996. https://doi.org/10.1016/j.microc.2020.104996.

46 Ghorbani, M., Pedramrad, T., Aghamohammadhasan, M. et al. (2019). Simultaneous clean-up and determination of Cu(II), Pb(II) and Cr(III) in real water and food samples using a magnetic dispersive solid phase microextraction and differential pulse voltammetry with a green and novel modified glassy carbon electrode. *Microchemical Journal* 147: 545–554. https://doi.org/10.1016/j.microc.2019.03.072.

47 Nasrollahi, S.S., Yamini, Y., and Mani-Varnosfaderani, A. (2022). A green approach for in-tube solid phase microextraction of acidic red dyes from juice samples using chitosan/poly vinyl alcohol electrospun nanofibers. *Journal of Food Composition and Analysis* 106: 104339. https://doi.org/10.1016/j.jfca.2021.104339.

48 Alsenedi, K.A., and Morrison, C. (2018). Determination of amphetamine-type stimulants (ATSs) and synthetic cathinones in urine using solid phase micro-extraction fibre tips and gas chromatography-mass spectrometry. *Analytical Methods* 10: 1431–1440. https://doi.org/10.1039/c8ay00041g.

49 Harati, F., Ghiasvanda, A., Dalvand, K., and Haddad, P.R. (2020). Fused-silica capillary internally modified with nanostructured octadecyl silica for dynamic in-tube solid-phase microextraction of polycyclic aromatic hydrocarbons from aqueous media. *Microchemical Journal* 155: 104672. https://doi.org/10.1016/j.microc.2020.104672.

50 Chen, T., and Xu, H. (2019). In vivo investigation of pesticide residues in garlic using solid phase microextraction-gas chromatography-mass spectrometry. *Analytica Chimica Acta* 1090: 72–81. https://doi.org/10.1016/j.aca.2019.09.011.

51 Tasmia, J., and Shah, M.R.J. (2020). Eco-friendly alginate encapsulated magnetic graphene oxide beads for solid phase microextraction of endocrine disrupting compounds from water samples. *Ecotoxicology and Environmental Safety* 190: 110099. https://doi.org/10.1016/j.ecoenv.2019.110099.

52 Xu, S., Li, H., Wu, H. et al. (2020). A facile cooling-assisted solid-phase microextraction device for solvent-free sampling of polycyclic aromatic hydrocarbons from soil based on matrix solid-phase dispersion technique. *Analytica Chimica Acta* 1115: 7–15. https://doi.org/10.1016/j.aca.2020.04.019.

53 Tungkijanansin, N., Alahmad, W., Nhujak, T., and Varanusupakul, P. (2020). Simultaneous determination of benzoic acid, sorbic acid, and propionic acid in fermented food by headspace solid-phase microextraction followed by GC-FID. *Food Chemistry* 329: 127161. https://doi.org/10.1016/j.foodchem.2020.127161.

54 Omarova, A., Baizhan, A., Baimatova, N. et al. (2021). New in situ solvothermally synthesized metal-organic framework MOF-199 coating for solid-phase microextraction of volatile organic compounds from air samples. *Microporous and Mesoporous Materials* 328: 111493. https://doi.org/10.1016/j.micromeso.2021.111493.

55 Moein, M.M., Abdel-Rehim, A., and Abdel-Rehim, M. (2015). Microextraction by packed sorbent (MEPS). *Trends in Analytical Chemistry* 67: 34–44. https://doi.org/10.1016/j.trac.2014.12.003.

56 Filippou, O., Bitas, D., and Samanidou, V. (2017). Green approaches in sample preparation of bioanalytical samples prior to chromatographic analysis. *Journal of Chromatography B* 1043: 44–62. https://doi.org/10.1016/j.jchromb.2016.08.040.

57 Kabir, A., Locatelli, M., and Ulusoy, H.I. (2017). Recent trends in microextraction techniques employed in analytical and bioanalytical sample preparation. *Separations* 4: 36–51. https://doi.org/10.3390/separations4040036.

58 Rasolzadeh, F., Hashemi, P., Haghjou, M.M., and Safdarian, M. (2019). Chlorella vulgaris microalgae as a green packing for the microextraction by packed sorbent of nitrofurantoin in urine. *Analytical and Bioanalytical Chemistry Research* 6: 419–429. https://doi.org/10.22036/ABCR.2019.164580.1297.

59 Florez, D.H.A., de Oliveira, H.L., and Borges, K.B. (2020). Polythiophene as highly efficient sorbent for microextraction in packed sorbent for determination of steroids from bovine milk samples. *Microchemical Journal* 153: 104521. https://doi.org/10.1016/j.microc.2019.104521.

60 Campestre, C., Locatelli, M., Guglielmi, P. et al. (2017). Analysis of imidazoles and triazoles in biological samples after MicroExtraction by packed sorbent. *Journal of Enzyme Inhibition and Medicinal Chemistry* 32: 1053–1063. https://doi.org/10.1080/14756366.2017.1354858.

61 Rosado, T., Gallardo, E., Vieira, D.N., and Barroso, M. (2020). Microextraction by packed sorbent as a novel strategy for sample clean-up in the determination of methadone and EDDP in hair. *Journal of Analytical Toxicology* 44: 840–850. https://doi.org/10.1093/jat/bkaa040.

62 Ares-Fuentes, A.M., Lorenzo, R.A., Fernández, P., and Carro, A.M. (2021). An analytical strategy for designer benzodiazepines and Z-hypnotics determination in plasma samples using ultra-high performance liquid chromatography/tandem mass spectrometry after microextraction by packed sorbent. *Journal of Pharmaceutical and Biomedical Analysis* 194: 113779. https://doi.org/10.1016/j.jpba.2020.113779.

63 Khesinaa, Z.B., Iartseva, S.D., Revelsky, A.I., and Buryaka, A.K. (2021). Microextraction by packed sorbent optimized by statistical design of experiment as an approach to increase the sensitivity and selectivity of HPLC-UV determination of parabens in cosmetics. *Journal of Pharmaceutical and Biomedical Analysis* 195: 113843. https://doi.org/10.1016/j.jpba.2020.113843.

64 Silveira, R.S., Rocha, B.A., Rodrigues, J.L., and Barbosa, F., Jr. (2020). Rapid, sensitive and simultaneous determination of 16 endocrine-disrupting chemicals (parabens, benzophenones, bisphenols, and triclocarban) in human urine based on microextraction by packed sorbent combined with liquid chromatography tandem mass spectrometry (MEPS-LC-MS/MS). *Chemosphere* 240: 124951. https://doi.org/10.1016/j.chemosphere.2019.124951.

65 Sorribes-Soriano, A., Sánchez-Martínez, S., Arráez-González, R. et al. (2020). Methylone determination in oral fluid using microextraction by packed sorbent coupled to ion mobility spectrometry. *Microchemical Journal* 153: 104504. https://doi.org/10.1016/j.microc.2019.104504.

66 Dinali, L.A.F., de Oliveira, H.L., Teixeira, L.S. et al. (2021). Mesoporous molecularly imprinted polymer core@shell hybrid silica nanoparticles as adsorbent in microextraction by packed sorbent for multiresidue determination of pesticides in apple juice. *Food Chemistry* 345: 128745. https://doi.org/10.1016/j.foodchem.2020.128745.

67 Souza, M.C.O., Rocha, B.A., Souza, J.M.O. et al. (2021). A fast and simple procedure for polybrominated diphenyl ether determination in egg samples by using microextraction by packed sorbent and gas chromatography–mass spectrometry. *Food Analytical Methods* 12: 1528–1535. https://doi.org/10.1007/s12161-019-01484-w.

68 Arcoleo, A., Bianchi, F., and Careri, M. (2021). A sensitive microextraction by packed sorbent-gas chromatography-mass spectrometry method for the assessment of polycyclic aromatic hydrocarbons contamination in Antarctic surface snow. *Chemosphere* 282: 131082. https://doi.org/10.1016/j.chemosphere.2021.131082.

69 Ahmed, H., Wahbi, A.A., Elmongy, H. et al. (2021). Determination and pharmacokinetics of omeprazole enantiomers in human plasma and oral fluid utilizing microextraction by packed sorbent and liquid chromatography-tandem mass spectrometry. *International Journal of Analytical Chemistry* 2021: 8845139. https://doi.org/10.1155/2021/8845139.

70 Rosado, T., Gallardo, E., Vieira, D.N., and Barroso, M. (2020). New miniaturized clean-up procedure for hair samples by means of microextraction by packed sorbent: determination of cocaine and metabolites. *Analytical and Bioanalytical Chemistry* 412: 7963–7976. https://doi.org/10.1007/s00216-020-02929-6.

71 Sartore, D.M., Medina, D.A.V., Costa, J.L. et al. (2020). Automated microextraction by packed sorbent of cannabinoids from human urine using a lab-made device packed with molecularly imprinted polymer. *Talanta* 219: 121185. https://doi.org/10.1016/j.talanta.2020.121185.

72 Kumar, R., Gaurav, H., Malik, A.K. et al. (2014). Efficient analysis of selected estrogens using fabric phase sorptive extraction and high-performance liquid chromatography-fluorescence detection. *Journal of Chromatography A* 1359: 16–25. https://doi.org/10.1016/j.chroma.2014.07.013.

73 Guedes-Alonso, R., Ciofi, L., Sosa-Ferrera, Z. et al. (2016). Determination of androgens and progestogens in environmental and biological samples using fabric phase sorptive extraction coupled to ultra-high performance liquid chromatography tandem mass spectrometry. *Journal of Chromatography A* 1437: 116–126. https://doi.org/10.1016/j.chroma.2016.01.077.

74 Samanidou, V., Kaltzi, I., Kabir, A., and Furton, K.G. (2016). Simplifying sample preparation using fabric phase sorptive extraction technique for the determination of benzodiazepines in blood serum by high-performance liquid chromatography. *Biomedical Chromatography* 30: 829–836. https://doi.org/10.1002/bmc.3615.

75 Locatelli, M., Kabir, A., Innosa, D. et al. (2017). A fabric phase sorptive extraction-high performance liquid chromatography-photo diode array detection method for the determination of twelve azole antimicrobial drug residues in human plasma and urine. *Journal of Chromatography B* 1040: 192–198. https://doi.org/10.1016/j.jchromb.2016.10.045.

76 Locatelli, M., Tinari, N., Grassadonia, A. et al. (2018). FPSE-HPLC-DAD method for the quantification of anticancer drugs in human whole blood, plasma, and urine. *Journal of Chromatography B* 1095: 204–213. https://doi.org/10.1016/j.jchromb.2018.07.042.

77 Alampanos, V., Kabir, A., Furton, K.G. et al. (2020). Fabric phase sorptive extraction combined with high-performance-liquid chromatography-photodiode array analysis for the determination of seven parabens in human breast tissues: application to cancerous and non-cancerous samples. *Journal of Chromatography A* 1630: e461530. https://doi.org/10.1016/j.chroma.2020.461530.

78 Tartaglia, A., Kabir, A., Ulusoy, S. et al. (2019). FPSE-HPLC-PDA analysis of seven paraben residues in human whole blood, plasma, and urine. *Journal of Chromatography B* 1125: 121707. https://doi.org/10.1016/j.jchromb.2019.06.034.

79 Locatelli, M., Furton, K.G., Tartaglia, A. et al. (2019). An FPSE-HPLC-PDA method for rapid determination of solar UV filters in human whole blood, plasma, and urine. *Journal of Chromatography B* 1118–1119: 40–50. https://doi.org/10.1016/j.jchromb.2019.04.028.

80 Alampanos, V., Kabir, A., Furton, K.G., and Samanidou, V. (2021). Magnet integrated fabric phase sorptive extraction of selected endocrine disrupting chemicals from human urine followed by high-performance liquid chromatography-photodiode array analysis. *Journal of Chromatography B* 1654: e462459. https://doi.org/10.1016/j.chroma.2021.462459.

81 Parla, A., Zormpa, E., Paloumpis, N. et al. (2021). Determination of intact parabens in the human plasma of cancer and non-cancer patients using a validated fabric phase sorptive extraction reversed-phase liquid chromatography method with UV detection. *Molecules* 26: 1526–1546. https://doi.org/10.3390/molecules26061526.

82 Lioupi, A., Kabir, A., Furton, K.G., and Samanidou, V. (2019). Fabric phase sorptive extraction for the isolation of five common antidepressants from human urine prior to HPLC-DAD analysis. *Journal of Chromatography B* 1118–1119: 171–179. https://doi.org/10.1016/j.jchromb.2019.04.045.

83 Tartaglia, A., Covone, S., Rosato, E. et al. (2022). Fabric phase sorptive extraction (FPSE) as an efficient sample preparation platform for the extraction of antidepressant drugs from biological fluids. *Advances in Sample Preparation* 1: 1–23. https://doi.org/10.1016/j.sampre.2022.100022.

84 Alampanos, V., Kabir, A., Furton, K.G. et al. (2019). Fabric phase sorptive extraction for simultaneous observation of four penicillin antibiotics from human blood serum prior to high performance liquid chromatography and photo-diode array detection. *Microchemical Journal* 149: e103964. https://doi.org/10.1016/j.microc.2019.103964.

85 Agadellis, E., Tartaglia, A., Locatelli, M. et al. (2020). Mixed-mode fabric phase sorptive extraction of multiple tetracycline residues from milk samples prior to high performance liquid chromatography-ultraviolet analysis. *Microchemical Journal* 159: 105437. https://doi.org/10.1016/j.microc.2020.105437.

86 Tartaglia, A., Kabir, A., D'Ambrosio, F. et al. (2020). Fast off-line FPSE-HPLC-PDA determination of six NSAIDs in saliva samples. *Journal of Chromatography B* 1144: e122082. https://doi.org/10.1016/j.jchromb.2020.122082.

87 Mazaraki, K., Kabir, A., Furton, K.G. et al. (2021). Fast fabric phase sorptive extraction of selected β-blockers from human serum and urine followed by UHPLC-ESI-MS/MS analysis. *Journal of Pharmaceutical and Biomedical Analysis* 199: e114053. https://doi.org/10.1016/j.jpba.2021.114053.

88 Tartaglia, A., Romasco, T., D'Ovidio, C. et al. (2021). Determination of phenolic compounds in human saliva after oral administration of red wine by high performance liquid chromatography. *Journal of Pharmaceutical and Biomedical Analysis* 209: e114486. https://doi.org/10.1016/j.jpba.2021.114486.

89 Locatelli, M., Tartaglia, A., Ulusoy, H.I. et al. (2021). Fabric-phase sorptive membrane array as a noninvasive in vivo sampling device for human exposure to different compounds. *Analytical Chemistry* 93: 1957–1961. https://doi.org/10.1021/acs.analchem.0c04663.

90 Płotka-Wasylka, J. (2018). A new tool for the evaluation of the analytical procedure: green analytical procedure index. *Talanta* 181: 204–209. https://doi.org/10.1016/j.talanta.2018.01.013.

91 Sereshti, H., Khorram, P., and Nouri, N. (2018). Recent trends in replacement of disperser solvent in dispersive liquid-liquid microextraction methods. *Separation & Purification Reviews* 48: 159–178. https://doi.org/10.1080/15422119.2018.1460851.

92 Saha, S., Singh, A.K., Keshari, A.K. et al. (2018). Modern extraction techniques for drugs and medicinal agents. In: *Ingredients Extraction by Physicochemical Methods in Food: Handbook of Food Bioengineering* (ed. A.M. Grumezescu and A.M. Holban), 65–106. London: Academic Press. https://doi.org/10.1016/B978-0-12-811521-3.00002-8.

93 Merone, G.M., Tartaglia, A., Rosato, E. et al. (2021). Ionic liquids in analytical chemistry: applications and recent trends. *Current Analytical Chemistry* 17: 1340–1355. https://doi.org/10.2174/1573411017666210331113712.

94 Abbott, A.P., Capper, G., Davies, D.L. et al. (2001). Preparation of novel, moisture-stable, Lewis-acidic ionic liquids containing quaternary ammonium salts with functional side chains. *Chemical Communications* 19: 2010–2011. https://doi.org/10.1039/B106357J.

95 Smith, E.L., Abbott, A.P., and Ryder, K.S. (2014). Deep eutectic solvents (DESs) and their applications. *Chemical Reviews* 114: 11060–11082. https://doi.org/10.1021/cr300162p.

96 Wang, T., Zhang, R., Gong, Z. et al. (2020). Poly (ionic liquids) functionalized magnetic nanoparticles as efficient adsorbent for determination of pyrethroids from environmental water samples by GC-MS. *Chemistry Select* 5: 91–96. https://doi.org/10.1002/slct.201904231.

97 Sahebi, H., Konoz, E., Ezabadi, A. et al. (2020). Simultaneous determination of five penicillins in milk using a new ionic liquid-modified magnetic nanoparticle based dispersive micro-solid phase extraction followed by ultra-performance liquid chromatography-tandem mass spectrometry. *Microchemical Journal* 154: 1–13. https://doi.org/10.1016/j.microc.2020.104605.

98 Pajewska-Szmyt, M., Buszewski, B., and Gadzała-Kopciuch, R. (2020). Supported ionic liquid adsorbent and ELSD–HPLC method as an alternative procedure for exogenous fatty acid analysis in breast milk. *Microchemical Journal* 157: 1–7. https://doi.org/10.1016/j.microc.2020.104961.

99 Garmangani, B., Ghaderi, E., and Amiri, A.A. (2021). Extraction of pioglitazone via dispersive liquid–liquid microextraction based on ionic liquids and its measurement in drug samples using high-performance liquid chromatography. *Journal of the Iranian Chemical Society* 18: 1741–1748. https://doi.org/10.1007/s13738-020-02146-z.

100 Zhao, J., Meng, Z., Zhao, Z., and Zhao, L. (2020). Ultrasound-assisted deep eutectic solvent as green and efficient media combined with functionalized magnetic multi-walled carbon nanotubes as solid-phase extraction to determine pesticide residues in food products. *Food Chemistry* 310: 125863. https://doi.org/10.1016/j.foodchem.2019.125863.

101 Liu, X., Chen, M., Meng, Z. et al. (2020). Extraction of benzoylurea pesticides from tea and fruit juices using deep eutectic solvents. *Journal of Chromatography B* 1140: 121995. https://doi.org/10.1016/j.jchromb.2020.121995.

102 Sereshti, H., Karami, F., and Nouri, N. (2021). A green dispersive liquid-liquid microextraction based on deep eutectic solvents doped with β-cyclodextrin: application for determination of tetracyclines in water samples. *Microchemical Journal* 163: 105914. https://doi.org/10.1016/j.microc.2020.105914.

103 Qiao, L., Sun, R., Yu, C. et al. (2021). Novel hydrophobic deep eutectic solvents for ultrasound-assisted dispersive liquid-liquid microextraction of trace non-steroidal anti-inflammatory drugs in water and milk samples. *Microchemical Journal* 170: 106686. https://doi.org/10.1016/j.microc.2021.106686.

104 Nemati, M., Farajzadeh, M.A., Mohebbi, A. et al. (2020). Development of a stir bar sorptive extraction method coupled to solidification of floating droplets dispersive liquid-liquid micro-extraction based on deep eutectic solvents for the extraction of acidic pesticides from tomato samples. *Journal of Separation Science* 43: 1119–1127. https://doi.org/10.1002/jssc.201901000.

105 Santana-Mayor, A., Herrera-Herrera, A.V., Rodríguez-Ramos, R. et al. (2021). Development of a green alternative vortex-assisted dispersive liquid–liquid microextraction based on natural hydrophobic deep eutectic solvents for the analysis of phthalate esters in soft drinks. *ACS Sustainable Chemistry & Engineering* 9: 2161–2170. https://doi.org/10.1021/acssuschemeng.0c07686.

106 Ortega-Zamora, C., González-Sálamo, J., Hernández-Sánchez, C., and Hernández-Borges, J. (2020). Menthol-based deep eutectic solvent dispersive liquid-liquid microextraction: a simple and quick approach for the analysis of phthalic acid esters from water and beverage samples. *ACS Sustainable Chemistry & Engineering* 8: 8783–8794. https://doi.org/10.1021/acssuschemeng.0c02603.

107 Triaux, Z., Petitjean, H., Marchioni, E. et al. (2020). Deep eutectic solvent–based headspace single-drop microextraction for the quantification of terpenes in spices. *Analytical and Bioanalytical Chemistry* 412: 933–948. https://doi.org/10.1007/s00216-019-02317-9.

108 Shahbodaghi, M., Faraji, H., Shahbaazi, H., and Shabani, M. (2020). Sustainable and green microextraction of organophosphorus flame retardants by a novel phosphonium-based deep eutectic solvent. *Journal of Separation Science* 43: 452–461. https://doi.org/10.1002/jssc.201900504.

109 Altunay, N., Elik, A., and Bingöl, D. (2020). Simple and green heat-induced deep eutectic solvent microextraction for determination of lead and cadmium in vegetable samples by flame atomic absorption spectrometry: a multivariate study. *Biological Trace Element Research* 198: 324–331. https://doi.org/10.1007/s12011-020-02064-4.

110 Shishov, A., Gerasimov, A., Nechaeva, D. et al. (2020). An effervescence-assisted dispersive liquid–liquid microextraction based on deep eutectic solvent decomposition: determination of ketoprofen and diclofenac in liver. *Microchemical Journal* 156: 104837. https://doi.org/10.1016/j.microc.2020.104837.

4

Impact of Green Approaches in Pharmaceutical Industries

Taruna Grover[1,2], *Rishita J. Chauhan*[3], *Anuradha K. Gajjar*[3], *Tejas M. Dhameliya*[4] *and Maulikkumar D. Vaja*[5]

[1] *Department of Chemistry, Lovely Professional University, Phagwara, Punjab, India*
[2] *Aarti Industries Research and Technology Center, Dhirubhai Ambani Knowledge City, Navi Mumbai, Maharashtra, India*
[3] *Department of Pharmaceutical Chemistry and Quality Assurance, L. M. College of Pharmacy, Ahmedabad, Gujarat, India*
[4] *Department of Pharmaceutical Chemistry, Institute of Pharmacy, Nirma University, Ahmedabad, Gujarat, India*
[5] *Department of Pharmaceutical Chemistry, Saraswati Institute of Pharmaceutical Sciences, Gandhinagar, Gujarat, India*

CONTENTS

4.1 Introduction

Paul Anastas and John C. Warner from the US Environmental Protection Agency (EPA) coined the term ‘green chemistry’ in 1998 along with the 12 principles leading to its foundation [1]. It has received the prominent recognition within the scientific community ever since. These principles of green chemistry (Table 4.1 and Figure 4.1) have pioneered its great contribution to the current stage of sustainability [2].

The adoption of life-cycle assessment in the design of green synthesis increases the production of greener ideas by providing extensive and thorough insights into the relationships among chemicals, processes, and environmental implications [5]. The reaction conditions such as heating, refluxing, steam cleaning, and so on should be optimised to meet the demand for green aspects [6]. After all, all these aspects have a huge impact on the pharmaceutical industry, claiming to contribute to the life expectancy and quality of life of human beings, and wherein industrial processes have affected the environment to a great degree [7].

Sustainable Approaches in Pharmaceutical Sciences, First Edition. Edited by Kamal Shah, Durgesh Nandini Chauhan, and Nagendra Singh Chauhan.

Table 4.1 The 12 principles of green chemistry.

1	Prevent waste	Design chemical synthetic processes in such a way that no waste is generated
2	Maximise the atom economy	The synthesis process should be designed in such a way that the maximum starting materials are incorporated into the structure of the final product
3	Design less hazardous chemical synthesis	Design a synthesis process in which chemicals used or side products generated in the process have very few or no toxic effects
4	Design safer chemicals and products	Chemicals and products should have little or no toxicity and be ecofriendly
5	Use safer solvents and reaction conditions	Circumvent the use of auxiliary chemicals, solvents, separation agents, and harsh reaction conditions. Always try to utilise safer solvents and mild reaction conditions
6	Increase energy efficiency	The energy required for chemical processes should be reduced and experiments conducted at ambient pressure and temperature
7	Use renewable feed stocks	Raw materials used in the process should be renewable rather than non-renewable
8	Avoid chemical derivatives	Avoid the use of protection and de-protection steps
9	Use catalysts, not stoichiometric reagents	Reduce waste by use of catalysts in reactions that can be reused. A catalyst is better than a stoichiometric reagent for chemical reactions
10	Design chemicals and products to degrade after use	Chemicals and products should be easily degraded after use so that they do not amass in the environment
11	Analyse processes in real time to prevent pollution	Real-time monitoring and control should be included in the synthesis process to minimise or eliminate the formation of hazardous by-products
12	Minimise the potential for accidents	Choose the chemicals used in a synthetic process to minimise hazards and risk of accidents such as explosions, fires, and releases to the environment

Source: Adapted from [3] and [4].

4.2 Metrics for Green Chemistry

4.2.1 Atom Economy (AE)

The efficiency of a reaction is measured by the total number of atoms in the reactants that appear in the final product:

$$AE = \frac{\text{molecular weight of product}}{\text{total molecular weight of reactants}} \times 100$$

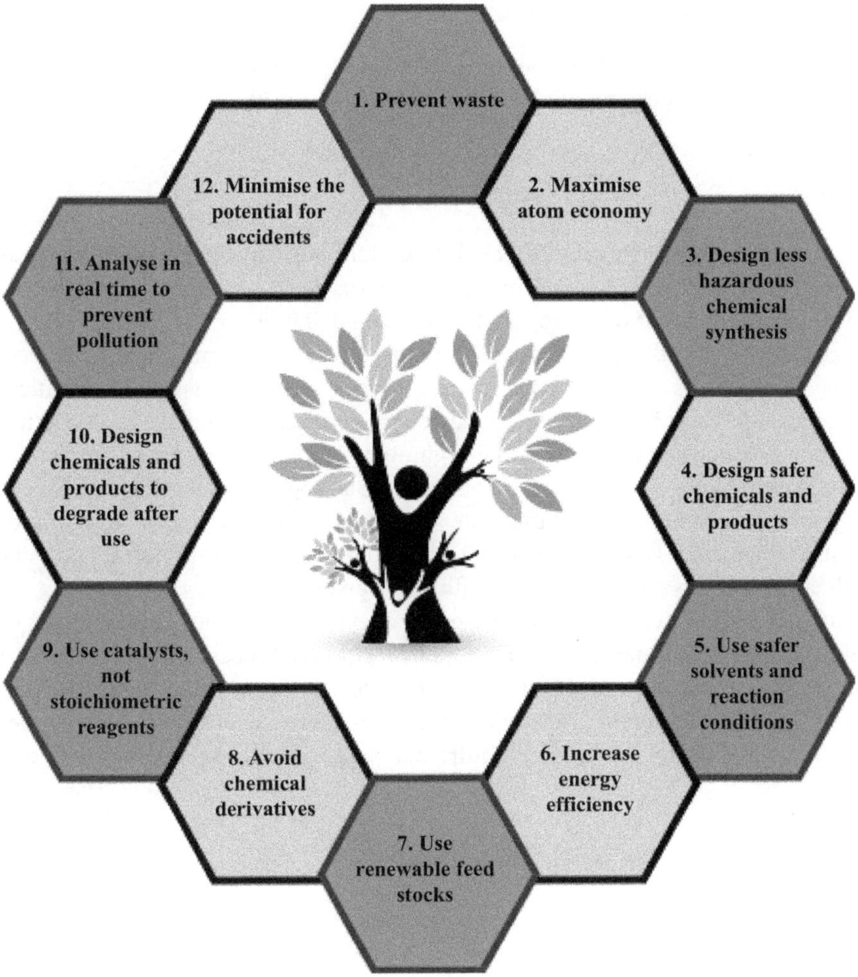

Figure 4.1 Green chemistry principles. *Source:* Adapted from [4].

4.2.2 Mass Intensity/Process Mass Intensity (MI/PMI)

PMI is defined as the total mass of materials that is used to produce a specified mass of product:

$$\text{Mass intensity} = \frac{\text{total mass in a process or process}|\text{step}}{\text{mass of product}}$$

All mass-based inputs are captured in this metric, such as catalysts, reagents, solvents, and work-up, in addition to stoichiometry and yield. It is referred to as MI for a single-step reaction or PMI for an entire synthetic process.

4.2.3 Environmental Factor (E Factor)

An environmental factor proposed by Sheldon in 1992 is represented by E. The E factor is a metric that focuses on waste generated per unit of product synthesised:

$$\text{E factor} = \frac{\text{Total mass of waste from process (Kg)}}{\text{Total mass of product (Kg)}}$$

Routine use of this type of matrix may still be difficult for pharmaceutical industry operations because there may be a lack of clarity depending on how 'total waste' is ultimately determined and which types of waste generation are included in it.

The main goal of green synthesis is to reduce energy waste, optimise consumption, and use renewable energy resources for the supply of power. Despite the fact that pharmaceutical companies are leading contributors to the world economy, most of them are not adopting green technology as set-up costs are high at the beginning. Therefore there are some barriers to adopting such technology. Green chemistry has large-scale applications in the pharmaceutical industry, which as one of the most dynamic areas always finds itself at the forefront of any substantial change, for instance in terms of improved feed stocks, innovative ideas, safer raw materials, and safer processes that save health, time, and cost (Tables 4.2 and 4.3).

Green synthesis is involved in process development and in the development of commercial routes for active pharmaceutical ingredients (APIs). Process chemists may face several challenges in this regard, including for raw materials like starting materials, reagents, synthetic methods, selection of best route, technologies to use that provide the target molecules at the right time for the project requirements, and loss of patent exclusivity due

Table 4.2 Green metrics, tools, and proactive management used for the production of active pharmaceutical ingredients.

Green metric	Advantages
Process mass intensity (PMI)	A lower PMI means reduction of the use of excess raw material and production cycle time
E factor	Correlation of the amount of waste generated with the synthesis of a particular amount of product
Electronic lab notebook (ELN)	An ELN reduces the use of paper
Atom economy	The atom economy gives the idea of maximum incorporation of all raw materials into the final products
Life-cycle analysis (LCA)	The LCA technique evaluates the environmental aspects and potential impacts associated with a product, process, or service
Green solvent selection guide	This encourages the use of green solvents
Reagent guide	This encourages the use of green chemicals that are ecofriendly
Solvent recovered and recycled	This reduces the cost of production and wastage of solvent

Source: Adapted from [4–22].

Table 4.3 Greener technologies.

Green technology	Advantages
Biotechnology competence fermentation/enzyme catalysis/ competence chemocatalysis/ biocatalysis	Greener, economical, fast, selective for specific manufacturing processes
Combining biocatalysis and homogeneous catalysis	Shortcut synthesis of a pharmaceutical intermediate
Microwave-assisted organic synthesis	Requires minimal time and energy
Integrated approach of chemistry, biology, and process technology	Reduction of the number of chemical steps to form the final product
Solid phase synthesis	Synthesis of multiple non-oligomeric organic molecules at the same time
Multicomponent/convergent synthesis	Saves time and energy
Hydrogenation technology	An easy reduction technique without using harmful reagents
Flow chemistry	Micro-reactor technology
	Successful multi-ton application with higher selectivity and less waste
	High productivity
	Process intensification towards sustainable manufacturing
	High selectivity GMP production
	Improved selectivity of particular isomers
	Less consumption of raw materials and energy (purification)
	Energy integration
	Intrinsic safety
	Reduced DSP effort
	Modular small units enable a switch from batch to continuous processing
	Avoidance of cryogenic cooling (energy), high heat, and mass transfer
Microprocess technology	Learning from nature
	Enhanced transfer by increased transfer area
	Enhanced transfer by decreased transfer distance
Eco-design toolkit	Used for green processes that guide the company to focus on the current vision and mission and reduce the negative impact in the future
Life-cycle analysis (LCA)	Many companies are diverting towards the biotechnology route for synthesis of compounds by LCA for sustainable development
'LCA light' tool for pharmaceutical intermediates	Green ICT is a tool in which computer programs are used for efficient and effective synthesis

(Continued)

Table 4.3 (Continued)

Green technology	Advantages
Proactive management	Telescoping and solvent recycling encourage innovation while integrating green chemistry and engineering into drug discovery, development, and manufacturing Defines and delivers tools for innovation

DSP, dynamic solvent process; GMP, good manufacturing practice; ICT, information and communications technologies. *Source:* Adapted from [4–22].

to the lifetime criteria of the patent. The overall objective of green synthesis is to develop the process that is most cost-effective for commercial production of an API.

Cost-effective processes involve less waste generation, including disposal of the waste, high yield, reagent/reactant utilisation factors, waste treatment, and cost of material to be used. During development these factors lead to improvement of the process and ease of operation, which makes the reaction process greener. In terms of metrics, reaction mass efficacy (RME) is responsible for increasing yield and using reagents more economically. This factor will also help to decrease waste over time, as waste is decreased with a more efficient work-up process and mapping, and it also helps to reduce solvent uses. Processes can be improved when green chemistry (methods, reagent/catalyst) is introduced. Biocatalysis is one of these greener methods and the use of catalysts has become a valuable technology for manufacturing sustainably in different chemical sectors, like pharmachemicals, fine chemicals, and other chemical divisions.

4.3 Case Studies of Active Pharmaceutical Ingredients

There are many examples related to green chemistry achievements, some of which are described in this section. (The authors declare no competing financial interests.)

4.3.1 Ibuprofen

Ibuprofen is the basis of painkillers like Motrin®, Brufen®, Advil®, and Nurofen®. It has had wide application since it was first synthesised by Boots Company in 1961. In the early stages, iso-butylbenzene was acylated to give isobutyl acetophenone by Friedel–Crafts acylation, followed by Darzens condensation, and oximate/hydrolysis or oxidation. This older route was complicated with a six-step reaction, a low atom economy (atom efficiency 40%), and intensive energy consumption. More than 50% of the raw materials used were wasted. Moreover, several other disadvantages were complicated purification, generation of inorganic salts, high cost, and detrimental effects on pollution.

During the 1990s, BASF and Hoechst Celanesee Company (BHC copartnership) developed a new route for the synthesis of ibuprofen. In this route carbonylation of 1-(4-isobutylphenyl)ethanol improves ibuprofen synthesis, as shown in Figure 4.2 [23]. In the traditional route, a stoichiometric amount of $AlCl_3$ is required for a high yield in the first

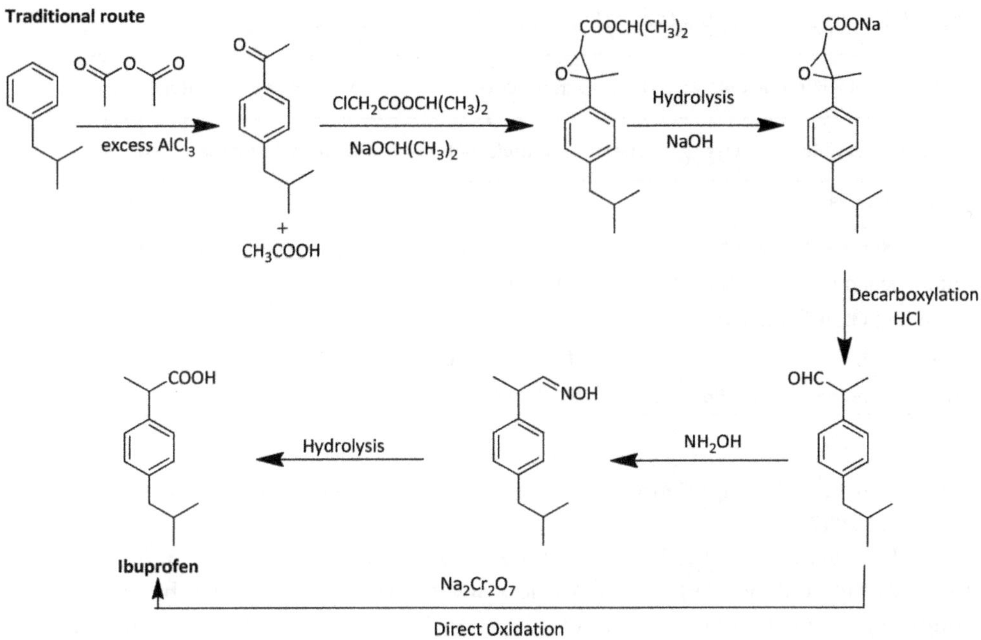

Figure 4.2 Traditional route of synthesis for ibuprofen.

step, which generates a large amount of $Al(OH)_3$ simultaneously (Figure 4.2), while in the BHC route a high yield is obtained by the hydrofluoric acid (HF) catalyst, and meanwhile the catalyst can be recovered and reused so that no waste is generated. Thus, the target product is acquired by only three steps in the new route, resulting in a great improvement of the atom economy (atom efficiency 77.4%) with energy savings and a shorter period of production. In addition to this, the other two steps in the new process use Raney nickel and palladium catalysts, which also can be recovered and reused. Furthermore, the by-product (acetic acid) is recovered, and thus the atom economy reaches 99% (Figure 4.3). Therefore, this new synthetic process could lead to a remarkable reduction in detrimental effects on pollution and production cost in comparison with the traditional route, thus representing an improved process with both environmental and economic benefits. The BHC process

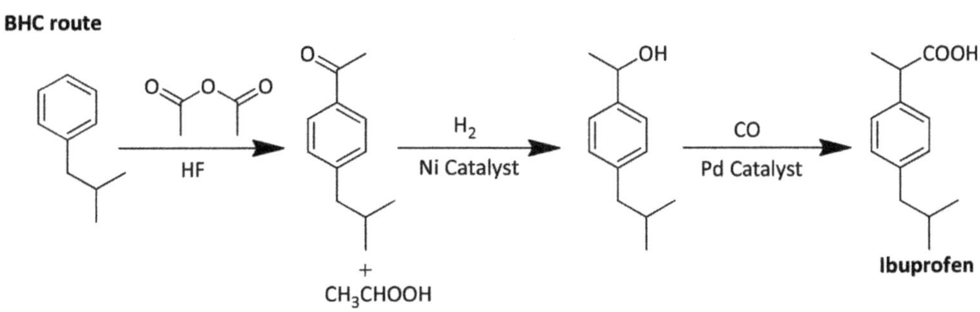

Figure 4.3 Hoechst (BHC) synthesis of ibuprofen.

Table 4.4 Comparison of Boots and Hoechst (BHC) synthesis processes.

Starting materials/reagent		Utilised in product		Not utilised in product	
Chemical formula	**Mol wt**	**Chemical formula**	**Mol wt**	**Chemical formula**	**Mol wt**
Boots process					
$C_{20}H_{42}NO_{10}ClNa$	514.5	$C_{13}H_{18}O_2$	206	$C_7H_{24}NO_8ClNa$	308.5
Atom economy = 206/(206 + 308.5) × 100% = 40%					
Hoechst (BHC) process					
$C_{15}H_{22}NO_4$	266	$C_{13}H_{18}O_2$	206	$C_2H_4O_2$	60
Atom economy = 206/(206 + 60) × 100% = 77.40%					

for the synthesis of ibuprofen was awarded the 'Presidential Green Chemistry Challenge Award' in 1997 [24].

The BHC synthetic route is much more easy and efficient compared to the traditional route. In this route waste generation is less and the yield also improves by up to 77.40% compared to the traditional route (Table 4.4). The advantages can be summarised as follows:

- Waste generation is less.
- Yield is improved by up to 77.40%.
- Less reagent is used compared to the traditional route.
- The atom economy is higher than with the traditional route.
- There is recycling and reuse of by-products, catalyst, and reagent.
- There is a shorter route of synthesis.

4.3.2 Sildenafil Citrate (Viagra)

Sildenafil citrate (Viagra) is used for the treatment of male erectile dysfunction. The first route of synthesis is shown in Figure 4.4. This route is not suitable for the environment. Later, a new route was reported to remove the adverse effect of the old route on the environment. The old and new green synthetic routes for sildenafil citrate are compared in this section.

Tin(II)chloride, which was used for the reduction of the nitro group in the old route, was replaced by H_2, Pd/C in the new green route, because tin chloride is a major environmental polluter that it is difficult to decompose. In the greener route, thionyl chloride is used in stoichiometric amounts as a solvent, which decreases the excess use of harmful thionyl chloride that was used in the old route. Hydrogen peroxide was replaced by KO^tBu in ^tBuOH in a greener route, because hydrogen peroxide causes skin irritation and can catch fire, especially when it is in contact with organic materials. In the greener route, oxalyl chloride was replaced by thionyl chloride for the synthesis of 2-ethoxybenzoyl chloride, because while using oxalyl chloride carbon monoxide was emitted from the reaction, which was very harmful to human health. The overall yield of sildenafil citrate increased to 75%, and the high yields minimised the detrimental effect on the environment (Figure 4.5) [25, 26].

Sildenafil citrate (Viagra) traditional route

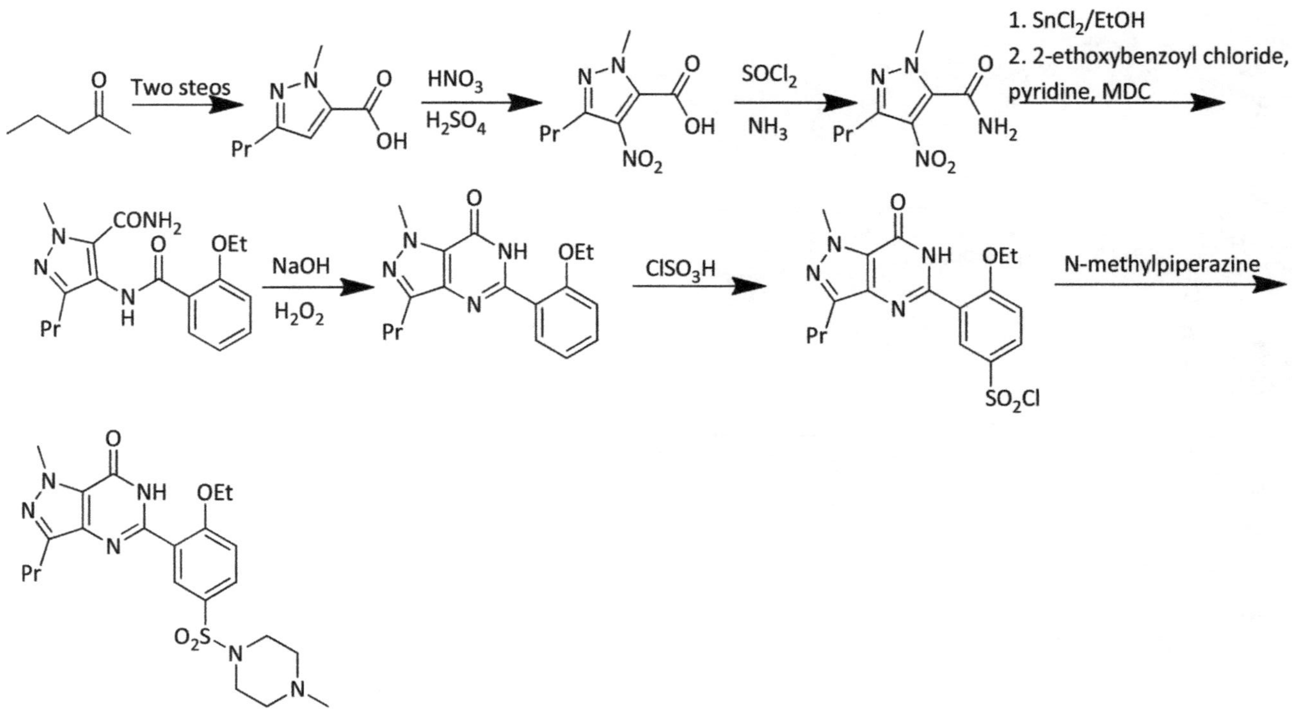

Sildenafil citrate (Viagra)

Figure 4.4 Traditional route of synthesis for sildenafil citrate.

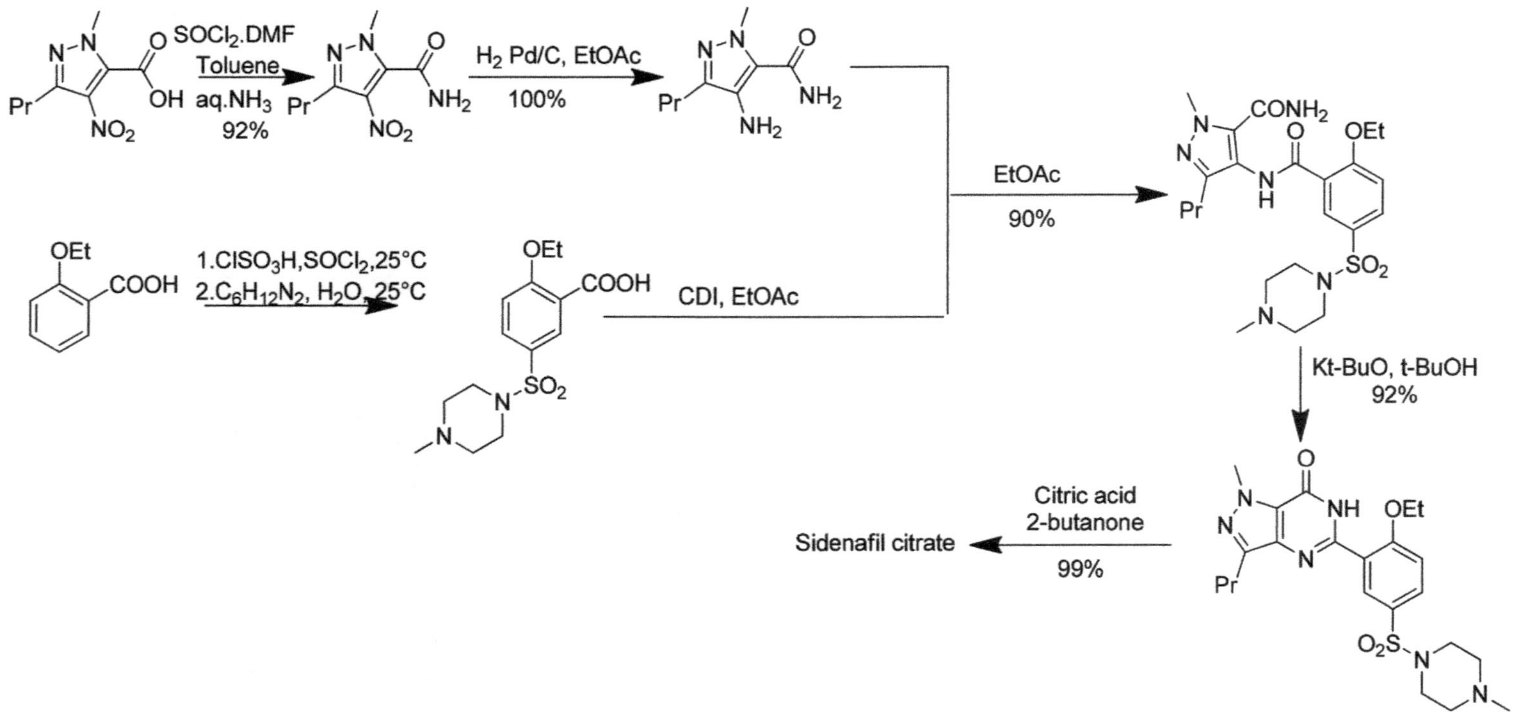

Figure 4.5 Greener route of synthesis for sildenafil citrate.

4.3.3 Talampanel (LY300164)

Talampanel (LY300164) is an oral drug for the treatment of seizure and it is a selective α-amino-3-hydroxy-5-methyl-4-isoxazole propionate (AMPA) receptor antagonist. Eli Lilly's greener process makes use of environmentally friendly processes such as a biocatalytic reduction and air oxidation. The old route of synthesis is a linear approach of eight steps and gave a 22% overall yield. There are several environmental disadvantages of this traditional route, like the use of chromium trioxide (it was the only acceptable oxidant for making the diketone at that time), borane, perchloric acid, and hydrazine (Figure 4.6). The disposal of 3 kg of chromium waste per kg of the product was a very difficult task because disposal generates a large quantity of waste. Hydrazine was used in the last step, which increases the chance of generating genotoxic impurities in the drug [27–31].

In the new route the required chirality was introduced at the beginning of the sequence. The chiral alcohol was prepared enzymatically instead of by the late-stage borane imine reduction. The resin-bound *Zygosaccharomyces rouxii* in water was used efficiently to provide the chiral alcohol in a remarkable 100% conversion, 99.9% enantiomeric excess (ee), and 96% isolated yield (Figure 4.7) [32–34].

The chiral alcohol was used in the cyclisation step directly to form the chiral cyclic ether. A new alternative route was developed to the oxonium salt route for oxidation that prevented the hard-won chirality. In the new route, the oxidation of the benzylic centre was carried out by air via base-mediated oxidation using NaOH in dimethyl sulfoxide to

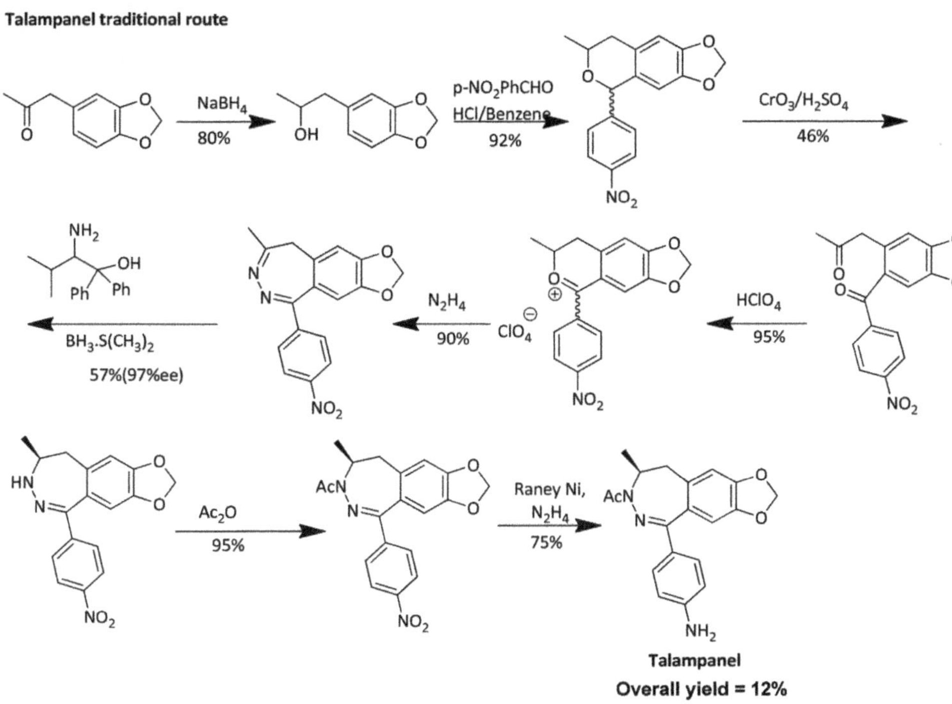

Figure 4.6 Traditional route of synthesis for talampanel.

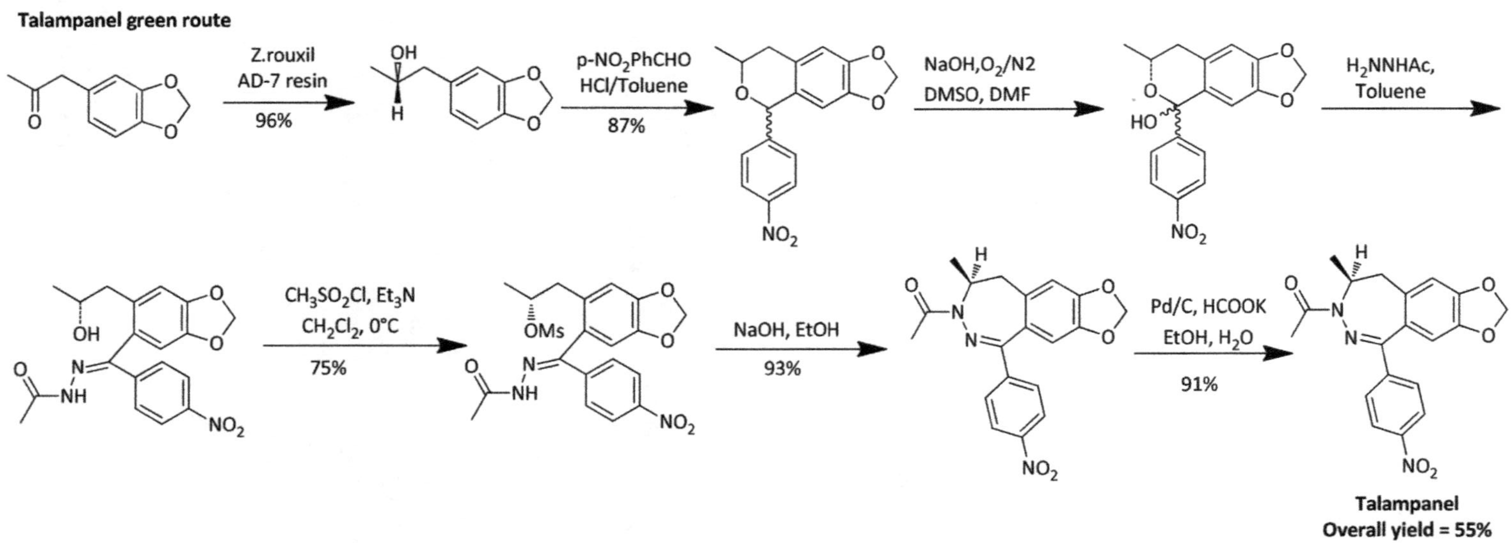

Figure 4.7 Greener route of synthesis for talampanel.

generate the hemiketal. It reacted with acetylhydrazine and formed the compound, which then reacted with triethylamine and mesylchloride. The crystalline mesylate salt was isolated in a 75% overall yield in a three-step reaction. The beauty of the new greener route is that hydrazine has been replaced by the less hazardous acetylhydrazine, chromium by air, and the persistent environmental pollutant perchloric acid to form the oxonium salt is totally avoided. The subsequent cyclisation formed the benzodiazepine in a 93% isolated yield [32, 33].

The greener route tripled the overall yield, substituted heavy metal-induced oxidation by air, reduced the number of steps, and developed a biocatalytic reduction for establishing the chiral centre.

4.3.4 Saxagliptin

Saxagliptin is used to treat type 2 diabetes. It is synthesised via asymmetrical synthesis. Chiral drugs can be synthesised using asymmetrical synthesis, hence application of the enzymes in such reactions has advantages over traditional chemical synthesis. Most chemoenzymatic reactions are stereoselective and can be carried out at atmospheric pressure and ambient temperatures, which typically reduces hazards and cost, and minimises the chances of the formation of undesired by-products. Generally enzymatic processes are carried out in water, using chemicals that are less toxic, and thus waste generation is minimised.

(*S*)-*N*-*BOC*-3-hydroxy adamantyl glycine is an important key intermediate for the synthesis of saxagliptin. It was prepared by an asymmetrical Strecker reaction in the traditional route and requires the highly toxic potassium cyanide (KCN) (Figure 4.8). The Bristol–Myers Squibb enzyme technology research group successfully generates the chiral centre by a modified phenylalanine dehydrogenase in the intermediate, which involves an enzymatic reductive amination of a keto acid. This greener route is beneficial because of the reduction of five steps to only one step, which ultimately reduces time, cost, and the possibility of accidents. This process eliminates the use of KCN and the expensive chiral reagent (*R*)-2-phenylglycinol, as well as poor oxidation using $KMnO_4$ in the final step, and the reductive amination uses water as a solvent. It also increases the isolated yield up to 81% with minimal side product formation (Figure 4.9) [35, 36].

4.3.5 Pregabalin (Lyrica)

(*S*)-(+)-3-Aminomethyl-5-methylhexanoic acid (pregabalin) is used to treat pain caused by fibromyalgia, or nerve pain in people with herpes zoster (post-herpetic neuralgia), diabetes (diabetic neuropathy), or spinal cord injury [37, 38].

The old synthesis of pregabalin involved Knoevenagel condensation of diethyl malonate and isovaleraldehyde, followed by cyanation that gives the intermediate. The intermediate on hydrolysis, decarboxylation, and reduction gave a racemic mixture of 3-aminomethyl-5-methylhexanoic acid. The resolution of the crude racemic pregabalin was carried out by using (*S*)-(+)-mandelic acid. This was a three-step crystallisation process and the overall yield of the reaction was about 20%. This synthetic route had several disadvantages, including high PMI (raw material input/API output) and high manufacturing costs because the undesired by-product (γ-amino acid enantiomer) could not be recycled (Figure 4.10) [39, 40].

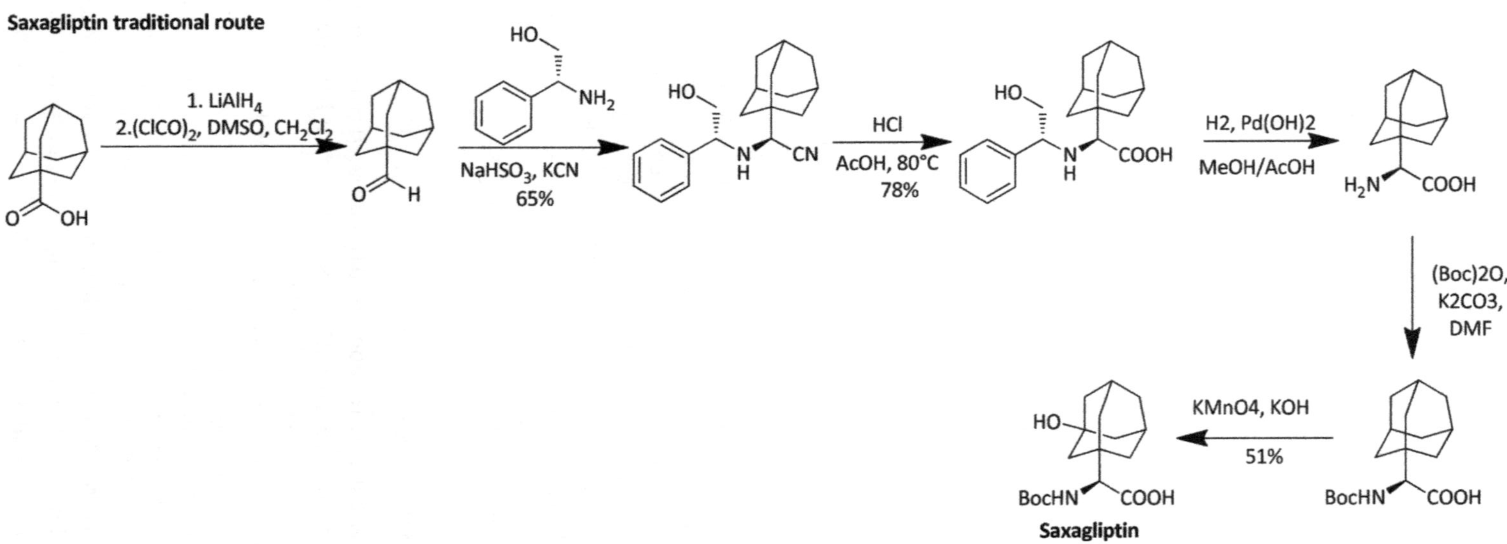

Figure 4.8 Traditional route of synthesis for saxagliptin.

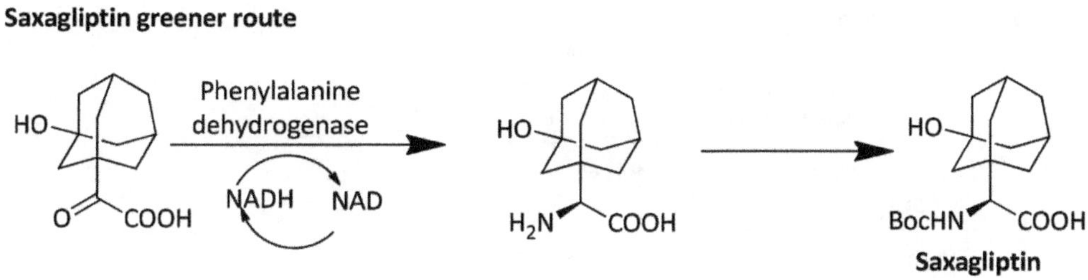

Figure 4.9 Greener route of synthesis for saxagliptin.

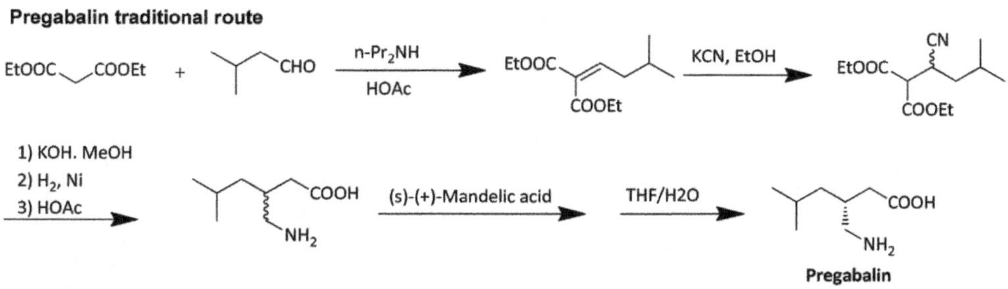

Figure 4.10 Traditional route of synthesis for pregabalin.

In the new route of synthesis, green chemistry and cost issues have been addressed by both chemocatalysis and biocatalysis. The new greener synthetic route is a biocatalytic method in which resolution is carried out by a lipolase-catalysed reaction of a cyanodiester to produce the desired single (*S*)-mono acid enantiomer in high-resolution yields (45%) and enantioselectivity (98% ee). The pregabalin was subsequently synthesised from this on decarboxylation, hydrolysis, and hydrogenation reaction. The undesired (*R*)-enantiomer could be easily racemised to cyanodiester. The yield of the reaction was improved to 40%, which is almost double the yield of the old chemical synthetic route. Furthermore, all three steps after the cyanodiester were carried out in water. As a result, the biocatalytic route is greener than the chemical synthetic route, with reduction of the E factor from 86 to 17.27. It is predicted that more than 10 million gallons of alcoholic solvents and nearly 2000 metric tonnes of raw material would be eliminated annually by this biocatalytic route for pregabalin (Figure 4.11) [41, 42].

4.4 Solvent Selection Guide

An absence of solvent is the best choice for green chemistry. But all reactions cannot be performed without using any solvent, so non-hazardous and ecofriendly solvents are required for performing green reactions. Pfizer offers a selection guide based on three key areas [18, 33, 43–49]:

- Worker safety, including reproductive toxicity, mutagenicity, carcinogenicity, skin absorption/sensitisation, and toxicity.
- Process safety, including static charge, potential for high emissions through high vapour pressure, potential for peroxide formation, flammability, and odour issues.

Pregabalin greener route

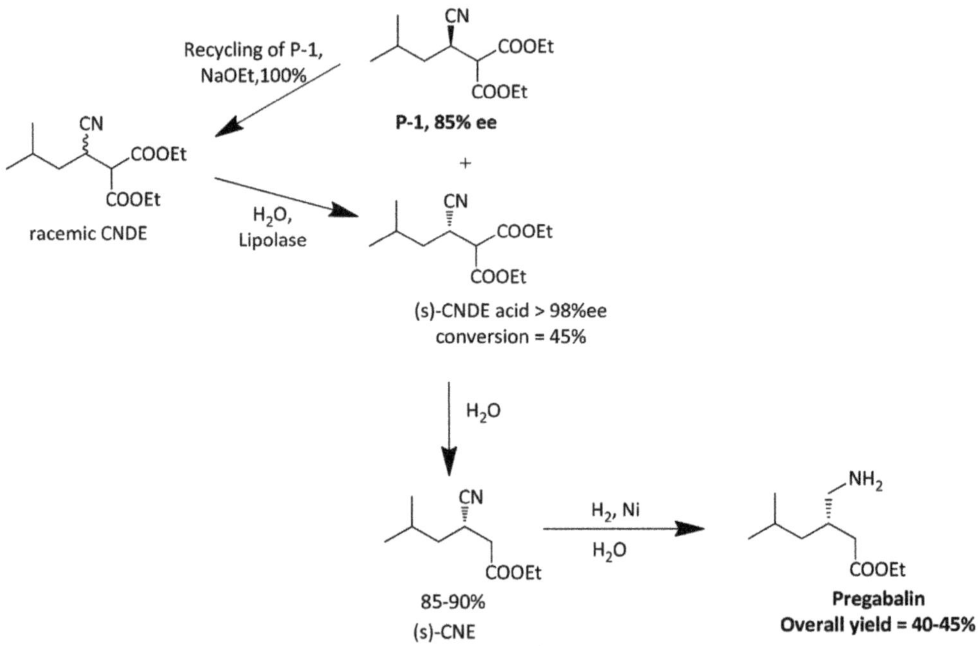

Figure 4.11 Greener route of synthesis for pregabalin.

- Environmental and regulatory considerations, including potential environment, health, and safety (EHS) regulatory restrictions, ecotoxicity, groundwater contamination, photoreactive potential, and ozone depletion potential.

The Center for Drug Evaluation and Research (CDER) of the US Food and Drug Administration (FDA) classify solvents into four classes organised by environmental hazard considerations and patient safety:

- *Class I solvents* (C_6H_6, CCl_4, $C_2H_4Cl_2$, 1,1-dichloroethylene, and 1,1,1-trichloroethane) are highly undesirable based on their deleterious environmental impact or unacceptable toxicity.
- *Class II solvents* are most commonly used organic solvents that have inherent toxicity such as methanol, acetonitrile, tetrahydrofuran, methylene chloride, toluene, and hexane.
- *Class III solvents* (acetic acid, acetone, ethanol, ethyl acetate, heptane, and dimethyl sulfoxide) have lower risk to human health and the lowest toxic potential.
- *Class IV solvents* (isooctane, 2-methyltetrahydrofuran, isopropyl ether, and petroleum ether) have insufficient toxicological data.

Hazardous, toxic, and flammable solvents should be replaced by alternative green solvents (Table 4.5).

Table 4.5 Unfavourable solvents and their alternatives.

Solvent	Unfavourable issues	Possible alternative solvents
Carbon tetrachloride, 1,2-dichloroethane, chloroform	Mutagenicity and environmental impact	Dichloromethane
Ethyl ether	Flammable	Methyl tert-butyl ether (MTBE)
Pentane	Flammable	Heptane
Benzene	Toxicity	Toluene
Dioxane	Teratogen	Tetrahydrofuran, 2-Me-THF
Hexamethylphosphoramide (HMPA)	Toxicity	*N*-methyl pyrrolidine
Isopropyl ether	Peroxide formation	MTBE
Ethylene glycol	Toxicity	1,2-propanediol

4.5 Barriers to the Adoption of Green Chemistry

There are some key barriers to the implementation of green chemistry in industry [9, 50]:

- Limited patent life.
- Regulatory requirements.
- Availability of green technologies.
- Technical barriers, i.e. no ecosystem is available for knowledge-based entrepreneurship.
- Commercialisation.
- Connection between green chemistry solution providers and industry.
- Understanding the basics of green chemistry principles.
- Short development cycle.
- Product quality.
- Lack of harmonised metrics.
- High cost for development.
- High chance of weakening a project because of high set-up costs.
- Seed capital and funding barriers.
- Intellectual property barriers.
- Regulatory barriers: changes in drug master file.
- Market barriers: business model, awareness.
- Human barriers: reluctance to change, culture, language.
- Scaling-up barriers: reproduction of result, availability of plant.
- Barriers created by previous generation of technology.
- Financial barriers: working capital for growth.

4.6 Electronic Lab Notebooks

Electronic lab notebooks (ELNs) are new software used for maintaining lab records. This leads companies towards a paperless approach so that there is no paper waste involved in maintaining lab records. It also saves time and space on maintaining paper files.

Industries are advised to add green metric calculations into their ELN templates. This aims to help a scientist think about how to reduce waste and treat it to convert it into non-hazardous materials. The E factor and PMI are the green metrics that are useful for comparing the environmental impact of different processes involved in a given compound [52]. Box 4.1 outlines a further approach for identifying key research areas in green chemistry.

Box 4.1 Process for identification and agreement on key green chemistry research areas

The process starts by collecting ideas from all the industries involved via a group discussion exercise. It is followed by a cross-company debate and assessment of the research areas. The output of one group discussion exercise is shown here. The ideas were classified into three categories:

1) Reactions that pharmaceutical industries currently use but where they would strongly prefer to use better and greener reagents.
   - Mitsunobu reactions.
   - OH activation for nucleophilic substitution.
   - Reduction of amides without $LiAlH_4$ or B_2H_6.
   - Bromination reactions.
   - Amide formation by avoiding poor atom economy reagents.
   - Ester hydrolysis.
   - Radical chemistry without Bu3SnH.
   - Nitration reactions.
   - Demethylation reactions.
   - Friedel–Crafts reactions on substrates that are unactivated.
   - Epoxidation.
   - Sulfonation reactions.
   - Wittig chemistry without Ph_3PO.
2) More aspirational reactions (reactions that industries would like to use, as they offer potentially cleaner synthetic processes to the current ones).
   - C–H activation of alkyl groups.
   - N-Centred chemistry circumventing azides, hydrazine, etc.
   - Asymmetrical hydrocyanation.
   - ROH + ArCl to give ROAr.
   - Oxygen nucleophiles with high reactivity.
   - Asymmetrical hydrogenation of unfunctionalised enamines/olefins/imines.
   - Aldehyde or ketone + 'X' + NH_3 to give a chiral amine.
   - Green sources of electrophilic nitrogen.
   - C–H activation of an aromatic system (cross-coupling reactions without the preparation of halo aromatics).
   - Asymmetrical hydroamination of olefins.
   - Asymmetrical hydrolysis of nitriles.
   - Asymmetric hydroformylation.
   - Organocatalysis.
   - New greener fluorination methods.

Box 4.1 (Continued)

3) Ideas outside of the reaction theme (concerned with use of solvents).
   - Replacements for polar aprotic solvents, DMAc, NMP, DMF, etc.
   - Alternatives to halogenated solvents.
   - Solvent-less reactor cleaning.

4.7 Applications of Green Chemistry in the Pharmaceutical Industry

Green chemistry has been used efficiently in the design of organic transformations such as oxidation of alcohols, biocatalysis, immobilisation of enzyme, and C–C bond formations [53]. There is a vast implementation of sustainable and green chemistry in commercial fields through bioresources, chemical manusfacturing, organic transformations, and so on. Some examples are discussed in this section.

4.7.1 Bioresources

For the last decade competition has arisen among scientists to look for the appropriate remedy for the effective use of bioresources. The alternatives to such bioresources have included nanocellulose, ionic liquids (ILs), catalysts, use of aqueous medium as a vehicle, supercritical CO_2 ($scCO_2$), and ultrasound irradiation. For instance, nanocellulose has been used effectively owing to its physical (feathery, higher surface area to volume ratio), chemical, or biological properties [54]. Further, the utilisation of ILs (liquid salts of cation and anion) [55] as potential solvents to overcome the constraints of organic solvents has been an emerging field to construct heterocycles in industrial organic transformations. The finely tuned, unique, and tempting physiochemical qualities of ILs offer a higher solvation capacity to dissolve the variety of biopolymers with significant thermal stability and low vapour pressure. Thus they can be modified to substitute for standard cellulose processing solvents/agents. Potential solvent retrieval with minimal loss and ability to be reused multiple times is one of the key benefits of employing ILs in nanocellulose treatment over the traditional method. On the other hand, if ILs are not handled effectively their hazards and expense may restrict their widespread application at an industrial scale.

Additionally, catalysts have advantages and physiologically mediated chemical processes, often known as biotransformation, have been promoted extensively in this regard. Using water as a solvent is safer because it is cheap and plentiful. On first impression, using aqueous solutions for processes was a promising idea, but in fact it masks the difficulty of extraction processes and it is not suitable for several processes, such as transesterification or amidation. Among other biocatalytic organic media, the majority of organic materials are only slightly soluble in water, which leads to environmental concerns about numerous volatile organic solvents and polar aprotic solvents. Here $scCO_2$ can be regarded as a suitable option to replace volatile organic solvents [56].

Powerful ultrasound irradiation has recently been used to improve the functional characteristics and bioactivity of natural polymers. In order to improve the gelling characteristics of natural polymers, ultrasound has been widely utilised. Considering gel toughness, cohesion, flexibility, stiffness, water retention ability, and degree of cross-linking, ultrasound techniques have yielded superior results. With the application of ultrasound to various products like goat milk, whey protein, and bovine gelatine, these characteristics have all been improved [57].

4.7.2 Chemical Manufacturing

The adoption of green chemistry among industrial sectors demands the utilisation of existing principles of green chemistry and measurement of green chemistry-related parameters, as well as the use of regenerative feed stocks to facilitate greater application of green chemistry. Manley and colleagues performed a survey of the implementation of green chemistry in the manufacturing of APIs and revealed that 5 of the 12 green chemistry principles are routinely incorporated in manufacturing of these APIs [58]. Gupta and Mahajan reviewed sustainable alternatives for the synthetic construction of medicinally important APIs such as atorvastatin, sitaglitptin, sildenafil, pregabalin, β-lactam antibiotics, simvastatin, saxagliptin, sertraline, imatinib, paclitaxel, oseltamivir, plavix, and valsartan, and rationalised the merits of these sustainable methods over traditional synthetic strategies for the wider benefit of chemistry communities [26].

The pharmaceutical industry has many difficulties in its efforts to increase sustainability and to reduce the cost of finished drug products needed for APIs. Paradoxically, this has opened up new avenues for incorporating the fundamentals of green chemistry throughout the process [59]. Some of these approaches involved in chemical manufacturing have been employed in oligonucleotide manufacturing [60], ILs [61], chemoenzymatic processes [62], continuous manufacturing using flow chemistry [63–65], and ultrasound [66].

4.7.3 Organic Transformations

For organic transformation reagents, catalysts, synthetic strategy, and artificial intelligence play a significant role in imparting greenness to the adopted protocols. Cp2TiCl has been demonstrated to be an excellent reagent for greener C–C and C–O bond formation, isomerisation, and deoxygenation procedures since it is extremely effective, discriminating, affordable, and ecologically benign [67]. One of the primary hurdles in chemistry is the creation of catalysts that are safe, ecological, and cost-effective. Nanostructure catalysts highlight green chemistry concepts and involve reactions like chemoselective oxidation and reduction, asymmetrical hydrogenation, linking operations, C–H activation, oxidative amination, cascade and sequential processes, and other organic modifications [68]. If the nanoscale structure is produced by sustainable chemistry, it has exceptional qualities [69]. The combination of nanochemistry and click chemistry introduces the model of an azidealkyne cycloaddition catalysed by copper, which is probably one of the most dependable and ubiquitous synthetic reactions in organic chemistry, with diverse implications [70]. As another example, zeolites are highly researched in green chemistry because of their unique properties such as morphological selectivity, heat resistance, regulated flexibility, recyclability, and ecofriendliness.

Greenness and sustainability as fundamental concepts of catalyst engineering also make it a beneficial alternative with significant practical relevance in asymmetrical organocatalysis. Two of the green chemistry principles, synthesis of new catalyts and a higher E factor, are efficiently met by organocatalysis [71]. Magnetic nanocatalysts do not just boost production yield, they can be reused numerous times without substantial loss of performance [72]. From the perspective of chalcone conversion, the use of ultrasonic irradiation is much more flexible and rapid than bioprocesses. Nevertheless, when contrasted to microwave irradiation, the processes are delayed, while there is no substantial change in results [73]. Ultrasonic radiation and the impact of combining it with a range of solvents, solvent-free, and perhaps other promising alternative sources such as microwaves and infrared rays, have transformed the process improvement part of synthetic organic processes [74]. Click chemistry's adaptability as well as its potential in new synthetic techniques are unique. The ability to produce copper-free click processes has resulted in the concept of 'bioorthogonal click chemistry', which has increased the effectiveness of this perspective in detection [75].

Many diverse attempts are now occurring in the domain of C–C coupling, with the goal of achieving simple and feasible approaches for generating carbon–carbon bonds in ecological situations with high outputs [76]. Because of its quick reactivity time, excellent yields, quality products, and purity, as well as a reduced rate of by-product formation, the microwave heating strategy has evolved into a novel green method in organic synthesis [77]. A handful of publications indicate that propargylamines can be successfully produced in metal-free circumstances. Propargylamines are an essential class of alkyne-linked amine compounds employed in heterocyclic and medicinal chemistry, and they have a significant effect as a pharmacophore in medicinal science [78].

4.8 Conclusion

The principles of green chemistry have been elaborated in this chapter by giving various examples and comparing them to conventional methods at the industrial level. Bioresources such as nanocellulose and ionic liquids have been explored to meet the sustainable demands of industry. Chemical manufacturing is becoming more opportune with the help of safer reagents, and catalysts that save time and cost and have been found to be friendly to the environment. Moreover, artificial intelligence has been applied to organic transformations and may be able to bring about a revolution in the field of green chemistry, where future scenarios are envisioned in Table 4.6.

Table 4.6 Future scenario for the chemical and pharmaceutical sectors.

Today's chemical and pharmaceutical sectors	Future chemical and pharmaceutical sectors
Fossil feed stocks	Renewable feed stocks
Covalent bonds	Weak, non-covalent interactions
Performance = maximise function	Performance = maximise function + minimise hazard
Large waste volume	Atom, solvent, and step economical processes
Conventional solvents	Low toxicity, inert, recyclable, easily separable, abundant green solvents, or solvent-free condition

(Continued)

Table 4.6 (Continued)

Today's chemical and pharmaceutical sectors	Future chemical and pharmaceutical sectors
Reactive, persistent, or hazardous chemical reagents and products	Benign chemical reagents and products
Waste treatment	Waste utilisation
Chemical production for increased profit	Maximum performance with minimum use of benign material
Material- and energy-consuming isolation process and purification	Self-separating systems
Catalysis using rare metals	Catalysis using enzymes, abundant metals, photons, or electrons

Source: Adapted from [51].

Acknowledgements

TMD and MDV thank Prof. Asit Kumar Chakraborti, Emeritus Fellow, School of Chemical Sciences, Indian Association for the Cultivation of Science (IACS), Jadavpur, Kolkata (India), for providing insightful knowledge on green chemistry through discussion, positive criticism, support, and guidance.

References

1 Kandepi, V.V.K.M., and Narender, N. (2012). Synthesis of N-heterocyclic compounds over zeolite molecular sieve catalysts: an approach towards green chemistry. *Catalysis Science & Technology* 2: 471–487.

2 Saleh, H.E.-D.M., and Koller, M. (2018). Introductory chapter: principles of green chemistry. In: *Green Chemistry*, ch. 1 (ed. H.E.-D.M. Saleh, and M. Koller), London: IntechOpen. http://www.doi.org/10.5772/intechopen.71191.

3 Ardila-Fierro, K.J., and Hernández, J.G. (2021). Sustainability assessment of mechanochemistry by using the twelve principles of green chemistry. *ChemSusChem* 14: 2145–2162.

4 Trost, B.M. (1991). The atom economy—a search for synthetic efficiency. *Science* 254: 1471–1477.

5 Kralisch, D., Ott, D., and Gericke, D. (2015). Rules and benefits of life cycle assessment in green chemical process and synthesis design: a tutorial review. *Green Chemistry* 17: 123–145.

6 Jiménez-González, C., Constable, D.J.C., and Ponder, C.S. (2012). Evaluating the 'greenness' of chemical processes and products in the pharmaceutical industry – a green metrics primer. *Chemical Society Reviews* 41: 1485–1498.

7 Dunn, P.J., Wells, A.S., and Williams, M.T. (2010). Future trends for green chemistry in the pharmaceutical industry. In: *Green Chemistry in the Pharmaceutical Industry* (ed. P.J. Dunn, A.S. Wells, and M.T. Williams), 333–355. Chichester: Wiley.

8 Zhang, T.Y. (2006). Process chemistry: the science, business, logic, and logistics. *Chemical Reviews* 106: 2583–2595.

9 Constable, D.J.C., Curzons, A.D., and Cunningham, V.L. (2002). Metrics to 'green' chemistry—which are the best? *Green Chemistry* 4: 521–527.

10 Sheldon, R.A. (2018). Metrics of green chemistry and sustainability: past, present, and future. *ACS Sustainable Chemistry & Engineering* 6: 32–48.

11 Roschangar, F., Sheldon, R.A., and Senanayake, C.H. (2015). Overcoming barriers to green chemistry in the pharmaceutical industry – the Green Aspiration Level™ concept. *Green Chemistry* 17: 752–768.

12 Prat, D., Wells, A., Hayler, J. et al. (2016). CHEM21 selection guide of classical – and less classical – solvents. *Green Chemistry* 18: 288–296.

13 Roschangar, F., Colberg, J., Dunn, P.J. et al. (2017). A deeper shade of green: inspiring sustainable drug manufacturing. *Green Chemistry* 19: 281–285.

14 Roschangar, F., Zhou, Y., Constable, D.J.C. et al. (2018). Inspiring process innovation via an improved green manufacturing metric: iGAL. *Green Chemistry* 20: 2206–2211.

15 DeVierno Kreuder, A., House-Knight, T., Whitford, J. et al. (2017). A method for assessing greener alternatives between chemical products following the 12 principles of green chemistry. *ACS Sustainable Chemistry & Engineering* 5: 2927–2935.

16 Constable, D.J.C., Dunn, P.J., Hayler, J.D. et al. (2007). Key green chemistry research areas—a perspective from pharmaceutical manufacturers. *Green Chemistry* 9: 411–420.

17 Caron, S. (ed.) (2020). *Practical Synthetic Organic Chemistry: Reactions, Principles, and Techniques*. Chichester: Wiley.

18 Alfonsi, K., Colberg, J., Dunn, P.J. et al. (2008). Green chemistry tools to influence a medicinal chemistry and research chemistry based organisation. *Green Chemistry* 10: 31–36.

19 Augé, J. (2008). A new rationale of reaction metrics for green chemistry. Mathematical expression of the environmental impact factor of chemical processes. *Green Chemistry* 10: 225–231.

20 Trost, B.M. (2002). On inventing reactions for atom economy. *Accounts of Chemical Research* 35: 695–705.

21 Andraos, J. (2006). On using tree analysis to quantify the material, input energy, and cost throughput efficiencies of simple and complex synthesis plans and networks: towards a blueprint for quantitative total synthesis and green chemistry. *Organic Process Research & Development* 10: 212–240.

22 Sheldon, R.A. (2017). The E factor 25 years on: the rise of green chemistry and sustainability. *Green Chemistry* 19: 18–43.

23 Elango, V., Murphy, M.A., Smith, B.L. et al. (1991). US Patent: method for producing ibuprofen. https://patents.google.com/patent/US4981995A/en.

24 Sharma, S., Das, J., Braje, W.M. et al. (2020). A glimpse into green chemistry practices in the pharmaceutical industry. *ChemSusChem* 13: 2859–2875.

25 Dunn, P.J., Galvin, S., and Hettenbach, K. (2004). The development of an environmentally benign synthesis of sildenafil citrate (Viagra™) and its assessment by green chemistry metrics. *Green Chemistry* 6: 43–48.

26 Gupta, P., and Mahajan, A. (2015). Green chemistry approaches as sustainable alternatives to conventional strategies in the pharmaceutical industry. *RSC Advances* 5: 26686–26705.

27 Sawant, R.T., and Waghmode, S.B. (2010). Organocatalytic approach to (S)-1-arylpropan-2-ols: enantioselective synthesis of the key intermediate of antiepileptic agent (−)-talampanel. *Synthetic Communications* 40: 2269–2277.

28 Erdélyi, B., Szabó, A., Birincsik, L., and Hoschke, Á. (2004). Process development of methylenedioxyphenyl-acetone chiral bioreduction. *Journal of Molecular Catalysis – B Enzymatic* 29: 195–199.

29 Erdélyi, B., Szabó, A., Seres, G. et al. (2006). Stereoselective production of (S)-1-aralkyl- and 1-arylethanols by freshly harvested and lyophilized yeast cells. *Tetrahedron: Asymmetry* 17: 268–274.

30 Easwar, S., and Argade, N.P. (2003). Amano PS-catalysed enantioselective acylation of (±)-α-methyl-1,3-benzodioxole-5-ethanol: an efficient resolution of chiral intermediates of the remarkable antiepileptic drug candidate, (−)-talampanel. *Tetrahedron: Asymmetry* 14: 333–337.

31 Simon, R.C., Busto, E., Richter, N. et al. (2014). Chemoenzymatic synthesis of enantiomerically pure syn-configured 1-aryl-3-methylisochroman derivatives. *European Journal of Organic Chemistry* 2014: 111–121.

32 Simić, S., Zukić, E., Schmermund, L. et al. (2022). Shortening synthetic routes to small molecule active pharmaceutical ingredients employing biocatalytic methods. *Chemical Reviews* 122: 1052–1126.

33 Cue, B.W., and Zhang, J. (2009). Green process chemistry in the pharmaceutical industry. *Green Chemistry Letters and Reviews* 2: 193–211.

34 Anderson, B.A., Hansen, M.M., Harkness, A.R. et al. (1995). Application of a practical biocatalytic reduction to an enantioselective synthesis of the 5H-2,3-benzodiazepine LY300164. *Journal of the American Chemical Society* 117: 12358–12359.

35 Hanson, R.L., Goldberg, S.L., Brzozowski, D.B. et al. (2007). Preparation of an amino acid intermediate for the dipeptidyl peptidase IV inhibitor, saxagliptin, using a modified phenylalanine dehydrogenase. *Advanced Synthesis and Catalysis* 349: 1369–1378.

36 Augeri, D.J., Robl, J.A., Betebenner, D.A. et al. (2005). Discovery and preclinical profile of saxagliptin (BMS-477118): a highly potent, long-acting, orally active dipeptidyl peptidase IV inhibitor for the treatment of type 2 diabetes. *Journal of Medicinal Chemistry* 48: 5025–5037.

37 Lauria-Horner, B.A., and Pohl, R.B. (2003). Pregabalin: a new anxiolytic. *Expert Opinion on Investigational Drugs* 12: 663–672.

38 Selak, I. (2001). Pregabalin (Pfizer). *Current Opinion in Investigational Drugs* 2: 828–834.

39 Burk, M.J., de Koning, P.D., Grote, T.M. et al. (2003). An enantioselective synthesis of (S)-(+)-3-aminomethyl-5-methylhexanoic acid via asymmetric hydrogenation. *Journal of Organic Chemistry* 68: 5731–5734.

40 Xie, Z., Feng, J., Garcia, E. et al. (2006). Cloning and optimization of a nitrilase for the synthesis of (3S)-3-cyano-5-methyl hexanoic acid. *Journal of Molecular Catalysis – B Enzymatic* 41: 75–80.

41 Felluga, F., Pitacco, G., Valentin, E., and Venneri, C.D. (2008). A facile chemoenzymatic approach to chiral non-racemic β-alkyl-γ-amino acids and 2-alkylsuccinic acids. A concise synthesis of (S)-(+)-pregabalin. *Tetrahedron: Asymmetry* 19: 945–955.

42 Martinez, C.A., Hu, S., Dumond, Y. et al. (2008). Development of a chemoenzymatic manufacturing process for pregabalin. *Organic Process Research & Development* 12: 392–398.

43 Byrne, F.P., Jin, S., Paggiola, G. et al. (2016). Tools and techniques for solvent selection: green solvent selection guides. *Sustainable Chemical Processes* 4: 7.

44 Prat, D., Hayler, J., and Wells, A. (2014). A survey of solvent selection guides. *Green Chemistry* 16: 4546–4551.

45 Tobiszewski, M., Tsakovski, S., Simeonov, V. et al. (2015). A solvent selection guide based on chemometrics and multicriteria decision analysis. *Green Chemistry* 17: 4773–4785.

46 Phan, T.V.T., Gallardo, C., and Mane, J. (2015). GREEN MOTION: a new and easy to use green chemistry metric from laboratories to industry. *Green Chemistry* 17: 2846–2852.

47 Prat, D., Pardigon, O., Flemming, H.-W. et al. (2013). Sanofi's solvent selection guide: a step toward more sustainable processes. *Organic Process Research & Development* 17: 1517–1525.

48 Dunn, P.J. (2012). The importance of green chemistry in process research and development. *Chemical Society Reviews* 41: 1452–1461.

49 Welton, T. (2015). Solvents and sustainable chemistry. *Proceedings of the Royal Society A: Mathematical, Physical and Engineering Sciences* 471: 20150502.

50 Mulvihill, M.J., Beach, E.S., Zimmerman, J.B. et al. (2011). Green engineering: a framework for sustainable technology development. *Annual Review of Environment and Resources* 36: 271–293.

51 Zimmerman, J.B., Anastas, P.T., Erythropel, H.C., and Leitner, W. (2020). Designing for a green chemistry future. *Science* 367: 397–400.

52 Bryan, M.C., Dillon, B., Hamann, L.G. et al. (2013). Sustainable practices in medicinal chemistry: current state and future directions. *Journal of Medicinal Chemistry* 56: 6007–6021.

53 Sheldon, R.A. (2012). Fundamentals of green chemistry: efficiency in reaction design. *Chemical Society Reviews* 41: 1437–1451.

54 Haron, G.A.S., Mahmood, H., Noh, M.H. et al. (2021). Ionic liquids as a sustainable platform for nanocellulose processing from bioresources: overview and current status. *ACS Sustainable Chemistry & Engineering* 9: 1008–1034.

55 Dhameliya, T.M., Nagar, P.R., Bhakhar, K.A. et al. (2022). Recent advancements in applications of ionic liquids in synthetic construction of heterocyclic scaffolds: a spotlight. *Journal of Molecular Liquids* 348: 118329.

56 Sheldon, R.A., and Woodley, J.M. (2018). Role of biocatalysis in sustainable chemistry. *Chemical Reviews* 118: 801–838.

57 Wang, X., Majzoobi, M., and Farahnaky, A. (2020). Ultrasound-assisted modification of functional properties and biological activity of biopolymers: a review. *Ultrasonics Sonochemistry* 65: 105057.

58 Giraud, R.J., Williams, P.A., Sehgal, A. et al. (2014). Implementing green chemistry in chemical manufacturing: a survey report. *ACS Sustainable Chemistry & Engineering* 2: 2237–2242.

59 Koenig, S.G., Bee, C., Borovika, A. et al. (2019). A green chemistry continuum for a robust and sustainable active pharmaceutical ingredient supply chain. *ACS Sustainable Chemistry & Engineering* 7: 16937–16951.

60 Andrews, B.I., Antia, F.D., Brueggemeier, S.B. et al. (2021). Sustainability challenges and opportunities in oligonucleotide manufacturing. *Journal of Organic Chemistry* 86: 49–61.

61 Siodmiak, T., Piotr Marszall, M., and Proszowska, A. (2012). Ionic liquids: a new strategy in pharmaceutical synthesis. *Mini-Reviews in Organic Chemistry* 9: 203–208.

62 Tao, J., Zhao, L., and Ran, N. (2007). Recent advances in developing chemoenzymatic processes for active pharmaceutical ingredients. *Organic Process Research & Development* 11: 259–267.

63 Baumann, M., Moody, T.S., Smyth, M., and Wharry, S. (2020). A perspective on continuous flow chemistry in the pharmaceutical industry. *Organic Process Research & Development* 24: 1802–1813.

64 Poechlauer, P., Colberg, J., Fisher, E. et al. (2013). Pharmaceutical roundtable study demonstrates the value of continuous manufacturing in the design of greener processes. *Organic Process Research & Development* 17: 1472–1478.

65 Ager, D.J. (2015). Popular synthetic approaches to pharmaceuticals. *Synthesis* 47: 760–768.

66 Levina, M., Rubinstein, M.H., and Rajabi-Siahboomi, A.R. (2000). Principles and application of ultrasound in pharmaceutical powder compression. *Pharmaceutical Research* 17: 257–265.

67 Castro Rodríguez, M., Rodríguez García, I., Rodríguez Maecker, R.N. et al. (2017). Cp2TiCl: an ideal reagent for green chemistry? *Organic Process Research & Development* 21: 911–923.

68 Chng, L.L., Erathodiyil, N., and Ying, J.Y. (2013). Nanostructured catalysts for organic transformations. *Accounts of Chemical Research* 46: 1825–1837.

69 Duan, H., Wang, D., and Li, Y. (2015). Green chemistry for nanoparticle synthesis. *Chemical Society Reviews* 44: 5778–5792.

70 Alonso, F., Moglie, Y., and Radivoy, G. (2015). Copper nanoparticles in click chemistry. *Accounts of Chemical Research* 48: 2516–2528.

71 Antenucci, A., Dughera, S., and Renzi, P. (2021). Green chemistry meets asymmetric organocatalysis: a critical overview on catalysts synthesis. *ChemSusChem* 14: 2785–2853.

72 Gebre, S.H. (2021). Recent developments in the fabrication of magnetic nanoparticles for the synthesis of trisubstituted pyridines and imidazoles: a green approach. *Synthetic Communications* 51: 1669–1699.

73 Rosa, G.P., Seca, A.M.L., Barreto, M.D.C., and Pinto, D.C.G.A. (2017). Chalcone: a valuable scaffold upgrading by green methods. *ACS Sustainable Chemistry & Engineering* 5: 7467–7480.

74 Dandia, A., Singh, R., and Bhaskaran, S. (2013). Multicomponent reactions and ultrasound: a synergistic approach for the synthesis of bioactive heterocycles. *Current Green Chemistry* 1: 17–39.

75 Musumeci, F., Schenone, S., Desogus, A. et al. (2015). Click chemistry, a potent tool in medicinal sciences. *Current Medicinal Chemistry* 22: 2022–2050.

76 Budarin, V.L., Shuttleworth, P.S., Clark, J.H., and Luque, R. (2011). Industrial applications of C–C coupling reactions. *Current Organic Synthesis* 7: 614–627.

77 Meera, G., Rohit, K.R., Saranya, S., and Anilkumar, G. (2020). Microwave assisted synthesis of five membered nitrogen heterocycles. *RSC Advances* 10: 36031–36041.

78 Ghosh, S., and Biswas, K. (2021). Metal-free multicomponent approach for the synthesis of propargylamine: a review. *RSC Advances* 11: 2047–2065.

5

Green Analytical Techniques Using Hydrotropy, Mixed Hydrotropy, and Mixed Solvency

Atish S. Mundada[1], *Dipak D. Patil*[2] *and Rajesh K. Maheshwari*[3]

[1] *SNJBs SSDJ College of Pharmacy, Neminagar, Chandwad, Nashik, Maharashtra, India*
[2] *K.K. Wagh College of Pharmacy, Nashik, Maharashtra, India.*
[3] *Department of Pharmacy, SGSITS, Indore, Madhya Pradesh, India*

CONTENTS

5.1 Introduction

Analytical chemistry, a crucial branch of chemistry, provides input related to the nature of chemical substances and their occurrence in organisms and in the environment through various analytical measures. It is impossible to understand a product's life cycle without chemical analysis of its components and degradation products. The standards and specifications followed for the use of chemicals in various industries are based on evidence obtained by analytical chemists and are further controlled by the chemical process. Sustainable development aims at decreasing the unfavourable aftereffects of the materials that we use and produce. At the same time, a leading concern is to change the way energy and aromatic chemicals are created from fossil fuels to make reproducible assets. Analytical chemistry is the only field that can validate the environmental friendliness of any novel method, process, or product.

The solubility of active ingredients, particularly low water solubility, poses enumerable challenges not only during drug discovery, but also in the initial and last stages of pharmaceutical development. Aqueous solubility is also associated with discharge and partition of the chemicals in the environment and thus it is considered an elementary parameter in the

Sustainable Approaches in Pharmaceutical Sciences, First Edition. Edited by Kamal Shah, Durgesh Nandini Chauhan, and Nagendra Singh Chauhan.

risk assessment of any chemical. The deployment of a combination of chemistry and high-throughput screening techniques in the invention of drugs has propelled the formation of high molecular weight new chemical entities (NCEs) that have greater lipid solubility. Aqueous solubility is critical for the mixing, circulation, and performance of organic chemicals within experiments, analytical systems, and the environment. It is always an uphill task to convert a poorly aqueous-soluble NCE into a final product for human use. Secondly, how to solubilise these NCEs is a tough question to be answered by chemists and formulation scientists, as solubilisation of NCEs dictates the utilisation of organic solvents.

There are many incorrect practices followed by analysts at some stage of either quantitative or qualitative laboratory experiments that might prove harmful not only to them but also to the environment. Foremost among these is the unrestrained dumping of organic vehicle wastes and unfortunately numerous organic vehicles possess substantial toxicity [1]. In addition, making use of unsafe chemical reagents has deleterious consequences on the environment. These days, ecological anxiety has become a burning issue in laboratory experiments and hence it is anticipated that all analytical tests should be safe and ecofriendly.

5.2 Green Chemistry

Green chemistry is the most striking notion in chemistry as it guarantees that subsequent inventions are more sustainable compared to existing ones. Exploitation of the 12 principles of green chemistry diminishes or eradicates the utilisation or creation of harmful chemicals in the planning, assembly, and functions of a chemical harvest [2]. A crucial area of green chemistry involves the elimination of vehicles in chemical practices or finding ecologically safe solvents as an alternative to dangerous solvents. Around 35% of synthesised drugs have an aqueous solubility issue, which thus demands the use of organic vehicles. It is the need of the hour to find ecofriendly and cost-effective alternatives to organic vehicles and this has led to the formation of new and commercial approaches [3]. The initiation of solvent-free processes as substitutes is obviously the first choice and if a solvent is a must for a particular process, then choosing a solvent that will have no or limited impact on the well-being of chemists and the environment is the best answer.

Various techniques have been exploited to solubilise poorly water-soluble medicaments [4, 5]. The utilisation of unconventional solvents is quickly growing and 'hydrotropy' technology is one of the most appealing green techniques that can lead to easy swaps from the typical universal organic solvents used in various processes.

5.3 Hydrotropes and Hydrotropy

The term hydrotropy was coined by Neuberg in 1916. Neuberg defined hydrotropes as the organic acid salts of metal that considerably enhance the aqueous solubility of organic substances at moderately elevated concentrations [6]. Neuberg's hydrotropic agent (Figure 5.1) generally has two fundamental portions: a hydrophilic portion made up of an anionic metal ion and a hydrophobic portion consisting of an aromatic ring/ring system. The metal ion portion boosts the water solubility, although the type of anion or metal ion in the hydrotrope usually demonstrates a trivial influence on this. Conversely, the

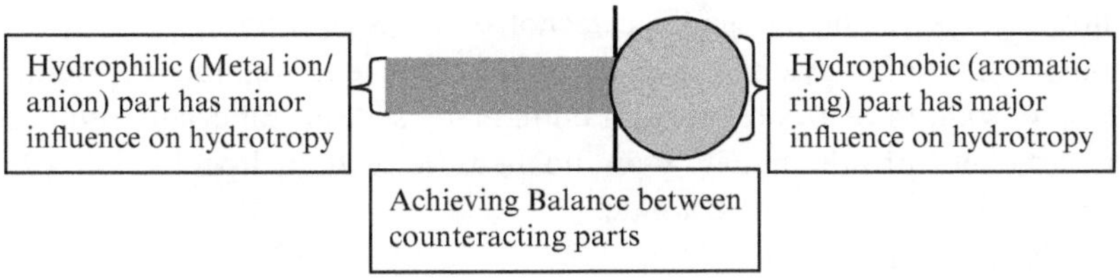

Figure 5.1 Hydrotropic agent.

planarity of the non-hydrophilic aromatic ring has been suggested as an imperative facet in the solubilisation process using a hydrotropic agent.

In 1985, Saleh and El-Khordagui explained that hydrotropes could be positively charged, negatively charged, or neutral, inorganic or organic, and non-micelle-forming molecules that may be solid or liquid in nature. Hydrotropes contain a very small hydrophobic portion compared to the surfactant and the equilibrium between the water-loving and the water-hating part controls the efficiency of hydrotropic solubilisation. The hydrotropic agents (solubilisers, additives, or enhancers) are ionic organic salts.

Hydrotropy is a molecular phenomenon wherein the water solubility of poorly soluble material is enhanced by incorporating a second solute (a hydrotrope) [7]. In simple terms, it is a solubility enhancement technique that augments the solubility of one solute by the presence of a large quantity of another solute [8, 9]. Hydrotropy not only assists in the segregation of a narrow boiling point isomeric agent from its mixture, but also enhances the speed of diverse reactions [10–13]. The phenomenon of hydrotropy is considered an exceptional and revolutionary solubilisation strategy as it shows effortless recovery of hydrotropes from the liquefied solute and the possibility of recycling such hydrotropic solutions [8].

5.3.1 Advantages of Hydrotropy

- Owing to its pH-independent solvent character, high solute selectivity, and non-requirement of an emulsification step, hydrotopy is considered as a better choice over alternative solubilisation processes like micellar solubilisation [14], co-solvents [15], and the salting-in method [16].
- The only requirement in hydrotropic solubilisation is mixing of the drug with the hydrotropic agent in water [17].
- Hydrotropy requires neither chemical alteration of an inadequately water-soluble medicament nor the use of any organic vehicle [17].
- Hydrotropy is a financially viable, harmless, and easy-to-use technique [17].

5.3.2 Classification of Hydrotropic Agents

The literature suggests that numerous hydrotropic agents could be employed for solubility augmentation of inadequately soluble medicaments. All these materials used as hydrotropes could be put up into the following categories [18–21]:

- *Urea and its derivatives*: e.g. urea and ethyl, butyl, and N,N-dimethyl derivatives of urea.
- *Organic metal salts and acids*: e.g. sodium salicylate, sodium glycinate, sodium ascorbate, sodium acetate, sodium and potassium citrate, sodium benzoate, benzoic acid.

- *Aromatic alcohols*: e.g. resorcinol, pyrogallol, catechol, α and β-naphthols.
- *Aromatic anionics*: e.g. sodium xylene sulfonate, sodium benzene sulphonate, sodium p-toluene sulfonate, sodium benzoate, sodium cinnamate, sodium salicylate, sodium-3-hydroxy-2-naphtholate, nicotinamides, p-amino benzoic acid hydrochloride, N,N-diethyl nicotinamide, N,N-dimethyl benzamide.
- *Aromatic hydrotropes*: e.g. caffeine, nicotinamides, N,N-dimethyl benzamide.
- *Aromatic cationics*: p-amino benzoic acid hydrochloride, caffeine, procaine HCl.
- *Aliphatic and linear compounds*: e.g. sodium alkanoate, urea, N,N-dimethyl urea, tertiary butyl alcohol.
- *Surfactants*: e.g. diacids, sodium dodecyl sulfate, dodecylated oxidibenzene, and many other anionic, cationic, non-ionic, and amphoteric surface-active agents.

5.3.3 Mechanism of Hydrotropic Solubilisation

In 1996, Coffman and Kildsig studied a riboflavin–nicotinamide mixture to understand the way a hydrotrope works and on the basis of spectral characters, established that there is no complex formation reaction involved between the drug and the hydrotropic agent [22]. Later it was shown that hydrotropes could be acting as a solubility-enhancing agent in the presence of their critical hydrotrope concentration, similar to surfactants but with a non-micellar property [23]. Various theoretical and experimental set-ups were tried to elucidate the mechanisms of hydrotropic solubilisation. The available projected ways can be summarised under three designs [20, 24]:

- *Self-aggregation potential*: e.g. sodium salicylate, sodium p-toluene sulfonate, sodium xylene sulfonate, etc.
- *Structure-breaker and/or -maker*: chaotropes, e.g. urea, guanidium chloride; or kosmotropes, e.g. polyhydric alcohol, trehalose, glycine, betaine, proline, etc.
- *Forming a micelle-resembling structure*: e.g. alkyl benzene sulfonate, alkyl sulfates, etc.

It is presumed that hydrotropic agents flock into the less rigid non-covalent congregation of non-polar microdomains to enhance the solubility of the hydrophobic candidates. Some scientists have commented that hydrotropic solubilisation resembles complexation, with a weak contact offered between solute and hydrotropic agent. In short, it can be said that the hydrotropic technique is a combined molecular event involving a mutual intermolecular interface and many complementary molecular pulls [25].

5.4 Hydrotropic Technology

Applications of hydrotropic agents in the field of pharmacy have been put into two groups on the basis of their use:

- Monohydrotropy or single hydrotropy, concerned with the application of single hydrotropic agents.
- Mixed hydrotropy, wherein two or more than two hydrotropic agents are used.

5.5 Pharmaceutical Analysis Using Monohydrotropy

Though the utilisation of a single hydrotropic agent appears to be easy and uncomplicated, the decision on the selection of the appropriate material may be intricate. The documented evidence suggests that monohydrotropic agents have been successfully used for the concurrent evaluation of drug pairs. The method of analysis to be selected depends on the conditions for the experiment and the category of the drug. The concept of hydrotropic solubilisation has been exploited by Maheshwari and his group in the estimation of numerous poorly aqueous-soluble drugs and the research findings have been well documented.

5.5.1 Thin-Layer Chromatography

Numerous non-polar organic vehicles like alkanes (hexane, heptane), aromatics (xylene, toluene, benzene), chloroform, ether, dichloromethane, cyclohexane, and polar solvents like acetone, ethyl acetate, butanol, and ethanol are being utilised for carrying out thin-layer chromatography (TLC) of a variety of drugs. Some organic solvents in that list are costly and generate poisons, and hence are considered to be toxic not only to the chemist but also to the environment. Hydrotropic solutions can be used as a mobile phase replacing these toxic organic solvents to perform TLC analysis of many poorly water-soluble compounds. The application of hydrotropic agents like urea and sodium benzoate has been shown to improve the solubility of some poorly water-soluble medicaments by Maheshwari et al. [26, 27]. Mangal et al. [28] proved the use of a 5.0 M solution of sodium salicylate as a hydrotropic agent in TLC analysis of omeprazole, whereas Jayronia et al. [29] effectively developed a novel, ecofriendly, simple, safe, and inexpensive TLC technique for model drugs like norfloxacin, erythromycin, and ciprofloxacin using sodium salicylate, sodium benzoate, and urea as hydrotropic agents in a mobile phase.

5.5.2 Titrimetric Analysis

The principle of hydrotropic solubilisation has been successfully exploited in titrimetric estimation to preclude the use of harmful organic solvents. Moreover, it has been observed and documented that organic solvents demonstrate inaccurate results in spectrophotometric evaluation of many medicaments due to the volatility of these solvents. Thus, the application of hydrotropy not only helps in overcoming this drawback, but also improves the solubility of certain poorly water-soluble drugs. The numerous titrimetric investigations of poorly aqueous-soluble drugs, in bulk as well as in solid dosage forms, carried out using a hydrotropic agent and thus avoiding the use of harmful and toxic organic solvents, have been summarised in Table 5.1.

5.5.3 Spectrophotometric Analysis

Today, about 35–40% of frequently used substances are found to have an aqueous solubility of less than 10 μM or 5 mg/mL at pH 7, which creates problems in the analytical evaluation or formulation of these types of drugs. Organic solvents that are expensive, toxic, as well as harmful to the environment are frequently employed for the spectrophotometric analysis of water-insoluble moieties. Furthermore, exposure to these organic solvents leads to

Table 5.1 Summary of hydrotropic agents used in titrimetric analysis.

Hydrotropic agent used	Drug	References
2.0 M sodium benzoate	Aspirin	[26]
	Frusemide	[30, 31]
	Ketoprofen	[32]
	Aceclofenac	[33, 34]
	Flurbiprofen	[35]
	Ibuprofen	[35]
	Benzoic acid	[36]
2.0 M sodium salicylate	Benzoic acid	[36]
	Aceclofenac	[37]
	Frusemide	[38]
	Ketoprofen	[39, 40]
0.5 M ibuprofen sodium	Frusemide	[41]
	Aspirin	[42]
	Aceclofenac	[43]
1.25 M sodium citrate	Aspirin	[26]
	Salicylic acid	[33]
	Ketoprofen	[39]
8.0 M urea	Salicylic acid	[33]
	Norfloxacin	[44]
1.0 M calcium disodium edetate	Salicylic acid	[45]
0.5 M ibuprofen sodium	Salicylic acid	[45]
1.5 M metformin HCl	Aspirin	[46]
2.0 M Nicotinamide	Salbutamol	[47]
2.0 M niacinamide	Aspirin	[48]
2.0 M sodium salicylate	Theophylline	[49]
2.0 M sodium saccharin	Salicylic acid	[50]
2.0 M sodium acetate	Ketoprofen	[33]
4.0 M sodium acetate	Aspirin	[26]

adverse effects like skin inflammation, eye irritation, nausea, headache, and sedation. Prolonged exposure may even lead to various harsh consequences like neurological disorders, mutagenic disorders, liver damage, chronic renal failure, and necrosis.

Researchers are persistently working in this direction to get an ecological solution for this issue and fortunately these harmful solvents can be substituted by some other ecofriendly sources. The spectrophotometric estimation of numerous poorly aqueous-soluble drugs precluding the employment of toxic organic vehicles has been carried out by Maheshwari and group as well as other researchers, and has been summarised in Table 5.2.

Table 5.2 Summary of hydrotropic agents used in spectrophotometric analysis.

Hydrotropic agent used	Drug	References
0.1 M citric acid	Lercanidipine	[51]
	Pioglitazone HCL	[52]
7.5 M N,N-dimethyl urea	Diclofenac sodium	[53]
	Gatifloxacin	[54]
	Naproxen	[55]
1.5 M metformin hydrochloride	Aspirin	[46]
	Gatifloxacin	[56]
	Famotidine	[57]
2.0 M niacinamide	Naproxen	[58]
	Indomethacin	[59]
	Nalidixic acid	[27]
	Norfloxacin	
	Tinidazole	
4.0 M sodium acetate	Lovastatin	[60]
	Cefixime	[61]
	Ketoprofen	[32]
	Tinidazole	[23]
	Amlodipine besylate	[62]
2.0 M sodium benzoate	Naproxen	[63]
	Ofloxacin	[26]
	Gatifloxacin	[56]
	Hydrochlorothiazide	[64]
	Indomethacin	
	Frusemide	[65, 66]
	Tinidazole	[23]
	Piroxicam	[67]
	Riluzole	[68]
	Lornoxicam	[69]
	Etoricoxib	[70]
1.25 M sodium citrate	Salicylic acid	[71]
	Cefixime	[61]
	Tinidazole	[23]
	Naproxen	[72]
5.0 M urea	Fluvoxamine	[73]
	Dextro-methorphan	[74]
	Amlodipine besylate	[62]
	Acyclovir	[75]
	Cefadroxil	[76]
	Lomefloxacin	[77]
	Ciprofloxacin	[78]

(Continued)

Table 5.2 (Continued)

Hydrotropic agent used	Drug	References
8.0 M urea	Cefixime	[61]
	Tinidazole	[23]
	Cephalexin	[79]
	Diclofenac sodium	[80]
	Terconazole	[81]
10 M urea	Hydrochlorothiazide	[82]
	Amoxicillin	[83]
	Paracetamol	[84]
1.0 M calcium disodium edetate	Benzoic acid	[85]
1.5 M ibuprofen sodium	Piroxicam	[86]
1.0 M lignocaine hydrochloride	Tinidazole	[87]
2.0 M potassium acetate	Ketoprofen	[88]
5.0 M potassium acetate	Amoxicillin	[89]
2.0 M sodium salicylate	Nifedipine	[90]

5.5.4 Simultaneous Spectrophotometric Estimation

A handful of investigations are known in the area of concurrent spectrophotometric estimation of poorly aqueous-soluble drugs. It has been well documented that a hydrotropic solubilisation technique has been successfully utilised and the outcomes of these analyses have been summarised in Table 5.3.

Table 5.3 Summary of simultaneous spectrophotometric estimation using hydrotropy.

Drug molecule(s)	Hydrotropic agent used	References
Norfloxacin and tinidazole	Urea	[91]
Atenolol and amlodipine besylate		[92]
Cefixime trihydrate and Oonidazole		[93]
Ciprofloxacin hydrochloride and tinidazole		[94]
Levofloxacin hemihydrate and ambroxol hydrochloride		[95]
Paracetamol and diclofenac sodium		[96]
Metronidazole and norfloxacin		[97]
Diclofenac sodium and rabeprazole sodium		[98]

Table 5.3 (Continued)

Drug molecule(s)	Hydrotropic agent used	References
Ibuprofen, flurbiprofen, naproxen	Sodium benzoate	[99]
Gabapentin, methyl-cobalamin		[100]
Esomeprazole and itopride	Metformin hydrochloride	[101]

5.6 Mixed Hydrotropy

In 2007, Maheshwari suggested a mixed hydrotropic solubilisation approach for solubility improvement of poorly water-soluble active pharmaceutical ingredients (APIs)/material [102]. As the name suggests, two or more hydrotropic agents are used at low concentration (instead of a single hydrotropic agent at higher concentration) to improve severalfold the water solubility of poorly water-soluble material [103]. The increase in solubility of poorly water-soluble APIs was measured through calculating the solubility enhancement ratio. This is the ratio of API solubility in a mixed hydrotropic solution to its solubility in water [102].

$$\text{Solubility enhancement ratio} = \frac{\text{Drug solubility in mixed hydrotropic solution}}{\text{Drug solubility drug in water}}$$

To enhance the solubility of poorly water-soluble drugs, a mixed hypotrophy approach was explored by many researchers, who found that it may lead to additive or synergistic effects on the solubility of the drug. The drugs analysed were hydrochlorothiazide [46], aceclofenac [104, 105], aceclofenac tablets [106], ketoprofen [107], ketoprofen tablets [53], nitazoxanide [108], metronidazole and miconazole nitrate [109], levofloxacin and ornidazole [110], acelofenac and paracetamol in bulk and tablet form [111], paliperidone in bulk and tablet form [112], nimesulide [113], indomethacin in bulk and capsule form [114], acyclovir in bulk and tablet form [115], and norfloxacin [116]. The spectrophotometric estimation of norfloxacin having low solubility was carried out using a mixed hydrotropic approach [116]. The details of the drug, mixed hydrotropic blend, and solubility increase are summarised in Table 5.4.

Table 5.4 Summary of mixed hydrotropy applications for spectroscopic estimation.

Material	Mixed hydrotropic blend	References
Aceclofenac	≥20% urea and 10% sodium citrate	[115]
Ketoprofen	30% urea and 30% sodium citrate	[107]
Hydrochlorothiazide	Niacinamide (8%) + sodium acetate (8%) + urea (8%) + sodium benzoate (8%) + sodium citrate (8%); total 40% hydrotropic agents	[46]
Nitazoxanide	1 M sodium benzoate and 1 M sodium salicylate	[108]

(Continued)

Table 5.4 (Continued)

Material	Mixed hydrotropic blend	References
Metronidazole and miconazole nitrate	40% urea and 10% sodium benzoate	[109]
Levofloxacin and ornidazole	2 M sodium acetate (50% w/w) + 8 M urea (50% w/w)	[110]
Paliperidone	20% sodium benzoate and 20% niacinamide	[112]
Nimesulide	25% sodium citrate + 30% phenol	[113]
Norfloxacin	20% urea + 20% sodium benzoate	[116]

Mixed hydrotropy solubilisation (MHS), including the mixed hydrotropic solid dispersion (MHSD) approach, has been exploited in formulation and development to reduce the high concentration of individual hydrotropic agents. Use of a single hydrotropic agent at high concentration may lead to toxicity issues. MHS reduces the concentration of an individual hydrotropic agent to the low side, leading to fewer toxicity issues. MHSD was reported to enhance the solubility of furosemide [25], acelofenac [117], nevirapine [118], and flupirtine maleate [119]. The drugs studied and the highest solubility obtained in optimised MHSD are shown in Table 5.5.

5.6.1 Discussion

A vast amount of work on solubility enhancement by hydrotropy and the mixed hydrotropy approach in formulation and analytical method has been carried out by Maheshwari, as already referenced. The different ultraviolet (UV)-visible spectroscopy analytical methods used for single-component analysis, multicomponent analysis using monohydrotropy, and the mixed hydrotropy approach were briefly reviewed in 2019 [20]. A book chapter by El Hamd et al., (2022) has summerised titrimetric and spectrophotometric methods of analytical measurements of poorly water soluble drugs using hydrotropic solubilisation approach [120].

The prevalence of monohydrotropy over mixed hydrotropy has been reported [20]. In most mixed hydrotropic approaches used for analytical method development of different drugs, urea hydrotrope has been used widely as one of the components. Researchers have

Table 5.5 Mixed hydrotropic solid dispersion (MHSD).

Drug	Highest solubility observed in MHSD	Ratio in MHSD	Concentration of hydrotropic agent blend (%)	References
Aceclofenac	Urea + sodium citrate	2 : 1	30	[117]
Furosemide	Urea + sodium citrate + sodium benzoate	15 : 5 : 20	40	[25]
Nevirapine	Lactose + citric acid	15 : 25	40	[118]
Flupirtine maleate	Sodium benzoate + niacinamide	1 : 1	20	[119]

reported hydrotrope concentration in units of % and M, but uniformity in the use of units is required. A design flow for hydrotropy, choice of hydrotrope, initial and final concentrations of hydrotrope, and initial ratio in a hydrotrope blend are the issues that need to be clarified for systematic use of mixed hydrotropy in analytical method development.

In cases of mixed hydrotropy solubilisation, MHSD was reported to improve the solubility of poorly water-soluble drugs. The total concentration of the blend of hydrotropic agents preferred by many authors was 40%. Specific guidelines for using mixed hydrotropy for formulation are missing. The choice of components of the hydrotropy blend, their initial and final concentrations, and toxicity concerns regarding hydrotrope use are unclear. It is possible to explore a design of experiment (DOE) approach in optimisation of the hydrotrope blend ratio.

5.7 Mixed Solvency

The mixed solvency concept was initiated by Maheshwari in 2009 based on the assumption that each material (solid, liquid, gas) in the universe has solubilising power [121]. Hydrotropy is a type of co-solvency [122]. The prepared blend is used to improve the solubility of a poorly water-soluble drug. Like in mixed hydrotropy, a blend of two hydrotropes is used to lower the concentration of a single hydrotropic agent. In mixed solvency, a blend/combination of hydrotrope, co-solvent, and water-soluble solid excipient is used, which shows mostly synergistic activity related to the solubility of a poorly water-soluble drug. The technique avoids the use of organic solvents for solubilisation, instead using solubilisers that do not cause any toxicity and are non-volatile [123].

Hydrotropes like urea, sodium benzoate, sodium ascorbate, and sodium citrate have been used. The different co-solvents explored were glycerine, PEG 200, PEG 300, PEG 400, and propylene glycol. The cyclodextrins, PEG 4000, and PEG 6000 were used as water-soluble solids.

The solubility of various poorly water-soluble drugs was improved by the mixed solvency approach, including salicylic acid [122], ketoprofen [123], tinidazole [124], ofloxacin and tinidazole [125], norfloxacin [126], diclofenac sodium [127], indomethacin [128], and nifedipine [129]. Details of the material, total concentration of solubiliser, blend with ratio of components, solubility increase, and contributory solubility are summarised in Table 5.6.

For the development of dosage forms like liquid/solution, injections, syrups, or topical solutions, the blends of water-soluble substances (hydrotropes, co-solvents, water-soluble excipients, etc.) can be made at safe concentrations of the individual solubiliser [122]. Ibuprofen syrup development was reported by a mixed solvency approach in which hydrotropes (disodium hydrogen phosphate, sodium citrate, potassium acetate, potassium citrate), propylene glycol, glycerine, and Tween® 80 were used [130]. Ibuprofen topical formulation using the mixed solvency concept was reported in which different combinations of hydrotropes and co-solvents were used, including sodium citrate, propylene glycol, urea, sodium acetate, and sodium caprylate. The maximum solubility of 95 mg/mL was observed in a blend of 5% sodium caprylate + 5% sodium citrate + 10% urea, which was explored for the topical solution and gel [131]. Diclofenac sodium lotion (topical formulation) was developed using the mixed solvency concept in which combinations of niacinamide (5% w/v), caffeine (5% w/v), glycerin, and sodium sulfite were used [132].

Table 5.6 Summary of mixed solvency applications.

Material	Total concentration of solubilisers (% w/v)	Blend with ratio of components	Contributory solubility of drug in blend (% w/v)	References
Salicylic acid	40	10% w/v glycerin, 10% w/v PEG 300, 10% w/v PEG 400, and 10% w/v sodium citrate	8.237	[122]
Ketoprofen	30	Sodium citrate (15%), PEG 400 (8%), and polyvinyl pyrolidine (7%)	Not calculated	[123]
Tinidazole	35	Phenol crystals and niacinamide 25 : 10	Not calculated	[124]
Norfloxacin	30	10% sodium caprylate, 10% sodium benzoate, and 10% niacinamide	Not calculated	[126]
Diclofenac sodium	1 M	0.6 M urea and 0.4 M sodium acetate	Not calculated	[127]
Indomethacin	30	10% sodium caprylate, 10% sodium benzoate, and 10% niacinamide	Not calculated	[128]
Nifedipine	40	25% phenol and 15% sodium benzoate	Not calculated	[129]

5.7.1 Discussion

Many UV-visible spectroscopy methods have been developed using a mixed solvency approach. For spectroscopic method development generally, organic solvents are preferred for the solubility of the drug. The disadvantages of organic solvents include environmental hazards, disposal after use, cost, and volatility. The mixed solvency blend overcomes these issues, which makes it a more ecofriendly and green approach for analytical method development.

Many researchers have reported blends using a mixed solvency system with the value of the total concentration of solubilisers constant at 30–40% w/v. However, there has been no rational experimentation to decide on the total blend concentration for solubility enhancement. The contributory solubility of the drugs in the blend (% w/v) was not calculated in many publications. A systematic approach to experimentation is therefore lacking. The different blends used in mixed solvency have not undergone systematic development via a rational approach. A proper justification for the use of the components in the blend is missing. There is an opportunity for researchers to systematically utilise the mixed solvency approach for spectrophotometric method development and formulation.

5.8 Conclusion

In conclusion, we can say that the application of green analytical techniques, specifically hydrotropy, mixed hydrotropy and mixed solvency concepts, has emerged as a promising and ecofriendly approach to overcome the challenges posed by conventional analytical methodologies. These progressive methods offer many advantages, including reduced waste generation, minimised hazardous chemical usage and improved analytical performance, making them highly attractive in the field of analytical chemistry.

References

1 Brautbar, N., and Williams, I.I.J. (2002). Industrial solvents and liver toxicity: risk assessment, risk factors and mechanisms. *International Journal of Hygiene and Environmental Health* 205: 479–491.
2 Anastas, P.T., and Warner, J.C. (1998). *Green Chemistry: Theory and Practice*. Oxford: Oxford University Press.
3 Namieśnik, J. (2001). Green analytical chemistry—some remarks. *Journal of Separation Science and Technology* 24: 151–153.
4 Vemula, V., Lagishetty, V., and Lingala, S. (2010). Solubility enhancement techniques. *International Journal of Pharmaceutical Sciences Review and Research* 5: 41–51.
5 Gajjar, K.T., Anuradha, K., and Savjani, J.K. (2012). Drug solubility: importance and enhancement techniques. *ISRN Pharmaceutics* 10: 195727.
6 Neuberg, C. (1916). Hydrotropy. *Biochemische Zeitschrift* 76: 107–176.
7 Saleh, A., and El-Khordagui, L. (1985). Hydrotropic agents: a new definition. *International Journal of Pharmaceutics* 24: 231–238.
8 Bauduin, P., Renoncourt, A., Kopf, A. et al. (2005). Unified concept of solubilization in water by hydrotropes and cosolvents. *Langmuir* 21: 6769–6775.
9 Kalyani, G., Bhuvaneswari, P., Hemalatha, B., and Padmalatha, K. (2022). Hydrotropy: a promising tool for solubility enhancement. *Asian Journal of Pharmacy and Technology* 12 (2): 146–150.
10 Agarwal, M., and Gaikar, V.G. (1992). Extractive separations using hydrotropes. *Journal of Separations Technology* 2 (2): 79–84.
11 Dhinakaran, M., Morais, A.B., and Nagendra, G.N. (2012). Separation of m/p-aminoacetophenone using hydrotropy. *Journal of Chemistry* 9: 504767.
12 Subbarao, C.V., Chakravarthy, I.P.K., Sai Bharadwaj, A.V.S.L., and Prasad, K.M.M. (2012). Functions of hydrotropes in solutions. *Chemical Engineering Technology* 35: 225–237.
13 Tavare, N.S., and Jadhav, V.K. (1999). Separation through crystallization and hydrotropy: the 6-aminopenicillanic acid (6-APA) and phenoxyacetic acid (PAA) system. *Journal of Crystal Growth* 198: 1320–1325.
14 Vinarov, Z., Katev, V., Radeva, D. et al. (2018). Micellar solubilization of poorly water soluble drugs: effect of surfactant and solubilizate molecular structure. *Drug Development and Industrial Pharmacy* 44 (4): 677–686.
15 Sajedi-Amin, S., Barzegar-Jalali, M., Fathi-Azarbayjani, A. et al. (2017). Solubilization of bosentan using ethanol as a pharmaceutical cosolvent. *Journal of Molecular Liquids* 232: 152–158.
16 Vilg, J.V., and Undeland, I. (2017). pH-driven solubilization and isoelectric precipitation of proteins from the brown seaweed Saccharina latissima—effects of osmotic shock, water volume and temperature. *Journal of Applied Phycology* 29 (1): 585–593.
17 Park, K., Acharya, G., Lee, J., and Lee, S., (2003). Pharmaceutical applications of hydrotropic agents, polymers thereof, and hydrogels thereof. US Patent, US 2003/0031715 A1.

18 Choudhary, A.N., and Nayal, S. (2019). A review: hydrotropy a solubility enhancing technique. *Pharmaceutical Innovation Journal* 8 (4): 1149–1153.

19 Lee, J., Lee, S.C., Acharya, G. et al. (2003). Hydrotropic solubilization of paclitaxel: analysis of chemical structures for hydrotropic property. *Pharmaceutical Research* 20: 1022–1030.

20 Patil, M.R., Ganorkar, S.B., Patil, A.S. et al. (2021). Hydrotropic solubilization in pharmaceutical analysis: origin, evolution, cumulative trend and precise applications. *Critical Reviews in Analytical Chemistry* 51 (3): 278–288.

21 Reddy, R.M., Srikanth, P.V.S., Bonthagarala, B., and Desu, P.K. (2013). A review on hydrotropy. *Journal of Pharmaceutical Research* 2: 5–6.

22 Coffman, R.E., and Kildsig, D.O. (1996). Hydrotropic solubilization—mechanistic studies. *Pharmaceutical Research* 13 (10): 1460–1463.

23 Maheshwari, R.K. (2006). Novel application of hydrotropic solubilization in the spectrophotometric analysis of tinidazole in dosage form. *Asian Journal of Chemistry* 18 (1): 640–644.

24 Dhapte, V., and Mehta, P. (2015). Advances in hydrotropic solutions: an updated review. *St. Petersburg Polytechnical University Journal: Physics and Mathematics* 1: 424–435.

25 Maheshwari, R., and Jagwani, Y. (2011). Mixed hydrotropy: novel science of solubility enhancement. *Indian Journal of Pharmaceutical Sciences* 73: 179–183.

26 Maheshwari, R.K., Chaturvedi, S.C., and Jain, N.K. (2005). Novel application of hydrotropic solubilizing additives in the estimation of aspirin in bulk sample and tablets. *International Journal of Pharmaceutical Excipients* 4 (3): 84–88.

27 Maheshwari, R.K., Chaturvedi, S.C., and Jain, N.K. (2006b). Novel spectrophotometric estimation of some poorly water soluble drugs using hydrotropic solubilizing agents. *Indian Journal of Pharmaceutical Sciences* 68 (2): 195–198.

28 Mangal, A., Bhadoriya, S.S., Verma, A., and Mishra, K.K. (2011). Novel application hydrotropic solubilization phenomenon in the thin layer chromatography analysis of omeprazole. *Journal of Current Pharmaceutical Research* 8 (1): 15–16.

29 Jayronia, S.Y.K., Sharma, B., Jain, S., and Maheshwari, R.K. (2013). Hydrotropy: a novel approach in estimation of poorly aqueous soluble drugs by TLC. *International Journal of Pharmacy and Pharmaceutical Science* 5 (2): 175–178.

30 Maheshwari, R., Sharma, S., Rai, N., and Rajput, M. (2010b). Simple titrimetric method to estimate ketoprofen in bulk using mixed hydrotropy. *Journal of Pharmacy Research* 3: 442–443.

31 Maheshwari, R.K. (2005). Analysis of frusemide by application of hydrotropic solubilisation phenomenon. *Indian Pharmacist* 4 (34): 55–58.

32 Maheshwari, R.K. (2006). A novel application of hydrotropic solubilization in the analysis of bulk samples of ketoprofen and salicylic acid. *Asian Journal of Chemistry* 18: 393–396.

33 Maheshwari, R.K. (2006). Application of hydrotropic solubilization in the analysis of aceclofenac. *Asian Journal of Chemistry* 18 (2): 1572–1574.

34 Maheshwari, R.K., Chaturvedi, S.C., and Jain, N.K. (2006). Titrimetric analysis of aceclofenac in tablets using hydrotropic solubilization technique. *Indian Drugs* 43: 516–518.

35 Maheshwari, R.K., Chaturvedi, S.C., and Jain, N.K. (2007). Novel application of hydrotropic solubilization in the analysis of some NSAIDs and their solid dosage forms. *Indian Journal of Pharmaceutical Sciences* 69 (1): 101–105.

36 Maheshwari, R.K., Rajpoot, M.S., Mathur, V. et al. (2009). Quantitative estimation of benzoic acid in bulk sample using sodium benzoate and sodium salicylate as hydrotropic solubilizing agent. *Journal of Pharmaceutical Research* 2: 1–7.

37 Maheshwari, R.K., and Moondra, S. (2010). A novel method for quantitative determination of aceclofenac in bulk drug and tablets using sodium salicylate as a hydrotropic solubilizing agent. *Journal of Advanced Pharmaceutical Technology* 1 (1): 78–82.

38 Maheshwari, R.K., Pandey, S.P., Gupta, H.M. et al. (2008). Analysis of frusemide by application of hydrotropic solubilization phenomenon in solid dosage form. *Asian Journal of Chemistry* 20 (1): 277–281.

39 Maheshwari, R.K., Kumar, S., Bhawsar, N., and Aansari, A. (2013). Tiitrimetric analysis of ketoprofen in the bulk of drug sample using sodium citrate as hydrotropic agent. *International Journal of Pharmaceutical and Biological Sciences* 4 (2): 58–61.

40 Tripathi, D., Chaudhary, N., Sharma, D.K., and Sahoo, J. (2021). An attempt to applying hydrotropy technique for titrimetric estimation of ketoprofen using sodium salicylate as hydrotrope. *Research Journal of Pharmacy and Technology* 14 (4): 2277–2279.

41 Maheshwari, R.K., and Ajmera, A. (2006). A novel application of hydrotropic solubilization in the quantitative analysis of bulk sample of ketoprofen and frusemide. *Asian Journal of Pharmaceutics* 1: 60–62.

42 Maheshwari, R.K., Saxena, M., Gahlot, M. et al. (2010). Novel application of hydrotropic solubilizing additives in the estimation of aspirin in tablets. *Indian Journal of Pharmaceutical Sciences* 72 (5): 649–651.

43 Maheshwari, R.K., Arif, D., Mittal, P. et al. (2008). A novel method for quantitative determination of aceclofenac in bulk drug and tablets using ibuprofen sodium as a hydrotropic solubilizing agent. *Journal of Applied Chemical Research* 5: 63–68.

44 Maheshwari, R.K. (2006). Application of hydrotropic solubilization phenomenon in spectrophotometric estimation of norfloxacin in tablets. *Indian Journal of Pharmaceutical Education and Research* 40 (4): 237–240.

45 Maheshwari, R.K., Chavada, V., Varghese, S., and Shahoo, K. (2008). Analysis of bulk sample of salicylic acid by application of hydrotropic solubilization method. *Indian Journal of Pharmaceutical Sciences* 70 (6): 823–825.

46 Maheshwari, R.K., Rajput, M.S., Sharma, S., and Nair, V. (2010). New spectrophotometric determination of hydrochlorothiazide in tablets using mixed hydrotropic solubilization technique. *Der Pharmacia Lettre* 2: 70–74.

47 Sundari, N., Radhika, T., Saranya, V., and Gandhi, N. (2012). Quantitative analysis of salbutamol bulk sample using nicotinamide hydrotrope. *International Journal of Pharmacy and Pharmaceutical Science Research* 2 (1): 16–19.

48 Maheshwari, R.K., Kumar, S., Ramchandani, U. et al. (2006). Quantitative determination of aspirin using hydrotropic solubilization technique. *Indian Pharmacist* 4: 124–126.

49 Jayakumar, C., Kumar, D., Nesakumar, D., and Gandhi, N. (2010). Quantitative analysis of theophylline bulk sample using sodium salicylate hydrotrope. *International Journal of Pharmacy and Pharmaceutical Science* 2 (3): 124–125.

50 Maheshwari, R.K., Rajpoot, M.S., and Nair, V. (2010). New quantitative estimation of salicylic acid bulk sample using sodium saccharin as hydrotropic solubilizing agent. *Journal of Pharmaceutical Research* 3 (1): 6–8.

51 Jain, R., Jain, N., Jain, D.K., and Jain, S.K. (2013). Eco-friendly quantitative estimation of lercanidipine hydrochloride: a novel approach using hydrotropic solubilization technique. *Bulletin of Pharmaceutical Research* 3 (1): 23–28.

52 Ramakrishna, K., Shiffali, R.D., and Kumar, P.A. (2013). Estimation of pioglitazone hydrochloride in bulk drug and pharmaceutical dosage forms by hydrotropy technique and oxidative-coupling reaction. *Asian Journal of Research in Chemistry* 6: 172–176.

53 Maheshwari, R., Amit, R., and Archana, A. (2010). New spectrophotometric method to determine ketoprofen in tablet dosage form using mixed hydrotropy. *International Journal of Chemical and Analytical Science* 1 (4): 62–63.

54 Jain, P.K., Abhilasha, T., Jain, A. et al. (2010). New spectrophotometric method for the estimation of gatifloxacin in tablets using N,N-di methyl urea as hydrotropic agent. *Journal of Global Pharma Technology* 2: 117–119.

55 Mahajan, R., Maheshwari, R.K., and Mahajan, S.C. (2010). Spectrophotometry estimation of naproxen using N,N dimethyl urea as hydrotropic agent. *Indian Pharmacist* 9 (4): 67–69.

56 Maheshwari, R.K., Gupta, H.M., Singh, M. et al. (2008). A novel application of hydrotropic solubilization in the spectrophotometric analysis of gatifloxacin in solid dosage form. *Asian Journal of Chemistry* 20 (1): 241–244.

57 Maheshwari, R.K., and Shukla, R.S. (2008). Quantitative spectrophotometric estimation of famotidine using hydrotropic solubilization technique. *Asian Journal of Chemistry* 20: 4221–4224.

58 Maheshwari, R.K., Lakkadwala, S., Vyas, R., and Ghode, P. (2010g). Spectrophotometric determination of naproxen tablets using niacinamide as hydrotropic solubilizing additive. *Journal of Current Pharmaceutical Research* 4: 11–14.

59 Maheshwari, R.K., Rathore, A., Agrawal, A., and Gupta, M.A. (2011). New spectrophotometric estimation of indomethacin capsules with niacinamide as hydrotropic solubilizing agent. *Pharmaceutical Methods* 2: 184–188.

60 Patil, D. (2012). Spectroscopic determination of lovastatin by hydrotropic solubilization technique. *International Journal of Pharmaceutical and Chemical Sciences* 1: 1491–1493.

61 Maheshwari, R.K. (2005). Spectrophotometric determination of cefixime in tablets by hydrotropic solubilization phenomenon. *Indian Pharmacist* 4 (36): 63–68.

62 Bernard, S., Mathew, M., and Senthilkumar, K.L. (2011). Spectrophotometric method of estimation of amlodipine besylate using hydrotropic solubilization. *Journal of Applied Pharmaceutical Science* 1 (9): 177–180.

63 Maheshwari, R.K., Wanare, G., Chahar, N. et al. (2009). Spectrophotometric estimation of naproxen tablets employing sodium benzoate as hydrotropic agent. *Indian Pharmacist* 71 (3): 75–77.

64 Maheshwari, R.K., and Tiwari, A. (2005). Spectrophotometric estimation of drugs using hydrotropic solubilization phenomenon. *Indian Pharmacist* 4 (39): 79–84.

65 Maheshwari, R.K. (2006). A novel application of hydrotropic solubilization in the spectrophotometric estimation of frusemide in tablets. *Pharma Review* 4 (24): 148–149.

66 Maheshwari, R.K., Deswal, S., Tiwari, D. et al. (2007). Novel spectrophotometric estimation of frusemide using hydrotropic solubilization phenomenon. *Indian Journal of Pharmaceutical Sciences* 69: 822–824.

67 Maheshwari, R.K. (2006). Novel application of hydrotropic solubilization in the spectrophotometric analysis of piroxicam in solid dosage form. *Indian Drugs* 43 (8): 683–685.

68 Saminathan, J., and Vetrichelvan, T. (2011). Validation of UV spectrophotometric method for determination of riluzole in pharmaceutical dosage form. *International Journal of Chemical Technology and Research* 3: 560–564.

69 Abraham, S., Deveswaran, R., Furtado, S. et al. (2014). Application of hydrotropic solubilization in spectrophotometric estimation of lornoxicam from tablets. *International Scholarly Research Notices* 2014: 810128.

70 Jat, R.K., Chhipa, R.C., and Sharma, S. (2010). Spectrophotometric quantification of etoricoxib in bulk drug and tablets using hydrotropic agent. *Pharmacophore* 1: 96–102.

71 Jhariya, A.N., Joshi, A., Parashar, A., and Nema, R. (2013). Application of sodium citrate as hydrotropic agent in spectrophotometric analysis of salicylic acid. *International Journal of Recent Advances in Pharmaceutical Research* 3: 36–38.

72 Kumar, P., Sunitha, A.D., Venkat Raju, G. et al. (2011). Novel spectrophotometric estimation of naproxen tablet formulations using sodium citrate as hydrotropic solubilizing agent. *Asian Journal of Research in Chemistry* 4: 845–847.

73 Jat, R.K., Chhipa, R.C., Sharma, S., and Ahmed, R. (2010a). Spectrophotometric estimation of fluvoxamine maleate in tablets using hydrotropic agent. *International Journal of Pharmaceutical Quality Assurance* 2 (4): 73–75.

74 Dahiya, J., Singh, A., Gupta, S.K., and Kumar, B. (2013). Spectrophotometric estimation of dextromethorphan in bulk drug using hydrotropic solubilization technique. *Asian Journal of Pharmaceutical Analysis* 3 (3): 90–93.

75 Aher, B.O., Jain, N.P., Jain, U.N. et al. (2015). Novel spectrophotometric estimation of acyclovir using hydrotropic solubilizing agent. *Innovational Journal of Chemistry* 1 (3): 22–32.

76 Shukla, R.S., Patel, A., Soni, M.L. et al. (2014). Quantitative spectrophotometric estimation of cefadroxil using hydrotropic solubilization technique. *Asian Journal of Pharmaceutics* 2: 146–147.

77 Jain, R., Jain, V., Jain, N. et al. (2012). Ecofriendly spectrophotometric method for quantitative estimation of lomefloxacin using hydrotropic approach. *Journal of Applied Pharmaceutical Science* 2 (4): 111–114.

78 Mishra, G.P., and Joshi, H.M. (2013). Quantitative estimation of ciprofloxacin in marketed formulation by hydrotropic techniques. *International Journal of Pharmaceutical and Life Sciences* 4: 3007–3009.

79 Maheshwari, R.K., Pandey, S.P., Apeksha, L. et al. (2006). Novel application of hydrotropic solubilization in the spectrophotometric analysis of cephalexin in solid dosage form. *Asian Journal of Chemistry* 18 (2): 1451–1454.

80 Maheshwari, R.K., Chavda, V., Sahoo, K., and Varghese, S. (2006). Novel application of hydrotropic solubilization in the spectrophotometric analysis of diclofenac sodium in solid dosage form. *Asian Journal of Pharmaceutics* 1: 30–32.

81 Srilakshmi, M., Devi, G.R., Sharmila, S., and Rahaman, S.A. (2013). Spectrophotometric determination of poorly water-soluble drug terconazole using hydrotropic solubilization technique. *Indo-American Journal of Pharmaceutical Research* 3: 3527–3534.

82 Maheshwari, R.K., Chaturvedi, S.C., and Jain, N.K. (2005). Application of hydrotropic solubilization phenomenon in spectrophotometric analysis of hydrochlorothiazide tablets. *Indian Drugs* 42 (8): 541–544.

83 Maheshwari, R.K. (2006). Spectrophotometric analysis of amoxycillin in tablets using hydrotropic solubilization technique. *Asian Journal of Chemistry* 18 (4): 3194–3196.

84 Maheshwari, R.K., Dewangan, A., Soni, P.K. et al. (2006). Novel application of hydrotropic solubilization in the spectrophotometric analysis of paracetamol tablet dosage form. *Asian Journal of Chemistry* 18 (4): 2879–2882.

85 Maheshwari, R., Rajput, M., and Sinha, S. (2010). New quantitative estimation of benzoic acid bulk sample using calcium disodium edetate as hydrotropic solubilizing agent. *Asian Journal of Pharmaceutical and Clinical Research* 3 (1): 43–45.

86 Maheshwari, R.K., Prasad, S., Pandey, P., and Wanare, G. (2010). Novel spectrophotometric analysis of piroxicam tablets using ibuprofen sodium as hydrotropic solubilizing agents. *International Journal of Pharmaceutical Sciences and Drug Research* 2 (3): 210–212.

87 Maheshwari, R.K., Rajput, M.S., and Sinha, S. (2009). Ecofriendly spectrophotometric estimation of tinidazole in tablets using lignocaine hydrochloride as a hydrotropic solubilizing agent. *Asian Journal of Pharmaceutics* 3: 319–321.

88 Pandey, S., and Maheshwari, R.K. (2010). A novel spectroscopic method for the estimation of ketoprofen in tablet dosage form using hydrotropic solubilization phenomenon. *Eastern Journal of Scientific Research* 6: 209–212.

89 Maheshwari, R.K., Deswal, S., Tiwari, D. et al. (2008). Analysis of amoxicillin by application of hydrotropic solubilization phenomenon in solid dosage form. *Asian Journal of Chemistry* 20 (1): 805–807.

90 Revathi, R., Ethiraj, T., Saravanan, V.S. et al. (2010). New spectrophotometric determination of nifedipine using hydrotropic solubilization. *International Journal of Pharmacy and Pharmaceutical Sciences* 2: 74–76.

91 Maheshwari, R.K., Maheshwari, R.B., and Bhatt, P. (2006). Simultaneous spectrophotometric estimation of norfloxacin and tinidazole in two component tablet formulations. *Asian Journal of Chemistry* 18 (2): 1481–1486.

92 Gurumurthy, V., Deveswaran, R., Bharath, S. et al. (2012). Application of hydrotropic solubilisation in simultaneous estimation of atenolol and amlodipine besylate. *Asian Journal of Research in Chemistry* 5 (1): 57–60.

93 Sharma, R., Pathodiya, G., Mishra, G.P., and Sharma, M. (2010). Simultaneous estimation and validation of cefixime trihydrate and ornidazole in bulk and tablets using hydrotropic solubilizing agents. *Journal of Pharmaceutical Research* 3: 2953–2955.

94 Sharma, R., Pathodiya, G., Mishra, G.P., and Sainy, J. (2011). A novel spectrophotometric method for quantitative determination of ciprofloxacin hydrochloride and tinidazole in tablets using hydrotropic solubilizing agent. *Journal of Pharmaceutical Research* 4: 859–861.

95 Mathew, C., Suman, B., Ajitha, M., and Babu, P.S. (2014). A green analytical method for the simultaneous estimation of levofloxacin hemihydrate and ambroxol hydrochloride using hydrotropy and first derivative UV spectroscopy. *Oriental Journal of Chemistry* 30: 1385–1389.

96 Sharma, M.C., and Sharma, S. (2011). Determination and validation of UV spectrophotometric method for estimation of paracetamol and diclofenac sodium in tablet dosage forms using hydrotropic solubilizing agents. *International Journal of Chemical Technology and Research* 3: 244–247.

97 Maliwal, D., Jain, A., Maheshwari, R.K., and Patidar, V. (2008). Simultaneous spectrophotometric estimation of metronidazole and norfloxacin in combined tablet formulations using hydrotropy. *Research Journal of Pharmacy and Technology* 1 (4): 357–361.

98 Gunji, R., Nadendla, R.R., and Ponnuru, V.S. (2012). Simultaneous UV spectrophotometric determination and validation of diclofenac sodium and rabeprazole sodium using hydrotropic agents in its tablet dosage form. *International Journal of Drug Development and Research* 4 (1): 316–324.

99 Maheshwari, R.K., Chaturvedi, S.C., and Jain, N.K. (2007). Novel application of hydrotropic solubilization in the analysis of some NSAIDs and their solid dosage forms. *Indian Journal of Pharmaceutical Sciences* 69: 101–106.

100 Sharma, M.C., Sharma, S., and Sharma, A.D. (2011). Simultaneous estimation and validation of gabapentin and methylcobalamin in tablet dosage form: hydrotropic approach. *Drug Invention Today* 3: 95.

101 Sharma, M.C., and Sharma, S. (2011a). Application of hydrotropic solubilization in spectrophotometric analysis of esomeprazole and itopride pharmaceutical combined tablet dosage forms. *Journal of Iranian Chemical Research* 4: 25–31.

102 Parihar, A. and Maheshwari, R.K. (2022). A review: green analytical application of hydrotropy and mixed hydrotropy in the field of TLC and HPLC. *International Journal of Research Publication and Reviews* 3: 1170–1178.

103 Maheshwari, R. (2007). Mixed hydrotropy in spectrophotometric analysis of poorly water-soluble drug. *Indian Pharmacist* 6: 66–67.

104 Maheshwari, R.K., and Indurkhya, A. (2010). Formulation and evaluation of aceclofenac injection made by mixed hydrotropic solubilization technique. *Iranian Journal of Pharmaceutical Research* 9: 233.

105 Vinnakota, S.A., Deveswaran, R., Bharath, S. et al. (2011). Application of mixed hydrotropic solubilization in spectrophotometric estimation of aceclofenac in tablets. *Journal of Current Pharma Research* 1: 223.

106 Shrivastav, R., Khare, A., Agrawal, S., and Patel, S. (2011). New titrimetric estimation of aceclofenac tablets using mixed hydrotropy. *International Journal of Pharmaceutical Sciences Review and Research* 11: 140–141.

107 Maheshwari, R., Rai, N., Sharma, S. et al. (2010). New titrimetric analysis of frusemide in bulk and tablets using mixed hydrotropy concept. *Drug Invention Today* 2: 223–225.

108 Sherje, A., Rahigude, A., Warma, S., and Vanshiv, S. (2010). Mixed hydrotropy in spectrophotometric analysis of nitazoxanide. *International Journal of ChemTech Research* 2: 1965–1969.

109 Kadam, S., Janjale, M.V., Akole, S., and Bhosale, S. (2012). Application of mixed hydrotropic solubilization technique for simultaneous spectrophotometric estimation of metronidazole and miconazole nitrate from different pharmaceutical dosage forms. *International Journal of Pharmaceutical and Biological Science Archive* 3: 93829160.

110 Jain, R., Jain, N., Maheswari, R.K., and Jain, S.K. (2013). Quantitative estimation of levofloxacin and ornidazole by UV spectrophotometer: a mixed hydrotropy solubilization approach. *International Journal of Pharmaceutical Sciences and Research* 4: 3073.

111 Mishra, G.P., Panigrahi, D., Joshi, H., and Meena, R. (2014). Simultaneous estimation and validation of acelofenac and paracetamol in bulk and tablets using mixed hydrotropic agents. *Chemical Science* 3: 664–669.

112 Remi, S., and Varkey, J. (2018). An eco-friendly novel spectrophotometric estimation and validation of paliperidone in bulk drug and their dosage forms by mixed hydrotropic solubilisation method. *Asian Journal of Pharmaceutical and Health Sciences* 8: 1996–2001.

113 Soni, M.K., and Sharma, K. (2019). An eco-friendly spectrophotometric analysis of poorly water-soluble drug (nimesulide) using the mixed hydrotropic concept. *Asian Journal of Pharmaceutical and Health Sciences* 9: 1281–2184.

114 Rathod, S.B., Salunke, P.A., Kulkarni, V.C. et al. (2018). Method development and validation of indomethacin in bulk drug and capsule formulation by using mix hydrotrophy. *Research Journal of Pharmaceutical Dosage Forms and Technology* 10: 175–178.

115 Patil, S., Barhate, S., Patil, A. et al. (2019). Novel mixed hydrotropic solubalisation technique for analytical method development and validation of acyclovir in bulk and tablet formulation by Spectrophotometry. *Asian Journal of Pharmaceutical Analysis* 9: 25–29.

116 Soni, K., and Sharma, K. (2022). Eco-friendly and economical spectrophotometric estimation of the low water-soluble drug (norfloxacin) applying the concept of mixed hydrotropy. *Journal of Health and Allied Sciences NU* 12: 263–266.

117 Maheshwari, R.K., and Indurkhya, A. (2010). Novel application of mixed hydrotropic solubilization technique in the formulation and evaluation of hydrotropic solid dispersion of aceclofenac. *Asian Journal of Pharmaceutics* 4: 235–238.

118 Madan, J.R., Kamate, V.J., Dua, K., and Awasthi, R. (2017). Improving the solubility of nevirapine using a hydrotropy and mixed hydrotropy based solid dispersion approach. *Polymers in Medicine* 47: 83–90.

119 Yadav, N.K., Shukla, T., Upmanyu, N. et al. (2018). Novel application of mixed hydrotropic solubilization technique in the formulation and evaluation of solid dispersion of flupirtine maleate. *Journal of Drug Delivery and Therapeutics* 8: 481–488.

120 El Hamd, M.A., El-Maghrabey, M.H., Almawash, S., and El-Shaheny, R.N. (2022). Green hydrotropic technology as a convenient tool for the handling of poor water-soluble candidates proceeding their economic analytical measurements. In: *Green Chemical Analysis and Sample Preparations: Procedures, Instrumentation, Data Metrics, and Sustainability*, ch. 6. (ed. M.H. El-Maghrabey, V. Sivasankar, and R.N. El-Shaheny), Cham: Springer International.

121 Maheshwari, R. (2009). Mixed-solvency. A novel concept for solubilization of poorly water-soluble drugs. *Journal of Technology and Engineering Science* 1: 39–43.

122 Maheshwari, R. (2010). Mixed-solvency approach—boon for solubilization of poorly water-soluble drugs. *Asian Journal of Pharmaceutics* 4 (1): 60–63.

123 Vittal, G.V., Deveswaran, R., Bharath, S. et al. (2012). Development of an analytical method for spectrophotometric estimation of ketoprofen using mixed co-solvency approach. *International Journal of Pharmaceutical Sciences* 3: 1053–1056.

124 Jain, D.K., Patel, V.K., Bajaj, S. et al. (2015). Novel approach for spectrophotometric estimation of solid dosage forms of tinidazole using solids (eutectic liquid of phenol and niacinamide) as solubilizing agent (mixed solvency concept). *World Journal of Pharmacy and Pharmaceutical Sciences* 4: 763–769.

125 Jain, S., Maheshwari, R., Nema, R.K., and Singhvi, I. (2017). Simultaneous estimation of ofloxacin and ornidazole in solid dosage form by uv-spectrophotometry using mixed solvency concept. *European Journal of Pharmaceutical and Medical Research* 4: 413–418.

126 Jain, S., Maheshwari, R., Nema, R.K., and Singhvi, I. (2018). New spectrophotometric estimation of norfloxacin in the tablets using mixed solvency approach. *World Journal of Pharmaceutical Research* 7: 1805–1813.

127 Suryawanshi, C., Dwivedi, S., Vaida, L., and Joshi, H.M. (2013). Quantitative estimation of diclofenac sodium in marketed formulation by using mixed solvency approach. *International Journal of Pharmacy and Life Sciences* 4: 3054–3056.

128 Jain, S., Maheshwari, R., Nema, R.K., and Singhvi, I. (2017). Development and validation of simple uv-spectrophotometric method of quantitation of indomethacin in solid dosage formulation using mixed solvency concept. *Pharma Innovation Journal* 6: 453–456.

129 Jain, S., Maheshwari, R., Nema, R.K., and Singhvi, I. (2017). Development and validation of simple uv-spectrophotometric method of quantitation of nifedipine in solid dosage formulations using mixed solvency concept. *World Journal of Pharmaceutical Research* 6: 2014–2021.

130 Thakur, A., Tripathi, D., Badwaik, H., and Nakhate, K. (2022). Ibuprofen syrup made by mixed solubilization technique: formulation and evaluation. *International Journal of Health Sciences* 6: 13015–13020.

131 Nagwanshi, K., Maheshwari, R., and Padiyar, A. (2022). Formulation and development of topical dosage form of ibuprofen using mixed solvency concept and its evaluations. *Annals of Pharma Research* 10: 610–624.

132 Padiyar, A., and Maheshwari, R.K. (2022). Formulation development of diclofenac sodium lotion using mixed solvency concept and in vitro evaluation. *Indian Drugs* 59: 24–30.

6

Application of Artificial Intelligence in Drug Design and Development

Somdutt Mujwar[1] *and Kamal Shah*[2]

[1] *Chitkara College of Pharmacy, Chitkara University, Rajpura, Punjab, India*
[2] *Institute of Pharmaceutical Research, GLA University, Mathura, UP, India*

CONTENTS

6.1 Introduction

Artificial intelligence (AI) is the process of developing cognitive properties in a non-living machine or device. Devices such as computers are trained on existing data in order to develop intelligent devices capable of decision-making based on their artificially developed cognition. AI is commonly used for devices or machines that have learning and problem-solving capabilities similar to those of the human brain [1]. Computers or computer-operated devices are trained to develop AI to execute human tasks of decision-making for resolving a specific issue. Problem-solving capabilities in humans are acquired through memory and learning experience, while AI is developed in a machine by training it on existing data to attain the desired skills to handle updated doubts and challenges [2, 3].

6.2 History of Artificial Intelligence

The history of AI goes back to 1963, when the Turing machine was developed by Alan Turing. From the mid-twentieth century to the 1980s the applicability of AI was symbolic in nature, limited to resolving issues of logic like robotics and playing chess. After that more sophisticated applications of AI came into existence, in which complex algorithms

Sustainable Approaches in Pharmaceutical Sciences, First Edition. Edited by Kamal Shah, Durgesh Nandini Chauhan, and Nagendra Singh Chauhan.

are developed to analyse existing data to develop correlations, which in turn are used to learn patterns required for decision-making and prediction of new properties [2].

6.3 Artificial Intelligence in the Field of Pharmaceuticals

Pharmaceutical scientists are facing challenges related to the development of potent therapeutic agents with optimised pharmacokinetics but minimal chance of the presence of toxic effects. Also, there is a high risk of a newly developed drug failing during the later stages of clinical trials, leading to a great loss of the valuable time of highly efficient scientific staff, the money of private firms or government agencies, as well as the never-ending efforts of the people involved [4–6].

The cost and time required in the development of novel therapeutic agents are major setbacks associated with the drug development process, as delay in the development of a specific medicine for the treatment of a specific disease will result in loss of life among patients suffering from that disease because of a lack of therapy or availability of subpotent therapeutic options. Consistent failure in the various steps of the drug development process results in a substantial increase of experimental cost because of repetition, as well as an increase in day-to-day expenditure of time [7–9].

Nowadays, success in the intense and complicated process of drug design and discovery largely depends on predictive analysis prior to the experimental research by applying AI-based analysis of existing data. In silico approaches like molecular docking, dynamic simulation, virtual screening, quantitative structure activity relationships, pharmacophore modelling, and pharmacokinetic profiling for drug design are largely based on the application of data analysis to predict the nature of the small chemical molecule by analysing its binding interaction with the macromolecular target as well as its stability over time [10–14].

The reliability of these approaches is mainly dependent on the availability as well as accuracy of the existing data. Thus, in the early days after the introduction of AI-based techniques for drug design and discovery, these techniques were not very fruitful because the data available were inaccurate as well as limited, leading to false-positive as well as true-negative predictions and the failure of the experimental procedure. However, today there is available a sufficient quantity of highly accurate data, because more prevalent and precise experimental techniques lead to more accurate predictive algorithms modelled by using highly efficient AI techniques based on deep learning and machine learning [1, 15, 16].

Drug design and development is a very long and complex process, which involves scientists belonging to diverse domains handling different types of experimental processes like pathophysiological analysis of the disease, selection of drug targets and validation of their involvement in the disease condition, screening of compounds, lead identification, optimisation of leads with intent to improve their affinity as well as reduce any associated toxic effects, dosage form design, preclinical and clinical trials, and the manufacturing process. All of these processes are interdependent and the accuracy of the resulting outcome for each step will severely affect the overall success of the ultimate molecule. Thus, each process should be handled with extreme care to avoid any type of inaccuracy in the final outcome. For these reasons, it is essential to use AI-based techniques to predict the success rate of the planned process [17–21].

6.4 Applications of Artificial Intelligence

Nowadays AI is widely applied in almost every domain of biological sciences related to therapeutics. It is based on training the computer program on existing experimental data, briefly described as the training set, to understand the existing patterns and their applicability in predicting the behaviour of new unknown data sets. Some of the general applications of AI in the field of pharmaceuticals and therapeutics are described next.

6.4.1 Drug Target Identification

It has always been a Herculean task to handle, store, analyse, and share big biological data. Biological data are highly complex and encode interesting information that needs to be decoded to be used for the development of novel therapeutics. But since they are vast in nature it was not possible to handle or analyse such biological data until the mid-twentieth century because of the lack of fast computing technologies.

By the early days of the twenty-first century the Human Genome Project was completed with the help of bioinformatics. This successfully revealed the whole human genome and opened the doors for utilisation of the related biological information for predicting the causes and associated macromolecular targets of various existing as well as upcoming human diseases. The genome data can be correlated with the occurrence and progression of certain diseases and can then be used to identify possible drug targets to develop novel therapeutics for their treatment. The biological data include the sequencing information of nucleic acids like DNA and RNA as well as various structural and functional proteins. The sequencing information on the macromolecules can be used to develop three-dimensional structure models of them to predict their functional role and involvement in the disease condition [17, 22–25]. In this way, important macromolecular targets with active involvement in a disease can be predicted by using systems biology to identify the protein network of the patient and compare it with those of normal healthy individuals to pinpoint overexpressed as well as underexpressed macromolecules in the diseased state.

6.4.2 Molecular Modelling

Molecular modelling is a technique in which biomolecular systems are modelled by mimicking the conditions present within the human body, like a similar temperature, pressure, pH, solvent system. Molecular modelling is performed with the intent of better understanding complex biological systems. Biological models are generally prepared by using AI-based computer programs. These computer programs are prepared by using certain mathematical algorithms that are based on existing experimental data and applying classical chemical and physical laws [22–24, 26]. Drug–receptor docking software is an excellent example of such a computer program that is trained on known experimental data of approved drugs against their macromolecular drug targets, and is further used to predict the behaviour of unknown new chemical compounds against their respective drug targets.

6.4.3 Pharmacokinetic Optimisation

Pharmacokinetics is defined as what the body does with an exogenously administered drug molecule, regulating critical processes related to its absorption, distribution, and metabolism, followed by its excretion. Pharmacodynamic interaction with the drug molecule is responsible for the generation of therapeutic effects in the human body, but the kinetics of the drug molecule is also equally important for execution of the therapeutic effect by maintaining the desired concentration of drug in the site of action. To do this it is necessary for the drug molecule to possess an optimum rate of absorption, distribution, metabolism, and excretion, as an increased rate may result in its quick elimination from the body without executing the intended therapeutic effect or only doing so for a very short span of time. Similarly, a slow rate of absorption and distribution may lead to an insufficient quantity of drug at the site of action to initiate the therapeutic effect. Also, a slow rate of metabolism and excretion may result in sustaining an active drug for a very long time in the human body, leading to the occurrence of certain undesirable and toxic effects [26–30].

The pharmacokinetic profile of a drug molecule is markedly regulated by its physicochemical properties. Lipinski et al. have correlated the pharmacokinetic profile of approved drugs with their physicochemical properties and concluded that the adsorption distribution, metabolism, as well as excretion of a drug molecule are greatly influenced by certain physicochemical properties like molecular weight, partition coefficient, topological polar surface area, hydrogen bond donor, and acceptor sites [31]. These properties are found to be directly linked with their permeability across the plasma membrane and this should be a rate-limiting step in most steps associated with their pharmacokinetic profile. Lipinski has also defined a specific range of physicochemical properties of a drug molecule, commonly termed Lipinski's rule of five, which states that a new drug should follow this filter to have drug-like behaviour with respect to its pharmacokinetics [31]. According to Lipinski's rule, a small chemical molecule should have a molecular weight less than or equal to 500 Dalton to behave like a drug molecule, as the molecular weight directly controls its size and the molecule should have a fixed bulk for easy movement across the plasma membrane. The partition coefficient should be in the range of −5 to +5 for optimum movement across the plasma membrane as well as sufficient distribution across the various compartments of the human body. The cellular membrane has both a lipophilic end as well as a hydrophilic tail embedded in the same structure, so a drug molecule should have a sufficient number of both hydrophilic as well as lipophilic functionalities for the smooth interaction required for permeability. The topological polar surface area is defined as the surface area covered by the polar functions present on the surface of the ligand molecule, as these polar functionalities directly contribute to the hydrophilicity of the compound. The ligand should have the presence of a defined quantity of hydrophilic polar functional groups required for its solubility as well as interactions with the polar layer of the plasma membrane [23, 27, 32–34]. Thus, according to Lipinski's rule, the topological surface area of a ligand should be within the range of 40–140 $Å^2$. Lipinski's rule also defines the number of hydrogen bond donor and acceptor sites required for the formation of hydrogen bonds. There should be up to 5 hydrogen bond donor sites and up to 10 hydrogen bond acceptor sites for optimum drug likeness.

6.4.4 Dosage Form Design

The type of ingredients and the quantity of those ingredients used while developing a dosage form play an important role in the rate of release of the active pharmaceutical ingredient present in that dosage form. Pharmaceutical dosage form design based on AI is a trending tactic that has been used by pharmaceutical scientists around the globe. Ingredient selection for dosage form design is a difficult task because of the availability of diverse types of ingredients with specific physical and chemical properties required for the preparation of a dosage form. While developing a dosage form the type of therapeutic response expected from that dosage – sustained release, delayed release, immediate release – should be clear. The nature of drug release from a dosage form largely depends on the nature and quantity of the excipients used [27]. Therefore, AI programs based on existing data are highly beneficial to predict the specific quantity of a specific excipient to be used in development of a dosage form intended for a specific type of drug release.

6.4.5 Drug–Receptor Interaction

The pharmacodynamic effect of a drug molecule is largely dependent on its interaction with the macromolecular target receptor, commonly known as drug–receptor interaction. Drug–receptor interaction is highly specific in nature and can play a crucial role in the development of new drug molecules. There are specific computational tools known as protein visualising tools that are primarily used for the visualisation as well as structural analysis of large macromolecular structures. This kind of computational software is primarily employed for structural analysis of large biomolecular structures, including the drug–receptor complex. The analysis of drug–receptor interaction at a molecular level discloses the number and types of chemical bonds present in the macromolecular complex [27]. The revealed drug–receptor interaction of an experimentally obtained macromolecular complex, either by X-ray crystallography or by nuclear magnetic resonance (NMR) techniques, can be highly valuable to develop a dataset based on the type of chemical interactions commonly observed within a drug–receptor complex, which can be further utilised to develop a drug–receptor docking simulation program, predict the binding conformation as well as preferred binding interactions of a newer ligand against a specific target macromolecule.

6.4.6 Establishing the Probable Mechanism of Action

AI-based computational programs for performing molecular docking and molecular dynamic simulation have been found to be extremely fruitful for identification of an unknown compound having affinity for the macromolecular target receptor. Also, these computational programs are broadly used for the prediction of the most potent compound with the highest affinity for a specific target receptor out of a series of structurally similar compounds. Furthermore, these computational techniques are used for establishing the most probable mechanism of action for a pharmacologically active compound with an unknown mechanism of action. Such compounds are screened against a series of macromolecular targets with established involvement in the specific disease conditions and, based on the predicted affinity of the compound against the specific macromolecular target, its mechanism can be established [3, 6, 35].

6.5 Conclusion

AI helps in speeding up the drug discovery process, as it assists in collecting, handling, analysing, integrating, and sharing the big biological data involved in the process with a high level of precision. AI also helps in predicting the biological behaviour of a new molecule to know whether it is going to possess therapeutic potency or not, and also to identify the associated problem that is supposed to be obstructing its pharmaceutical impact. There are numerous advantages of using AI in drug discovery and development, like reduction of process time, cost-cutting, reduction of number of staff involved, and most importantly increase in the success rate to get potent therapeutics to the market within the expected timeframe. Because of the benefits of the AI-based drug discovery process over the traditional wet lab-based hit-and-miss methods, it is essential to use AI in the drug discovery regime prior to moving to experimental procedures.

References

1 Gupta, R., Srivastava, D., Sahu, M. et al. (2021). Artificial intelligence to deep learning: machine intelligence approach for drug discovery. *Molecular Diversity* 25 (3): 1315–1360. https://doi.org/10.1007/s11030-021-10217-3.
2 Arabi, A.A. (2021). Artificial intelligence in drug design: algorithms, applications, challenges and ethics. *Future Drug Discovery* 3 (2): FDD59.
3 Agrawal, N., Mujwar, S., Goyal, A., and Gupta, J.K. (2022). Phytoestrogens as potential antiandrogenic agents against prostate cancer: an *in silico* analysis. *Letters in Drug Design & Discovery* 19 (1): 69–78.
4 Wen, H., Jung, H., and Li, X. (2015). Drug delivery approaches in addressing clinical pharmacology-related issues: opportunities and challenges. *AAPS Journal* 17 (6): 1327–1340. https://doi.org/10.1208/s12248-015-9814-9.
5 Jain, R., and Mujwar, S. (2020). Repurposing metocurine as main protease inhibitor to develop novel antiviral therapy for COVID-19. *Journal of Structural Chemistry* 31 (6): 2487–2499.
6 Kaur, A., Mujwar, S., and Adlakha, N. (2016). In-silico analysis of riboswitch of Nocardia farcinica for design of its inhibitors and pharmacophores. *International Journal of Computational Biology Drug Design* 9 (3): 261–276.
7 Lu, R.-M., Hwang, Y.-C., Liu, I.-J. et al. (2020). Development of therapeutic antibodies for the treatment of diseases. *Journal of Biomedical Science* 27 (1): 1–30.
8 Minaz, N., Razdan, R., Hammock, B.D. et al. (2019). Impact of diabetes on male sexual function in streptozotocin-induced diabetic rats: protective role of soluble epoxide hydrolase inhibitor. *Biomédecine & pharmacothérapie* 115: 108897. https://doi.org/10.1016/j.biopha.2019.108897.
9 Mujwar, S. (2021). Computational bioprospecting of andrographolide derivatives as potent cyclooxygenase-2 inhibitors. *Biomedical Biotechnology Research Journal* 5 (4): 446.
10 Fidan, O., Mujwar, S., and Kciuk, M. (2022). Discovery of adapalene and dihydrotachysterol as antiviral agents for the Omicron variant of SARS-CoV-2 through computational drug repurposing. *Molecular Diversity* 27: 463–475. https://doi.org/10.1007/s11030-022-10440-6.

11 Mujwar, S. (2021). Computational repurposing of tamibarotene against triple mutant variant of SARS-CoV-2. *Computers in Biology and Medicine* 136: 104748. https://doi.org/10.1016/j.compbiomed.2021.104748.
12 Mujwar, S., and Harwansh, R.K. (2022). In-silico bioprospecting of taraxerol as a main protease inhibitor of SARS-CoV-2 to develop therapy against COVID-19. *Structural Chemistry* 33 (5): 1517–1528. https://doi.org/10.21203/rs.3.rs-1308726/v1.
13 Mujwar, S., and Kumar, V. (2020). Computational drug repurposing approach to identify potential fatty acid-binding protein-4 inhibitors to develop novel antiobesity therapy. *Assay Drug Development Technologies* 18 (7): 318–327.
14 Mujwar, S., Sun, L., and Fidan, O. (2022). In silico evaluation of food-derived carotenoids against SARS-CoV-2 drug targets: crocin is a promising dietary supplement candidate for COVID-19. *Journal of Food Biochemistry* 46 (9): e14219. https://doi.org/10.1111/jfbc.14219.
15 Mujwar, S., Deshmukh, R., Harwansh, R.K. et al. (2019). Drug repurposing approach for developing novel therapy against mupirocin-resistant Staphylococcus aureus. *Assay Drug Development Technologies* 17 (7): 298–309. https://doi.org/10.1089/adt.2019.944.
16 Mujwar, S., Shah, K., Gupta, J.K., and Gour, A. (2021). Docking based screening of curcumin derivatives: a novel approach in the inhibition of tubercular DHFR. *International Journal of Computational Biology and Drug Design* 14 (4): 297–314.
17 Álvarez-Machancoses, Ó., and Fernández-Martínez, J.L. (2019). Using artificial intelligence methods to speed up drug discovery. *Expert Opinion on Drug Discovery* 14 (8): 769–777.
18 Mujwar, S., and Tripathi, A. (2022). Repurposing benzbromarone as antifolate to develop novel antifungal therapy for Candida albicans. *Journal of Molecular Modeling* 28 (7): 193.
19 Mujwar, S., and Pardasani, K.R. (2015). Prediction of riboswitch as a potential drug target and design of its optimal inhibitors for Mycobacterium tuberculosis. *International Journal of Computational Biology and Drug Design* 8 (4): 326–347.
20 Mujwar, S., and Pardasani, K.R. (2015). Prediction of riboswitch as a potential drug target for infectious diseases: an in silico case study of anthrax. *Journal of Medical Imaging and Health Informatics* 5 (1): 7–16.
21 Pradhan, P., Soni, N.K., Chaudhary, L. et al. (2015). In-silico prediction of riboswitches and design of their potent inhibitors for H1N1, H2N2 and H3N2 strains of influenza virus. *Biosciences Biotechnology Research Asia* 12 (3): 2173–2186.
22 Koromina, M., Pandi, M.-T., and Patrinos, G.P. (2019). Rethinking drug repositioning and development with artificial intelligence, machine learning, and omics. *Omics* 23 (11): 539–548.
23 Shah, K., Mujwar, S., Gupta, J.K. et al. (2019). Molecular docking and in silico cogitation validate mefenamic acid prodrugs as human cyclooxygenase-2 inhibitor. *Assay Drug Development Technologies* 17 (6): 285–291. https://doi.org/10.1089/adt.2019.943.
24 Shah, K., Mujwar, S., Krishna, G., and Gupta, J.K. (2020). Computational design and biological depiction of novel naproxen derivative. *ASSAY Drug Development Technologies* 18 (7): 308–317.
25 Kciuk, M., Gielecińska, A., Mujwar, S. et al. (2022). Targeting carbonic anhydrase IX and XII isoforms with small molecule inhibitors and monoclonal antibodies. *Journal of Enzyme Inhibition and Medicinal Chemistry* 37 (1): 1278–1298.
26 Fleming, N. (2018). Computer-calculated compounds. *Nature* 557 (7707): S55–57.

27 Yang, X., Wang, Y., Byrne, R. et al. (2019). Concepts of artificial intelligence for computer-assisted drug discovery. *Chemical Reviews* 119 (18): 10520–10594.

28 Soni, N., Pardasani, K.R., and Mujwar, S. (2015). Insilico analysis of dietary agents as anticancer inhibitors of insulin like growth factor 1 receptor (IGF1R). *Journal of Pharmaceutical Sciences* 7 (9): 191–196.

29 Sharma, K.K., Singh, B., Mujwar, S., and Bisen, P.S. (2020). Molecular docking based analysis to elucidate the DNA Topoisomerase IIβ as the potential target for the ganoderic acid: a natural therapeutic agent in cancer therapy. *Current Computer Aided Drug Design* 16 (2): 176–189. https://doi.org/10.2174/1573409915666190820144759.

30 Kciuk, M., Gielecińska, A., Mujwar, S. et al. (2022). Cyclin-dependent kinases in DNA damage response. *Biochimica et Biophysica Acta. Reviews on Cancer* 1877 (3): 188716.

31 Lipinski, C.A. (2004). Lead-and drug-like compounds: the rule-of-five revolution. *Drug Discovery Today: Technologies* 1 (4): 337–341.

32 Kciuk, M., Mujwar, S., Szymanowska, A. et al. (2022). Preparation of novel pyrazolo[4, 3-e]tetrazolo[1, 5-b][1, 2, 4]triazine sulfonamides and their experimental and computational biological studies. *International Journal of Molecular Sciences* 23 (11): 5892.

33 Kciuk, M., Gielecińska, A., Mujwar, S. et al. (2022). Cyclin-dependent kinase synthetic lethality partners in DNA damage response. *International Journal of Molecular Sciences* 23 (7): 3555.

34 Benet, L.Z., Hosey, C.M., Ursu, O., and Oprea, T.I. (2016). BDDCS, the rule of 5 and drugability. *Advanced Drug Delivery Reviews* 101: 89–98. https://doi.org/10.1016/j.addr.2016.05.007.

35 Mishra, I., Mishra, R., Mujwar, S., Chandra, P., and Sachan, N. (2020). A retrospect on antimicrobial potential of thiazole scaffold. *Journal of Heterocyclic Chemistry* 57 (6): 2304–2329.

7

Green Chemistry in the Development of Functionalised Hydrogels as Topical Drug-Delivery Systems

Maha Mohammad AL-Rajabi[1,2] and Teow Yeit Haan[3,4]

[1] *Faculty of Chemical Engineering & Technology, Universiti Malaysia Perlis (UniMAP), Arau, Perlis, Malaysia*
[2] *Centre of Excellence for Biomass Utilization (CoEBU), Universiti Malaysia Perlis (UniMAP), Arau, Perlis, Malaysia*
[3] *Department of Chemical and Process Engineering, Faculty of Engineering and Built Environment, Universiti Kebangsaan Malaysia, Bangi, Selangor Darul Ehsan, Malaysia*
[4] *Research Centre for Sustainable Process Technology (CESPRO), Faculty of Engineering and Built Environment, Universiti Kebangsaan Malaysia, Bangi, Selangor Darul Ehsan, Malaysia*

CONTENTS

7.1 Introduction

A drug-delivery system (also known as a drug-delivery medium, device, or vehicle) is defined as a formulation that introduces a therapeutic agent, active ingredient, or drug into the body and enhances its safety and efficaciousness by regulating its release profile [1]. Such a system acts as an interface between the drug and the patient, and may assume the form of either a formulation of the drug or a device used to deliver the drug. It is crucial to recognise this differentiation between the drug and the device, as it forms the basis for regulatory control of drug-delivery systems by supervisory agencies [1]. The process of drug delivery comprises the encapsulation of a drug for administration, from which its active ingredients are released, followed by their distribution across cellular membranes to the intended anatomical sites [1].

Drug-delivery systems may be categorised according to their routes of administration: systemic or topical. Systemic drug delivery introduces active ingredients into the systemic circulation of the human body in order to reach the diseased organs. This includes the oral, parenteral, or pulmonary (inhalation) routes [1]. Conversely, topical drug delivery introduces a

Sustainable Approaches in Pharmaceutical Sciences, First Edition. Edited by Kamal Shah, Durgesh Nandini Chauhan, and Nagendra Singh Chauhan.

drug-delivery system to the human body through direct administration to the diseased organs. Under this mode of localised treatment, the drug is not targeted for systemic delivery; instead, topical drug delivery involves the ophthalmic, rectal, vaginal, or dermatological routes [2].

The human skin represents a crucial route of drug delivery, given that it is one of the most accessible anatomical parts [3]. As the body's largest organ, it measures about 1.7 m^2 and accounts for about 10% of the total body mass. The skin primarily functions as a barrier between the body and the environment, offering protection against chemicals, ultraviolet radiation, microbes, and allergens, and retaining moisture. Additionally, it is involved in homeostasis, controlling both blood pressure and body temperature. The skin further aids in sensing and detecting environmental stimuli including temperature, pressure, and pain. Though ideal for drug delivery, the skin hinders the penetration of most chemical compounds. Anatomically, the human skin comprises four parts: the stratum corneum, viable epidermis, dermis, and subcutaneous tissues. Other anatomical features include sweat glands and hair follicles [1].

Dermatological or topical conditions have been reported as one of the top 15 disorders for which prevalence and medical spending have risen over the last decade [3]. The outcome of topical drug therapy is governed by the choice of drug-delivery system. Advances in biomedical sciences, alongside a growing market for dermatological products, have promoted the development of improved topical drug-delivery systems [3]. Topically delivered drugs are numerous, such as corticosteroids, antifungals, antivirals, antibiotics, antiseptics, anaesthetics, and antineoplastics [2].

Drug delivery represents a challenge in topical pharmaceuticals for treating burn wounds, ulcerations, and lesions. Conventional topical dosage forms are classified into semi-solids (ointments, creams, and pastes); liquids (lotions, emulsions, suspensions, and solutions) [4, 5]; and solids (conventional dry dressings and gauzes) (Figure 7.1).

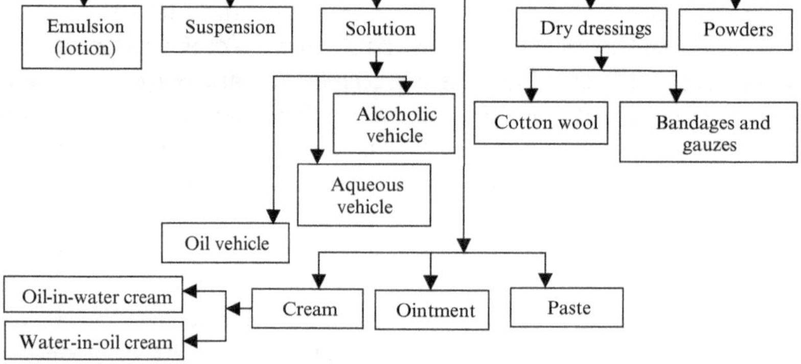

Figure 7.1 Typical examples of conventional topical drug-delivery media. *Source:* Maha AL-Rajabi, data adapted from [6].

Since the 1950s, drug-delivery systems have undergone continuous progress, with the ultimate objective of providing and sustaining therapeutic concentrations of a drug at the intended biological site [7]. Among various modern drug-delivery media, hydrogels have offered promising potential. Their merits are twofold. First, they are able to retain water in substantial volumes (up to 99% of their mass) [8]. Secondly, they spontaneously respond to extraneous triggers including temperature [9], pH [10], ionic strength [11], light [12], and electric and magnetic fields [13]. Thermo-responsive or temperature-sensitive polymers represent the most widely explored group of environmentally sensitive polymers, given their ease of control and preparation and their practical applications [14]. In this regard, their thermal sensitivity makes them ideal for formulating functionalised thermo-responsive hydrogels. Notably, the phenomenon of phase transition is observed for thermo-responsive polymers at specific temperatures, at which they undergo a sudden change in solubility. Accordingly, given their phase transition at physiological temperatures, thermo-responsive hydrogels have found much potential in biomedical applications, especially for topical delivery of pharmaceuticals [15].

Sustainable or green chemistry is an area for which the primary focus is on the design of chemical processes and products that minimise the deployment and generation of hazardous substances. With rising concerns over sustainability across the globe, the adoption of green chemistry as exemplified by the development of functionalised hydrogels represents a feasible and promising step. Such adoption can be undertaken in a wide range of contexts, such as deploying renewable and sustainable resources, and preferring safer solvents and less hazardous chemicals in synthesising hydrogels. Among available sustainable and renewable polymers used in hydrogel synthesis, cellulose is the most favourable, given its natural abundance, low cost, biodegradability, and biocompatibility. In this chapter, the use of bio-cellulose in synthesising functionalised hydrogels is detailed.

7.2 Conventional Topical Drug-Delivery Systems

The most conventional and established topical drug-delivery medium is the semi-solid dosage form, for which the classification is unfortunately vague and ill-defined [6]. A cream has been suggested to be defined as a semi-solid, emulsion-derived formulation, comprising less than 50% of polyethylene glycol or hydrocarbons as the medium, and more than 20% water and volatiles [16]. Creams can be classified into the oil-in-water formulation, for which water is the continuous phase (i.e. vanishing creams), and the water-in-oil formulation, for which oil is the continuous phase (i.e. oily creams). Vanishing creams are appropriate for water-soluble drugs, while their oily counterparts are appropriate for lipid-soluble ones [17].

On the other hand, an ointment is usually defined as a formulation comprising more than 50% polyethylene glycol or hydrocarbons as the medium and less than 20% water. Ointments act as the vehicle for topical delivery of active ingredients, offer skin protection, and act as an emollient [18]. They typically contain a drug emulsified, dissolved, or dispersed in an ointment-derived carrier; additionally, they are greasy [19]. The last type of semi-solid dosage form, a paste, can be viewed as a semi-solid formulation with approximately 20–50% finely dispersed solids in an oily medium of stiff consistency [20].

A liquid dosage form is another important conventional drug-delivery medium. Emulsions, also known as lotions, usually contain a water-based medium, with the water and volatiles exceeding 50% by proportion [16]. On the other hand, topical suspensions are defined as a two-phase medium consisting of 0–20% of solids dispersed in a liquid [4], which is typically water or alcohol based. Topical solutions, the last liquid dosage form, are defined as a homogeneous, translucent liquid medium for topical drug delivery. Topical solutions typically contain an alcohol- or water-based vehicle, although this role is at times played by an oil-based vehicle. Such solutions may contain a gelling agent for thickening their consistency [21].

Besides semi-solid and liquid formulations, solid dosage forms have also proven effective in topical drug delivery. They can be classified into powders and dry dressings. Powders are inert and insoluble solids, with utility in covering ulcers and wounds, absorbing moisture, decreasing friction, and discouraging microbial growth [22]. On the other hand, wound appliances and dressings constitute a significant segment of the global market for wound treatment. Conventional dressings with differing degrees of absorbency, as exemplified by bandages, gauzes, and cotton wool, have presented practical value in wound management [23].

Table 7.1 summarises the appearances, advantages, and disadvantages of conventional topical drug delivery media. Generally, topical semi-solid and liquid preparations register suboptimal retention on skin or wound surfaces, for which multiple applications are thus warranted [24]. Moreover, traditional drug-delivery media present inconvenience in administration: some dosage forms have to be rubbed in topically to disperse the formulation [25], causing pain, inflammation, and irritation. Notwithstanding their ease of application, traditional dry dressings do not support the moisture-rich condition essential for wound healing [26]. Furthermore, conventional methods have been associated with haphazard kinetics, under which drug release can be inappropriately rapid and excessive topical concentrations may induce toxicity [27]. To overcome such shortcomings, a viable alternative dosage form – hydrogels – has been introduced [26].

7.3 Hydrogels

Hydrogels are three-dimensional intermeshing structures of chemically or physically cross-linked polymeric chains of either synthetic or natural origin. Given their ability to swell/de-swell and be absorbed, hydrogels can release substantial amounts of retained water, solvents, or bodily fluids without themselves being dissolved [33]. The first study on hydrogels in 1960 revolved around polyhydroxyethylmethacrylate, which demonstrated a high swelling ratio and was used in biomedical application [34].

7.3.1 Methods of Synthesising Hydrogels

Common approaches to synthesising hydrogel involve cross-linking by chemical or physical means (Figure 7.2) [35–38]. Physically cross-linked hydrogels result from molecular entanglement and other forces (Figure 7.3). These forces contribute to the cross-linking through hydrogen bonding, amphiphilic graft and block polymers (hydrophobic interactions), crystallisation, and electrostatic interactions (Figure 7.4, A–D). The chief advantage

Table 7.1 Appearance, advantages, and disadvantages of conventional topical drug-delivery media.

Conventional topical drug-delivery medium	Appearance and sensation	Pros	Cons	References
Semi-solids				
Cream	Opaque, thick, not greasy to mildly greasy; tendency to mostly evaporate or be absorbed on topical application	Appropriate for use on most skin areas; tendency to cause less irritation Most appropriate for sensitive and/or dry skin Offers moisturising and emollient effects Can be spread more easily and are less oily than ointments	May cause a greasy feel, given its thickness Less moisturising than ointments Suboptimal retention on the wounds or skin surfaces Inconvenient application	[16, 18, 24, 25, 28, 29]
Ointment	Clear or opaque, thick, greasy; tendency not to evaporate or be absorbed on topical application	Appropriate for very dry skin Typically free from preservatives Offers greater potency and better drug permeation Efficacious on lesions with thickened skin Enhances skin hydration and maintains temperature	Water insoluble, thus can be challenging to wash off Can be viewed as greasy or messy to use Greasy or oily texture, thus can be less cosmetically or aesthetically appealing Cannot be spread easily Suboptimal retention on wounds or skin surfaces Inconvenient application	[16, 18, 24, 25, 29]
Paste	Opaque, thick, greasy to mildly greasy; good adhesion to the skin, affording a protective barrier	Less greasy and more absorptive than ointments Does not soften and flow easily	Usually inappropriate for hairy anatomical parts, given its stiffness	[18, 20, 30]

(Continued)

Table 7.1 (Continued)

Conventional topical drug-delivery medium	Appearance and sensation	Pros	Cons	References
Liquids				
Emulsion (lotion)	Opaque, non-viscous, non-greasy; tendency to rapidly evaporate with a cooling effect on topical application	Appropriate for all skin types Feels less weighty Favoured for large or hairy intertriginous anatomical parts (e.g. armpits, feet, and groin) Affords a cooling effect when the water-based phase vaporises Convenient application to hairy areas Can be spread easily	May irritate the skin (e.g. excessive drying and burning) Less moisturising than ointment or cream	[16, 18]
Topical suspension	Shaking required prior to use, given sedimentation of solids	Affords a soothing, cooling effect to skin on application Convenient application	More drying than ointment or cream Alcohol-derived formulations may sting, especially for skin with eczema or abrasions Requires to be shaken prior to use	[16, 22]
Topical solution	Clear, non-viscous	Easy to spread Leaves minimal residue Very simple to produce	Alcohol-derived formulations may irritate skin (dryness or stinging) Messy application Does not offer skin protection Less moisturising	[16, 22]

Solids				
Powders	Mixed or dry solids	Action is dry and absorption of fatty acids produces a deodorant and releasing effect	Light, fluffy powders may be inhaled by patients if proper care is not taken Drying effects are often seen for powders	[31, 20]
Dry dressing	Fine mesh gauze with a supplement to enhance occlusion with non-adherent characteristics	Promotes dryness of the wound through airing and evaporation of exudates and wards off microbes Convenient to use	Does not support a moisture-rich condition for wounds to heal Dressing changes are frequently required There has to be intact skin surrounding the site being dressed, which may not be the case for large donor sites, e.g. burns Wound contraction may be hindered by dressing-induced occlusion Dressing removal disruptive of formation of new epithelia	[23, 26, 32]

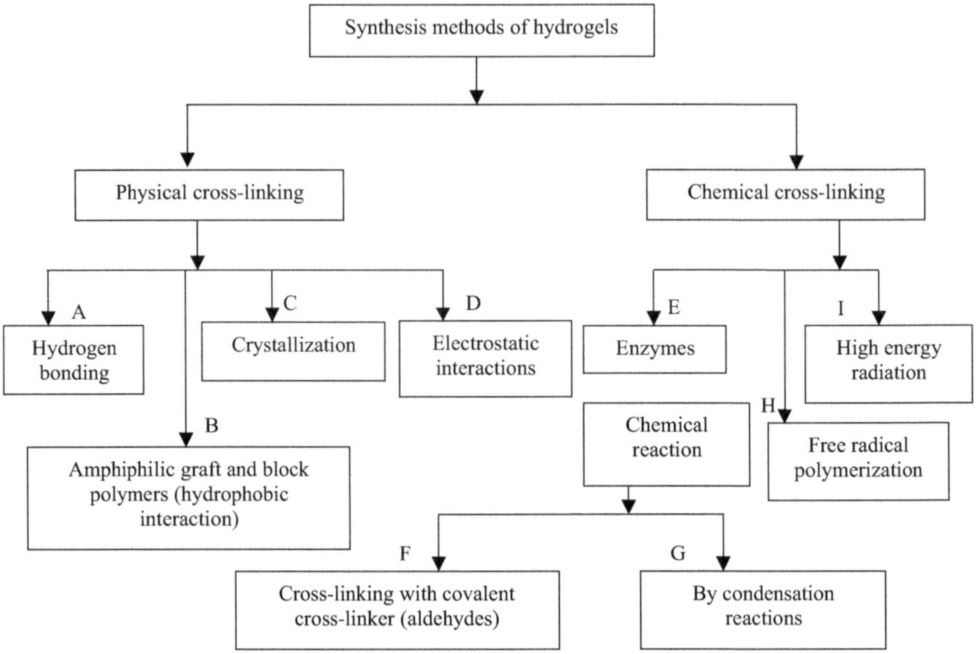

Figure 7.2 Synthesis methods of hydrogels. *Source:* Maha AL-Rajabi, data adapted from [36].

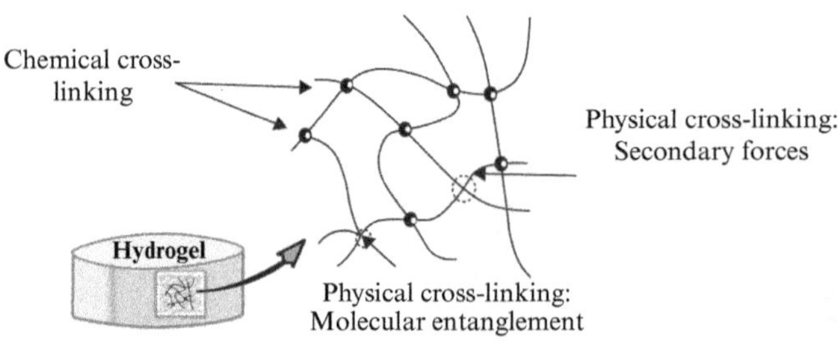

Figure 7.3 Physical and chemical cross-linking of hydrogel. *Source:* Ullah, F. et al., 2015 / Reproduced with permission from Elsevier.

of physically cross-linked hydrogels is their biocompatibility, given the lack of toxic chemical cross-linkers [39]. Additionally, the preparation conditions required for their synthesis are relatively mild [36]. However, notable shortcomings include the inconsistent performance of the hydrogels and the often reversible physical cross-linking [39]. Conversely, chemically cross-linked hydrogels formed by non-reversible cross-linking can be synthesised using enzymes, different cross-linking agents, free radical polymerisation, and high-energy radiation (Figure 7.4, E–I) [35, 39, 40]. Unlike their physically cross-linked counterparts, chemically cross-linked hydrogels are stable against degradation and register improved mechanical properties [41]. However, cross-linking agents have their drawbacks, given their potential toxicity, environmental implications, and likelihood of undesirable reactions with bioactive substances in the hydrogel matrices [42].

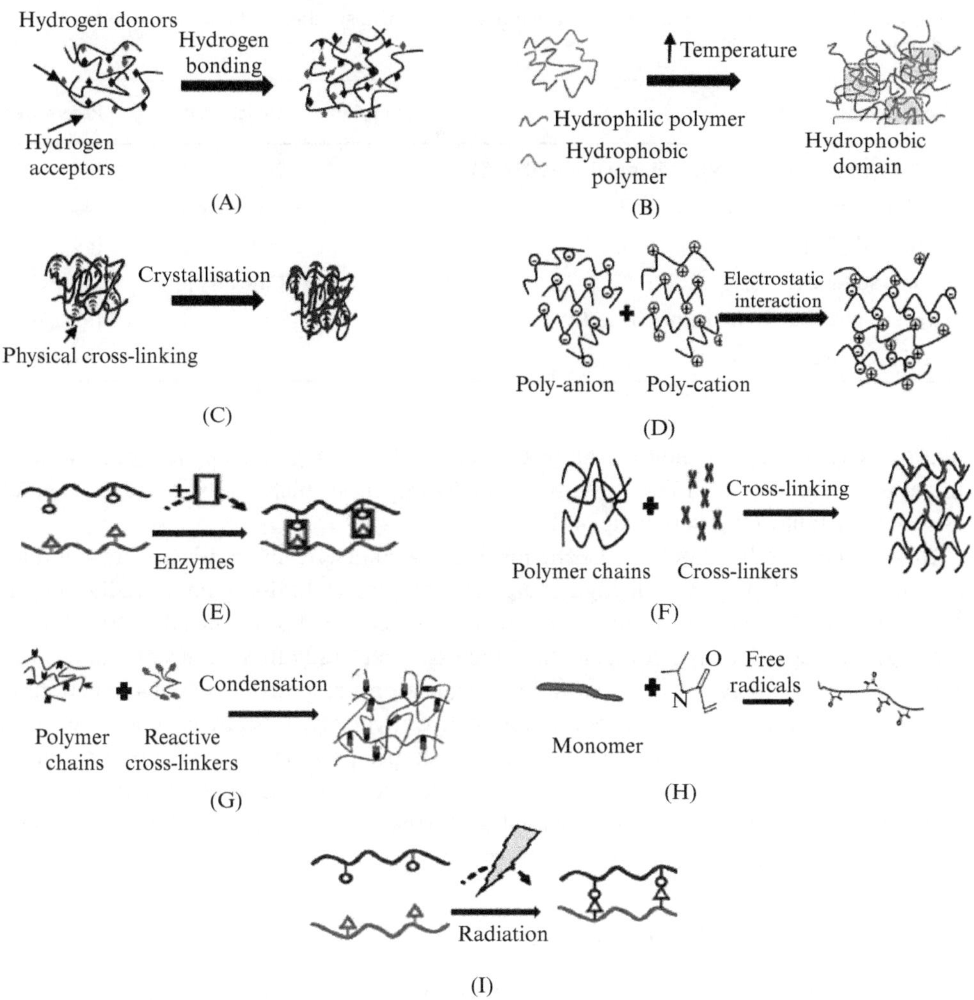

Figure 7.4 Hydrogels formed by (A–D) physical and (E–I) chemical cross-linking: (A) hydrogen bonding; (B) amphiphilic grafting and blocking of polymers (hydrophobic interaction); (C) crystallisation; (D) electrostatic interaction; (E) enzymes; (F) covalent cross-linker; (G) condensation reaction; (H) free radical polymerisation; and (I) high-energy radiation. *Source:* Adapted from [39] with permission from the Royal Society of Chemistry and from [46] with permission of Elsevier.

Table 7.2 shows the LD_{50} of the most common chemical cross-linking agents in the synthesis of hydrogels. The approach adopted to study their acute toxicity is based on the Global Harmonised System of classification, labelling, and packaging of substances, according to the oral LD_{50} lethal dose (50% test population). Based on the acute toxicity estimates (ATEs) (mg/kg body weight), the following categories are used: category 1 (ATE ≤5), fatal on ingestion; category 2 (ATE 5–50), fatal on ingestion; category 3 (ATE 50–300), toxic on ingestion; category 4 (ATE 300–2000), harmful on ingestion; category 5 (ATE 2000–5000), may be harmful on ingestion; and LD_{50} >5000 mg/kg not classified [43]. It is important to consider the toxicity of the cross-linkers prior to their use in the synthesis of

Table 7.2 LD_{50} of commonly used cross-linking agents in the synthesis of chemically cross-linked hydrogels.

Cross-linking agent	LD_{50} (mg/kg)	Toxicity category	References
1,2,3,4-butanetetracarboxylic dianhydride (BTCA)	1720	Category 4	[47]
Epichlorohydrin (ECH)	90–175	Category 3	[44, 48]
Citric acid (CA)	5400	Not classified	[49]
Divinyl sulfone (DVS)	32	Category 2	[50, 51]
Ethylene glycol diglycidyl ether (EGDE)	460	Category 4	[52, 53]
Succinic anhydride (SA)	1.7–9	Category 1/2	[54, 55]

hydrogels, especially for biomedical, pharmaceutical, and hygienic applications. Notably, the most common cross-linker in synthesising hydrogels is epichlorohydrin (ECH), which as shown in Table 7.2 is very toxic [44].

To overcome the drawbacks of the chemical cross-linkers, irradiation-based cross-linking may instead be deployed with high-energy irradiation, including gamma radiation and electron beam (e-beam). Gamma radiation is cost-effective at lower doses (<80 kGy) and for large and high-density hydrogels. Nonetheless, such irradiation causes random formation of radicals on polymeric chains and hydrogen atoms responsible for such reactions as grafting and intermolecular cross-linking [45]. Conversely, e-beam is mostly used for smaller and low-density hydrogels and for linear-shaped products such as wires and tubing [42]. All in all, cross-linking by radiation is considered more useful because the extent of cross-linking is controlled by the dose applied; furthermore, it is power efficient and neat, with no undesirable residues in the products [42].

7.3.2 Classification of Hydrogels

Hydrogels may be distinguished based on different parameters: sources, polymeric composition, configuration, type of cross-linking, appearance, and electrical charge (Figure 7.5). Depending on their material sources, hydrogels can be of natural – collagen, alginate, gelatine, chitosan, and cellulose – or synthetic origin – poly(vinyl alcohol), polyethylene glycol (PEG), poly(ethylene glycol)-poly(lactone)-poly(ethylene glycol), poly(methacrylamide), poly(acrylic acid), and polyamides [35, 37, 56]. Another classification revolves around their sensitivity to stimuli: stimuli-sensitive (smart, intelligent, or physiologically responsive hydrogels) and non-stimuli-responsive [57]. Based on network electrical charge, hydrogels can be grouped into neutral, anionic, cationic, and ampholytic [37, 58]. Based on physical structure, they can be divided into amorphous, crystalline, and semi-crystalline [59, 60]. Additionally, swelling capacity can be used to classify hydrogels: superabsorbent hydrogels can absorb water or fluids of up to 10–1000 times their weight, while superporous ones swell within minutes to their equilibrium swollen state [59, 61]. Cross-linking based on synthetic strategies is another such parameter: hydrogels exhibit either physical or chemical cross-linking [38]. Lastly, polymeric compositions can be used for categorisation: homopolymeric (comprising one type of monomer), copolymeric (cross-linking two

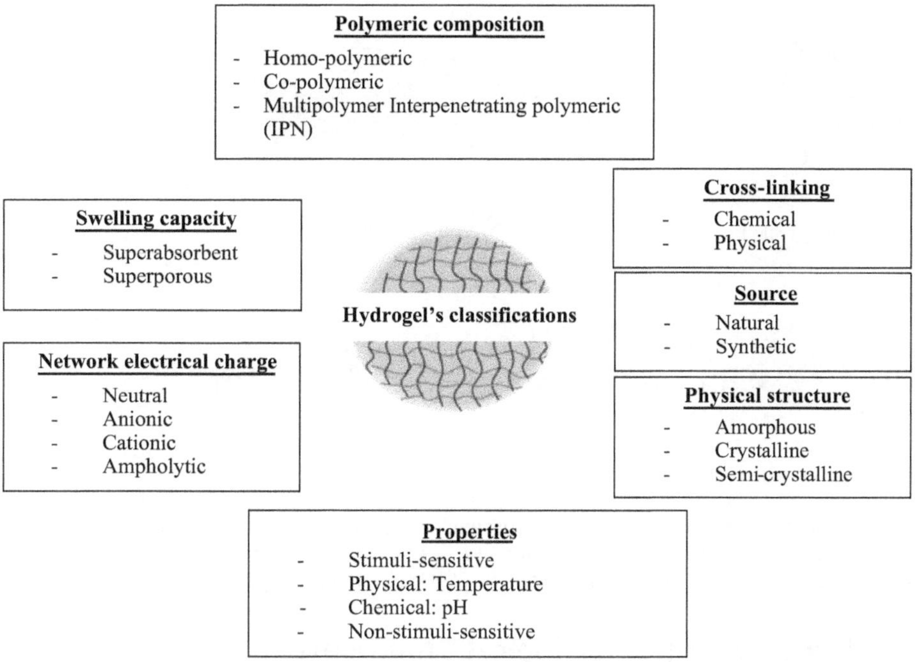

Figure 7.5 Hydrogel classifications based on different parameters. *Source:* Adapted with permission from [62]

dissimilar monomers, of which at least one is hydrophilic), and multipolymer interpenetrating polymeric (comprising two independent, cross-linked polymeric components in a lattice structure) [58, 59].

7.3.3 Drug-Transport Mechanisms of Hydrogels

The manifold drug-release mechanisms from hydrogels include diffusion-, swelling-, chemical-, and erosion-controlled modalities [63] (Figure 7.6). Of these, diffusion-controlled release represents a widely adopted mechanism: drug molecules in different sizes entrapped in hydrogel matrices can distribute themselves by diffusion, subject to the mesh size of the matrices [64, 65].

In diffusion-controlled release, the mechanism is governed by aspects such as the extent of cross-linking, chemical properties of monomers, and intensity of environmental stimuli. The mesh size of hydrogels (when swollen) typically measures between 5 nm and 100 nm [67]. Thus, drugs that are smaller than the mesh size diffuse freely, whereas macromolecules will be subjected to sustained release if the hydrogels are not judiciously engineered for the intended diffusion kinetics [68]. In the chemically controlled modality, chemical reactions in the hydrogel matrices govern drug release, including hydrolysis of polymeric chains, enzyme-assisted degradation, or other drug-polymer reactions [69]. Finally, under the erosion-controlled mechanism, drug release is determined by the rate at which the hydrogels are eroded away [65].

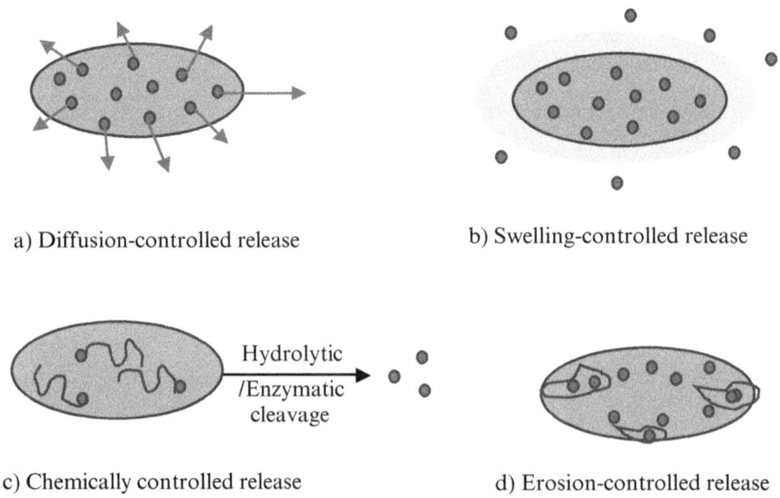

Figure 7.6 Drug-release mechanisms from hydrogel: (A) diffusion-controlled release; (B) swelling-controlled release; (C) chemically controlled release; and (D) erosion-controlled release. *Source:* Adapted from Ghasemiyeh & Mohammadi-Samani, 2019 [63]; Mohammed et al., 2017 [66].

7.4 Tailored Hydrogels for Topical Drug Delivery

Over the last few decades, tailored or intelligent hydrogels with smart, sensitive, or environmentally responsive properties have received considerable attention from researchers, given their spontaneous responsiveness to external stimuli. In topical drug delivery, crucial stimuli include pH [10], redox potential [70], enzymatic activity [71], and temperature [72].

For pH-responsive hydrogels, the choice between acidic and basic polymers depends on the pH of the application sites [73]. For human skin, the normal pH ranges from 4 to 6; however, disturbances may occur in the context of atopic dermatitis [74] and wound healing, where the pH could be elevated to 7.6 [75]. Given the association of some dermatological conditions with pH imbalance of the skin, pH-sensitive hydrogels have been investigated for controlled drug delivery [75].

For redox-responsive hydrogels, efforts have focused on their development for topical drug delivery. It is well established that inflammation leads to the undesirable production of reactive oxygen species and other oxidants, with consequent imbalance in the oxidative state. Reactive oxygen species often cause redox adaptation in view of the continuous oxidative imbalance, thus upregulating antioxidant molecules such as glutathione. Since disulfide bonds are sensitive to glutathione, there have been investigations into incorporating them in hydrogels for smart topical applications [76].

Another important type of hydrogel is the enzyme-responsive hydrogel, used in localised drug delivery for inflamed skin. Inflammation has been found to be crucial to wound healing and many skin diseases. During the process, immune cells migrate to the sites of infection and produce various biomolecules to neutralise the detrimental stimuli. Specifically, neutrophils reach these microenvironments most rapidly. When activated for degranulation, they release numerous enzymes including human neutrophil elastase. As its pronounced presence signifies the occurrence of specific biological events (i.e. disorders or lesions), the elastase represents an ideal trigger for site-based drug release [77].

Most notably, the use of temperature as a stimulus has attracted much attention. Motivated by the fact that thermal variations are naturally present, efforts have been underway to develop thermo-responsive materials over recent years. A detailed discussion of such thermo-responsive materials in topical drug-delivery systems is presented in the following sections.

7.4.1 Thermo-responsive Polymers

Temperature-sensitive or thermo-responsive polymers represent a widely explored class of environmentally sensitive polymers, given their ease of control and preparation and their practical applications [14]. Such thermo-responsive polymers undergo phase transition at specific temperatures with resultant changes in their solubility, thus underlining their suitability for preparing thermo-responsive hydrogels. In this context, a lower critical solution temperature (LCST) polymer refers to a polymer that becomes insoluble when heated, while an upper critical solution temperature (UCST) polymer refers to one that becomes soluble [78]. Figure 7.7 depicts the phase diagrams of thermo-responsive polymers with LCST and UCST polymers such as neutral poly(N-acryloyl glycinamide) [79], dimethylpolysiloxane [80], poly(sulfobetaine) [81], and poly(methacrylamide) [82]. Such UCST polymers have highly polar zwitterionic groups capable of strong intermolecular interactions [83].

Polymers with LCST are deployed chiefly for formulating drug-delivery systems [85]. Table 7.3 outlines some common thermo-responsive polymers with LCST. Among such polymers in thermo-responsive hydrogels, Pluronic F127 (PF127) has been widely used given its promising potential as a hydrogel material. At temperatures below the phase transition temperature (room temperature), PF127 remains in the sol phase; above the transition temperature (body temperature), it morphs into the gel phase [86]. Given its phase transition, PF127 can be applied to the skin to fill wounds or burn surfaces in the sol phase [27], and then transforms into a rigid hydrogel. Additionally, PF127 not only is non-toxic [87], but also has been endorsed by the US Food and Drug Administration (FDA) for pharmaceutical application [88, 89]. However, as a thermo-responsive polymer, PF127 cannot be employed on its own for preparing hydrogels given its insufficient mechanical robustness [90]. This therefore warrants the addition of another polymer to the hydrogel network.

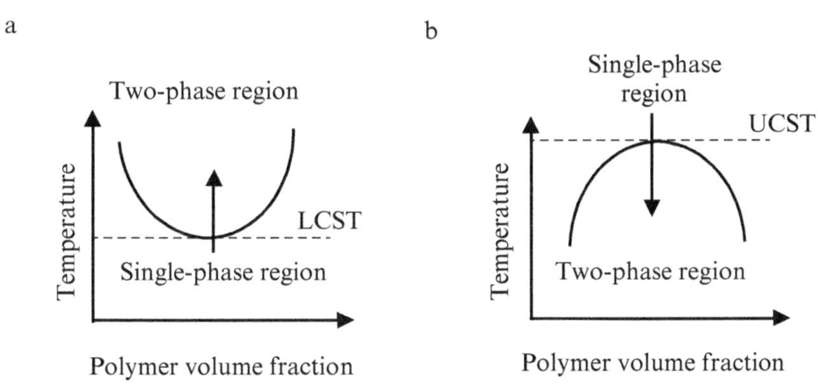

Figure 7.7 Phase diagram of thermo-responsive polymers with (A) lower critical solution temperature (LCST) and (B) upper critical solution temperature (UCST). *Source:* Adapted with permission from [84].

Table 7.3 Most common thermo-responsive polymers with lower critical solution temperature (LCST).

Thermo-responsive polymer	Abbreviation	LCST (°C)	References
Poly(ethylene oxide)-poly(propylene oxide)-poly(ethylene oxide)	PEO–PPO–PEO, Pluronic	20–85	[87, 91]
Poly(ethylene glycol)	PEG	106–115	[92, 93]
Poly(propylene glycol)	PPG	10–40	[94, 95]
Poly(N-isopropylacrylamide)	PNIPAm/PNIPAAm	32	[96, 97]
Poly(methyl vinyl ether)	PMVE	28–34	[98, 99]
Poly(N-vinyl caprolactam)	PNVC/PVCL	30–50	[100, 101]
Methyl cellulose	MC	60–80	[65, 101]
Hydroxypropyl cellulose	HPC	41	[102, 103]

7.4.2 Importance of Thermo-responsive Hydrogels in Topical Drug Release

Thermo-responsive hydrogels have been extensively developed for biomedical applications, particularly as a topical drug-delivery system, because of their controllable, accurate, and sustained modality in attaining optimal doses at local sites for effective treatment [65]. The sustained release through such a modality is termed long-acting or delayed release, in contrasted to rapid or traditional drug-release profiles (Figure 7.8). A sustained-release

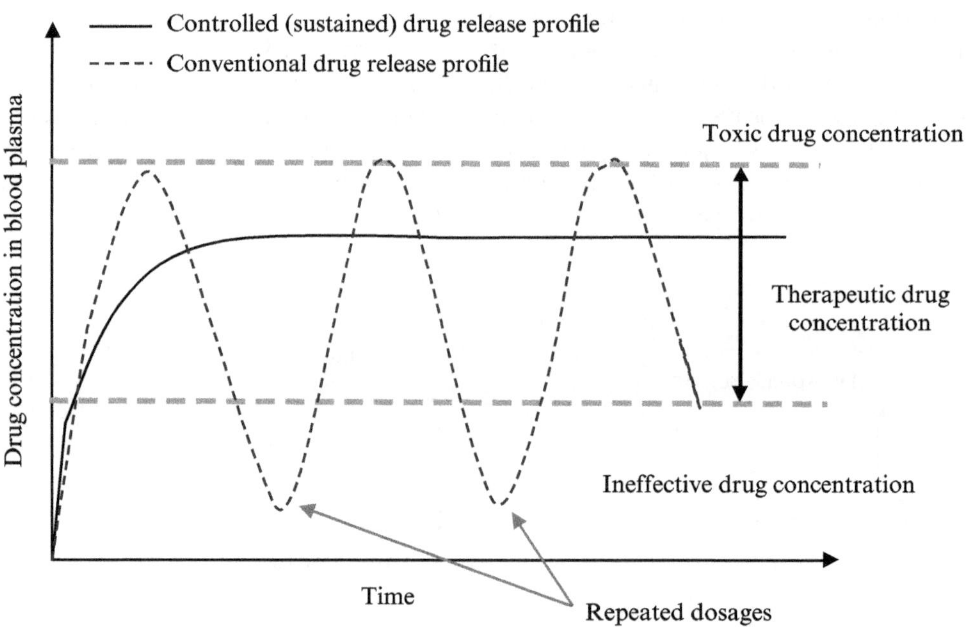

Figure 7.8 Typical drug-release profiles for controlled (sustained) drug release and conventional drug release. *Source:* Versypt 2015 [104] / Reproduced with permission from Ashlee Nicole Ford Versypt.

Table 7.4 List of drug molecules delivered by thermo-responsive hydrogels with sustained release.

Thermo-responsive hydrogel	Drug molecules incorporated	Sustained-release duration	References
PF127 and N,N,N-trimethyl chitosan hydrogel	Docetaxel	1 month	[105]
PF127 and alginate hydrogel	Cisplatin	6 hours	[106]
PF127 and alginate hydrogel	Selegiline	48 hours	[107]
PNIPAAm-b-poly(L-alanine) (PNIPAAm-b-Pala)	Doxorubicin	20 hours	[108]
PF127, N,N,N-trimethyl chitosan (TMC), polyethylene glycolated hyaluronic acid (PEG-HA)	Gallic acid	5 days	[109]
PF127 and α-tocopheryl polyethylene glycol 1000 succinate	Paclitaxel and doxorubicin	3 days	[110]
PF127 and hyaluronic acid	Cisplatin and carboplatin	6 hours	[88]
PF127 and cellulose	Silver sulfadiazine	24 hours	[72, 111]

profile has numerous advantages: it promotes sustained duration of drug action, prolongs the dosing interval, minimises fluctuations in the plasma level of the drug, improves drug utilisation, and finally results in a lower incidence of adverse drug effects [1].

A wide range of drugs can be delivered via thermo-responsive hydrogels, such as proteins, DNA, and antibiotics [15]. Apart from the ease of drug loading and injectability in the sol phase, there are additional benefits of using thermo-responsive hydrogels such as localised drug application and a sustained-release profile. Table 7.4 outlines various drug molecules investigated for sustained release from thermo-sensitive hydrogels.

7.5 Adoption of Green Chemistry in Developing Functionalised Hydrogels

Green chemistry is defined as the engineering of chemical processes and products to minimise the deployment and production of hazardous substances. Under this paradigm, sustainability is to be attained at the molecular level; thus, it is unsurprising that green chemistry has found application in many industries [112]. A guiding framework based on the 12 principles of green chemistry has been proposed for devising new chemical processes and products: it applies comprehensively to aspects of the process life cycle, including the raw materials used, process safety and efficiency, and characteristics of products and reagents used (toxicity and biodegradability) [113]. Those 12 principles are preventing waste, atom economy, safer chemical synthesis, designing less hazardous chemicals, designing less harmful solvents and auxiliaries, advocating efficiency in energy usage, using renewable feedstock, reducing unnecessary derivatisation, catalysis, designing for degradation, analyses for preventing pollution in real time, and safer chemistry for preventing accidents [112].

The sustainability of a product or process is the result of complex interactions of environmental, technological, and economic factors that can be challenging to predict. Accordingly, guides are required in selecting potentially viable or useful avenues for further research and development. Against this background, green metrics should be deployed to measure the environmental sustainability of the product or process including its life-cycle analysis (LCA), atom economy, and mass-based metrics (environmental factor and effective mass yield) [113].

With escalating concerns about sustainability across the globe, it is important to examine the adoption of green chemistry in developing functionalised hydrogels. Unfortunately, green metrics have not been highlighted in functionalised hydrogels. In this section, the adoption of green chemistry for functionalised hydrogels is discussed, with a focus on deploying renewable materials in producing them with safer reagents.

7.5.1 Renewable Materials in Synthesising Functionalised Hydrogels

The deployment of materials of renewable and sustainable origins constitutes a vital component of next-generation practice in many industries. The increasing preference for such materials is contributed to by numerous rationales, including the necessity for sustainable growth, effective resource management, a low carbon footprint, and improved functional properties of the materials [114]. Innovation-driven sustainable resources (such as materials from recycling, wastes, co-products, and bio sources) are feasible for producing hydrogels to lessen the reliance on non-renewable resources [115].

In contrast to renewable and sustainable resources, petroleum-based materials used in hydrogel synthesis are expensive, toxic, and non-biodegradable [116]. Thus, the use of hydrogels generated from such undesirable materials is anticipated to cause downstream waste-disposal problems [117]. Hence, for environmental conservation and minimal ecological repercussions, a more sustainable engineering practice is warranted to develop innovative natural polymer-based hydrogels to replace existing synthetic ones for drug delivery [118]. Against this background, advances in the adoption of natural polymers such as cellulose and gelatine have expanded the modalities of hydrogel synthesis.

Natural polymers used to synthesise hydrogels are commonly of naturally occurring origins [119]. Compared to their synthetic counterparts, natural hydrogels offer notable advantages: lack of toxicity, biocompatibility, and biodegradability [120, 121]. Additionally, they are known for their remarkable swelling behaviours, mechanical similarity to natural tissues, and ease of use for surgical grafts [122]. These properties make them ideal for many areas, particularly in drug formulations and tissue engineering. Among natural polymers used in synthesising hydrogels, cellulose is found in the greatest abundance in green flora, aquatic animals, and microorganisms [123, 124].

7.5.1.1 Cellulose and Its Derivatives as a Green Polymer for Hydrogel Synthesis

Interactions in the macromolecules of cellulose are non-covalent in nature, such as the interplay of van der Waals forces and hydrogen bonding. Its intramolecular interactions (in the same chain) are attributed to the OH–O hydrogen bonding, whereas its intermolecular ones (between chains) stem from not only the interplay of van der Waals forces, but also the weaker CH–O hydrogen bonding (Figure 7.9) [125]. As a whole, hydrogen-bonding networks lead to regions of differing hydrophilicity and hydrophobicity on the ring planes [126].

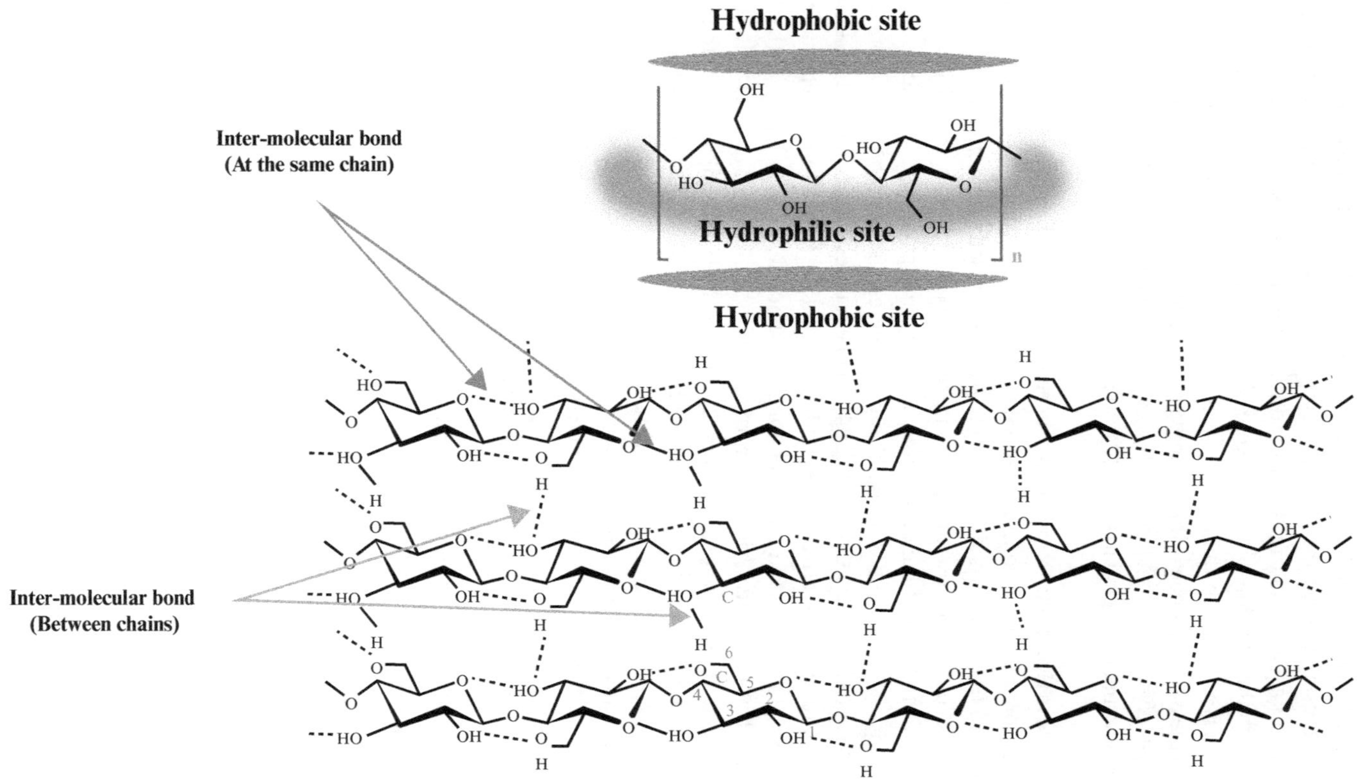

Figure 7.9 The molecular structure of cellulose shows the inter/intramolecular bonds and the hydrophobic/hydrophilic sites.
Source: Adapted with permission from [126].

The hydroxyl moieties on the cellulose chains can be chemically modified to enhance solubility and reactivity [127, 128]. From such modification, cellulose derivatives can be obtained for preparing cellulose-derived hydrogels. Converting cellulose into cellulose derivatives solves the difficulty of using untreated cellulose, whose structure, crystallinity, and rigidity render it barely soluble in aqueous and most other solvents. Such conversion of cellulose entails the esterification or etherification of its hydroxyl moieties; the extent of these processes is expressed through the degree to which the hydroxyl groups are substituted [129]. Table 7.5 depicts the structures of the most common cellulose derivatives. Cellulose-derived hydrogels have attracted much interest, given their remarkable physical and chemical properties, high swelling ratio, soft consistency, and biodegradability [129, 130].

7.5.1.2 Cellulose Hydrogels from Renewable and Sustainable Resources

The industrial production of commercial cellulose is performed through acidic hydrolysis of cellulose derived from cotton and wood [132]. Although wood represents the main industrial source of bio-cellulose, the cost-effective sourcing of wood is challenging, given the competition from the furniture and building industries, pulp and paper sectors, and combustion of wood for energy. Thus, there has been heightened interest in identifying other renewable and sustainable sources for bio-cellulose [133, 134]. Viable sources include bio-cellulose-rich materials such as natural plant-derived fibres and lignocellulosic fibres. More specifically, sources of bio-cellulose can be classified into fruit fibres (coconut and oil palm), grasses (bamboo and bagasse), cereal straws (wheat, rice, and corn), leaf fibres (pineapple and curaua), seed fibres (kapok), and bast fibres (flax, jute, and kenaf). Most of these natural sources are considered agricultural waste, representing a potential source of renewable materials to produce environmentally friendly products such as hydrogels [135, 136].

Notably, the choices of the sources of lignocellulosic fibres and of process parameters will govern the characteristics of the resultant bio-cellulose, such as its molecular weight, surface area, particle size, crystallinity, and porosity [134, 137]. Such variances in the bio-cellulose will in turn contribute to the dissimilar characteristics of bio-cellulose hydrogels. Table 7.6

Table 7.5 Chemical structures of most common cellulose derivatives.

Cellulose derivative	Substituent group®)
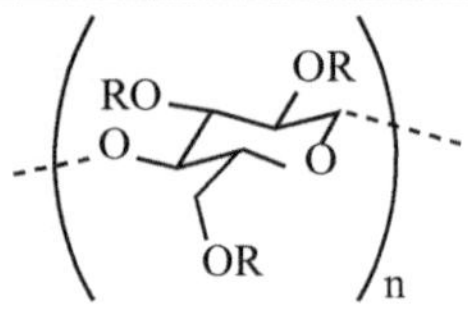	
Methyl cellulose (MC)	H, CH_3
Ethyl cellulose (EC)	H, CH_2CH_3
Hydroxyethyl cellulose (HEC)	H, $[CH_2CH_2O]_nH$
Hydroxypropyl cellulose (HPC)	H, $[CH_2CH(CH_3)O]_nH$
Hydroxyethylmethyl cellulose (HEMC)	H, CH_3, $[CH_2CH_2O]_nH$
Hydroxypropylmethyl cellulose (HPMC)	H, CH_3, $[CH_2CH(CH_3)O]_nH$
Carboxymethyl cellulose (CMC)	H,CH_2COONa

Source: Adapted from [131].

Table 7.6 Bio-cellulose hydrogels synthesised from cellulose extracted from lignocellulosic fibres.

Natural fibres	Pre-treatment	Solvent used	Cross-linking method	Results	References
Oil palm empty fruit bunches (OPEFB)	Sulphuric acid	LiOH/urea or NaOH/urea aqueous solution	Chemical cross-linking using ECH cross-linker	High transparency (93.74%) and high porosity hydrogel	[138]
OPEFB	–	NaOH/urea aqueous solution	Chemical cross-linking using ECH cross-linker	High swelling index (21491.0%)	[139]
OPEFB	–	NaOH/urea aqueous solution	Chemical cross-linking using ECH cross-linker	Percentage of swelling 80,000% Mixed with CMC	[140]
Rice straw	Alkaline-acid pulping treatment then bleaching	NaOH solution	Heterogeneous reaction with acrylic acid/MBA (cross-linker)/KPS (initiator)	High swelling ratio (> 3000%), a promising application in the agriculture field	[141]
Rice straw	Acid followed by alkali step	KOH solution	Heterogeneous reaction with acrylic acid/MBA (cross-linker)/KPS (initiator)	Swelling ratio 2.35 g/g	[142]
Rice husk	Alkaline pulping treatment then bleaching	Water	Gamma irradiation at 30 kGy	Swelling ratio 1108–3135%	[141]
Sugarcane bagasse	Alkali treatment, bleaching processes, and acid hydrolysis	NaOH/urea aqueous solution	Chemical cross-linking using ECH cross-linker	High swelling ratio (1567%), used for drug-delivery system Showed biocompatibility and antibacterial activity	[143]
Oil palm frond	–	Urea/NaOH solution	MBA (cross-linker), KPS (initiator) microwave polymerisation	Swelling index 1814%, efficient adsorbent for future applications	[144]
Bamboo fibres	–	NaOH– NaOH/urea aqueous solution and DMAc/LiCl solution	Physical cross-linking	High tensile strength of hydrogel 21–66 N/mm^2 Th hydrogel exhibited good cytocompatibility for cell cultivation scaffold	[145]

(Continued)

Table 7.6 (Continued)

Natural fibres	Pre-treatment	Solvent used	Cross-linking method	Results	References
Bamboo pulp	–	NaOH/urea aqueous solution	APS (initiator) Monomers AA and AM, MBA (cross-linker), and N-isopropylacrylamide (NIPPAm)	Temperature/pH sensitive for potential oral drug-delivery applications	[146]
Wheat straw	Extraction by benzene/ethanol, sodium chlorite treatment, NaOH and HCl acid treatment	NaOH/PEG aqueous solution	Physical cross-linking	Low-density cellulose aerogel (40 mg/cm^3) and large specific surface area (101 m^2/g) In addition, strong absorptive capacity for oil and dye solutions	[147]
Kenaf	NaOH, acetic acid, and sodium chlorite	NaOH/urea aqueous solution	Chemical cross-linking using ECH cross-linker	High transparent hydrogel	[148]
Soybean residue	–	NaOH aqueous solution	Chemical cross-linking, UV radiation with poly(acrylic acid)	Maximum adsorption capacity 1.43–2.04 mmol/g	[149]

AA, acrylic acid; AM, acrylamide; APS, ammonium persulfate; CMC, carboxymethyl cellulose; DMAc, N,N-dimethylacetamide; ECH, epichlorohydrin; KPS, potassium persulfate; LiCl, lithium chloride; MBA, N,N′-methylenebisacrylamide; OPEFB, oil palm empty fruit bunch; PEG, polyethylene glycol; UV, ultraviolet.

outlines the varying characteristics of hydrogels prepared from bio-cellulose involving different types of lignocellulosic fibre (as the source), pre-treatment methods, solvents, and cross-linking methods.

The use of bio-cellulose extracted from agricultural wastes has offered much promising potential in expanding the modalities of hydrogel synthesis. However, some shortcomings of the bio-cellulose hydrogels shown in Table 7.6 are noteworthy. First, their lack of functionalisation may lead to problematic drug-loading, retention, and drug-release control kinetics for their application in delivering pharmacological compounds. Secondly, they are characterised by a flat stagnant sheet structure, which is unable to completely cover uneven wounds or burn surfaces; the resultant exposure may heighten the risk of site infection.

Of note is that green synthesis has been investigated for fabricating thermo-responsive cellulose-derived hydrogels [72]. In AL-Rajabi and Haan's research, oil palm empty fruit bunch (OPEFB)-extracted cellulose was directly incorporated with PF127, without the need for modifying the cellulose, use of chemical solvents, or cross-linkers, through simultaneous homogenisation and polymerisation. Some insights deserve attention. First, the authors' synthesis involved no complicated fabrication and incurred no wastage of the materials used. This not only minimised undesired by-products, but also represented a greener and more sustainable approach to synthesising hydrogels. Secondly, the use of OPEFB, an agricultural biomass, as the renewable source to produce thermo-responsive cellulose-derived hydrogel offered a solution to the bottleneck of the agricultural industry. The production of hydrogels from OPEFB dovetails with one of the United Nations-endorsed sustainable development goals (SDGs), responsible consumption and production. Such innovative production reduces waste generation and also converts waste into high-demand pharmaceutical products through sustainable practice in the life cycle for the materials.

7.5.1.3 Thermo-Responsive Hydrogels from Natural Polymers for Drug Delivery

Table 7.7 summarises thermo-responsive hydrogels synthesised from natural polymers (such as cellulose, chitosan, and gelatine) for drug delivery. The reversible sol–gel transition property of methyl cellulose (MC), a cellulose derivative, is attributed to its hydroxyl moieties, which are partially replaced by methoxy moieties. In an aqueous medium, it transitions from its sol phase to its gel form, depending on the increases in temperature, followed by hydrophobic interactions. The gelation behaviour of MC-derived hydrogels could be regulated by varying the molecular weight of the MC, degree of substitution, concentration, and presence of additives [150]. The practical utility of MC-derived hydrogels has been copiously reported in the literature. Thermo-responsive cellulose-derived hydrogels synthesised from MC and kappa-carrageenan showed LCST and UCST (known as a double gel), which offered potential in drug formulations [151]. In tissue engineering, injectable thermo-responsive hydrogels derived from MC and chitosan were studied, demonstrating LCSTs that approximated the body temperature [152]. Moreover, MC and xanthan gum have been investigated in the preparation of injectable thermo-responsive hydrogels [153]. The materials had a remarkable shear-thinning property at room temperatures and formed thermo-responsive hydrogels at 37 °C. Additionally, their biocompatibility and biodegradability make them ideal for sustained drug delivery.

Apart from xanthan gum, other cellulose derivatives and polymers have been investigated. In one study, MC, carboxymethyl cellulose (CMC), polyethylene glycol (PEG), and chitosan

Table 7.7 Thermo-responsive hydrogels from natural polymers for drug delivery.

Thermo-responsive hydrogel	Cellulose derivative/nano concentration	Drug molecules incorporated	Application	References
HPMC, chitosan, and glycerophosphate	16% w/w	Vancomycin hydrochloride antibiotic	Local treatment of osteomyelitis	[156]
PF127 and MC	15% w/w	Docetaxel anticancer drug	Cancer treatment	[158]
		Insulin	Diabetes treatment	[159]
CMC and gelatine	1.24% w/w	Lidocaine	Transdermal drug therapy	[157]
PF127 and CMC	2% and 4% w/w	Chinese herbal medicine	Textile-based transdermal therapy	[89, 163]
PF127 and cellulose nano-crystals	0.8–1.2% w/v	Pilocarpine hydrochloride drug	Ophthalmic drug delivery	[160]
PNIPAAm and CMC	10% w/w	Lysozyme enzyme	Protein drug delivery	[162]
PNIPAAm and cellulose nano-crystals	1–5% w/v	Metronidazole	Wound infections	[9]

CMC, carboxymethyl cellulose; HPMC, hydroxypropylmethyl cellulose; MC, methyl cellulose.

sulfate were combined to produce injectable thermo-responsive hydrogels, which were found to effectively reduce adhesion formation and address adhesiolysis-related difficulties [154]. In another study, chitosan was combined with hydroxypropylmethyl cellulose (HPMC) and glycerol to prepare thermo-responsive hydrogels, which gelled within 15 minutes at 37 °C [155]. The findings further suggested their biodegradability, low cytotoxicity, and controlled drug-release profile. Furthermore, HPMC was deployed in preparing thermo-responsive hydrogels with chitosan and glycerophosphate as a vehicle for vancomycin, an antibiotic [156]. The resultant hydrogels lowered both the rate of release and the total amount of vancomycin release, implying favourable controlled-release kinetics for such localised antimicrobial therapy. Lastly, CMC and gelatine were combined in formulating thermo-responsive hydrogels for transdermal therapy with lidocaine, an anaesthetic [157].

PF127 has also been used with MC, CMC, or cellulose nano-crystals. Thermo-responsive hydrogels from the combination of MC and PF127 have been deployed to deliver docetaxel, an antineoplastic drug, demonstrating sustained drug release [158]. Likewise, such hydrogels have been used for insulin, demonstrating a sustained blood insulin level over 10 days [159]. Additionally, a PF127 thermo-responsive polymer was combined with CMC, a cellulose derivative, to produce a thermo-responsive vehicle for Chinese herbal medicine in the topical treatment of atopic dermatitis [155]. The hydrogels favourably registered an LCST approximating the body temperature [155]. Lastly, cellulose nano-crystals, another form of cellulose, have also been used alongside PF127 for ophthalmic drug delivery for pilocarpine, a cholinergic agent, with a remarkable sustained release profile and bioavailability [160].

Poly(N-isopropylacrylamide) (PNIPAAm) represents another crucial polymer used widely in formulating thermo-responsive cellulose-derived hydrogels. Its combination with MC produced a thermo-responsive hydrogel that not only would gel near the body temperature, but also had enhanced mechanical strength [161]. In addition, its co-formulation with CMC has been reported for synthesising thermo-responsive hydrogels to deliver lysozymes [162]. Lastly, the combination of PNIPAAm with cellulose nano-crystals registered an LCST of 36.2 °C in the delivery of metronidazole, an antibiotic for wound infections [9].

7.5.2 Green Chemistry in the Synthesis of Thermo-Responsive Hydrogels

In general, approaches employed to synthesise thermo-responsive hydrogels are similar to those discussed in Section 7.3.1. However, certain types of thermo-responsive polymers warrant specific methods to synthesise thermo-responsive hydrogels (Table 7.8).

Thermo-responsive hydrogels are further categorised based on their constituent materials. They can be synthesised directly from stimulus-responsive cellulose derivatives, such as MC and hydroxypropyl cellulose (HPC) [164, 165]. Alternatively, they can be synthesised through combining natural polymers (such as chitosan, gelatine, cellulose derivatives, or nano-cellulose/nano-crystals) with other thermo-responsive polymers [85].

The objectives of combining cellulose with thermo-responsive polymers are manifold. First, given its partial crystallinity, cellulose mechanically strengthens the resultant thermo-responsive hydrogels [9]. Secondly, it improves the biocompatibility and biodegradability of the hydrogels. Finally, the use of such a combination mitigates the production costs of the hydrogels. The investigations and use of biomass-based materials have become progressively crucial, in view of the industry-wide goals of attaining cost-effectiveness and alleviating environmental risks.

7.5.3 Green Chemistry in Different Preparation Methods

The role of solvents represents an active aspect in green chemistry. Accounting for the majority of mass wasted in synthesis, solvents present a crucial challenge to green chemistry, especially considering their toxicity, inflammability, and corrosive risks. Furthermore, their volatile and soluble nature has resulted in air, water, and land pollution, posed health risks to workers, and led to accidents. To overcome these, recovery and reuse are often implemented; however, such processes incur much energy consumption, are operationally complex (e.g. distillation), and face the risks of being cross-contaminated. Against this background, various new 'green' answers such as water have been proposed. In this regard, the use of water as a solvent in synthesising thermo-responsive hydrogels has been advocated for greener synthesis (Table 7.8).

While chemical cross-linking yields mechanically robust hydrogels, a necessary step is the removal of the toxic cross-linkers from the hydrogels. Accordingly, physical cross-linking is relatively safer as a non-toxic alternative [36]. Moreover, from the perspective of green chemistry, the cold method for synthesising thermo-responsive hydrogels is considered superior to chemical cross-linking. However, not all important thermo-responsive polymers can be synthesised via physical cross-linking, thus necessitating the unavoidable use of chemical cross-linking.

Table 7.8 Thermo-responsive hydrogel synthesis methods.

Thermo-responsive polymer	Synthesis method	Solvent	Thermo-responsive polymer concentration	Reference
PEO–PPO–PEO	Physical cross-linking: cold method (hydrophobic interaction)	Water	15–35% w/v	[167, 168]
PEG	Physical cross-linking: cold method (hydrophobic interaction)	Water	2–10% w/w	[159]
MC	Physical cross-linking: cold method One-pot synthesis using precursor salts	Water	1–8% w/v	[101, 159]
PPG	Chemical cross-linking: ring-opening polymerisation and side-chain modification	Anhydrous DMF	2.5–5% w/v	[169]
PNIPAm/ PNIPAAm	Chemical cross-linking: free radical polymerisation Initiator APS and accelerator TEMED	Water	10 w/v%	[9]
PNVC/PVCL	Chemical cross-linking: frontal polymerisation cross-linker BIS and initiator TETDPPS	DMSO	2.5–6% w/v	[166]

APS, ammonium persulfate; BIS, N,N-methylene-bis-acrylamide; DMF, N,N-dimethylformamide; DMSO, dimethyl sulfoxide; MC, methyl cellulose; PEG, polyethylene glycol; PEO–PPO–PEO, poly(ethylene oxide)–poly(propylene oxide)–poly(ethylene oxide); PNIPAm/PNIPAAm, poly(N-isopropylacrylamide); PNVC/PVCL, poly(N-vinylcaprolactam); PPG, polypropylene glycol; TEMED, 1,2-di-(dimethylamino) ethane; TETDPPS, trihexyltetradecylphosphonium persulfate.

Among chemical polymerisation methods to synthesise thermo-responsive hydrogels, frontal polymerisation takes advantage of the exothermic nature of the reaction to convert the monomers into the polymer. In this context, the reaction liberates heat and generates a self-sustaining polymerising part along the reactor. In contrast to conventional free radical polymerisation, frontal polymerisation offers green benefits in producing hydrogels: short reaction times, low energy consumption, simple protocols, and the lack of need for special apparatuses and for solvents [166].

7.5.4 Green Chemistry in Different Thermo-Responsive Polymers

Various thermo-responsive polymers can be highlighted from the perspective of green chemistry. While the use of cellulose derivatives as these polymers is considered greener than that of synthetic polymers, some aspects have hindered their application. Cellulose derivatives such as MC have been known to form thermo-responsive hydrogels with LCSTs of 60–80 °C, which are unsuitable for topical drug-delivery systems. Moreover, PNIPAAm-based thermo-responsive hydrogels are non-biodegradable and are characterised by the presence of hazardous amide-based substances when treated with strong acids; their biocompatibility has also been questionable. These reasons underlie their unsuitability for real drug-delivery systems.

Efforts have thus been underway to identify alternative greener polymers. Among these, poly(N-vinylcaprolactam) (PNVCL) is a promising candidate, given its biodegradability, aqueous solubility, non-adhesiveness, non-toxicity, and stability against hydrolysis [166, 170]. In addition to PNVCL, PF127-based thermo-responsive hydrogels are a viable alternative for drug-delivery systems. Not only do PF127-based hydrogels undergo sol–gel transformation at the body temperature, their biodegradability and non-cytotoxicity have been demonstrated. Some evidence has suggested that PF127 composites used for thermo-responsive hydrogels afforded a better drug-release profile and improved applicability [164].

7.6 Conclusion

Numerous topical drug-delivery systems are available, each with its advantages and disadvantages. Hydrogels represent an advanced system for topical drug delivery with the potential to replace conventional methods. Hydrogels tailored for responding to specific factors triggered during topical drug delivery have received much attention. While green chemistry with sustainable materials is the future of materials science, the development of functionalised hydrogels has not adopted it. In this context, cellulose derived from agricultural biomass represents an abundantly available, biodegradable, and renewable material that should be utilised in synthesising tailored hydrogels. Apart from sustainable raw materials, future research should focus on the synthesis of tailored hydrogels with greener solvents and less toxic chemical cross-linkers. Progress in developing novel, stimulus-sensitive hydrogels with sustainable, green resources ideal for practical use is envisioned to revolutionise the field of green chemistry.

Acknowledgments

The authors wish to gratefully acknowledge the financial support for this work from Geran Translasional UKM (TR-UKM).

References

1 Jain, K.K. (2020). Drug delivery systems. *Methods in Molecular Biology* 2059: 1–54. https://doi.org/10.1007/978-1-4939-9798-5_1.
2 Ueda, C.T., Shah, V.P., Derdzinski, K. et al. (2009). Topical and transdermal drug products. *Pharmacopeial Forum* 35 (3): 750–764.
3 Kaur, J., Kaur, J., Jaiswal, S., and Gupta, G.D. (2016). Recent advances in topical drug delivery system. *Indo American Journal of Pharmaceutical Research* 6 (7): 6353–6369.

4 Buhse, L., Kolinski, R., Westerberger, B. et al. (2005). Topical drug classification. *International Journal of Pharmaceutics* 295 (1–2): 101–112. https://doi.org/10.1016/j.ijpharm.2005.01.032.

5 Narasimha Murthy, S., and Shivakumar, H.N. (2010). Topical and transdermal drug delivery. In: *Handbook of Non-Invasive Drug Delivery Systems* (ed. V.S. Kulkarni), 1–36. Burlington, MA: William Andrew. https://doi.org/10.1016/b978-0-8155-2025-2.10001-0.

6 Benson, H.A.E., and Watkinson, A.C. (2012). *Transdermal and Topical Drug Delivery Principles and Practice*. Chichester: Wiley.

7 Li, C., Wang, J., Wang, Y. et al. (2019). Recent progress in drug delivery. *Acta Pharmaceutica Sinica B* 9 (6): 1145–1162. https://doi.org/10.1016/j.apsb.2019.08.003.

8 Ilochonwu, B.C., Urtti, A., Hennink, W.E., and Vermonden, T. (2020). Intravitreal hydrogels for sustained release of therapeutic proteins. *Journal of Controlled Release* 326: 419–441. https://doi.org/10.1016/j.jconrel.2020.07.031.

9 Zubik, K., Singhsa, P., Wang, Y., Manuspiya, H., and Narain, R. (2017). Thermo-responsive poly(n-isopropylacrylamide)- cellulose nanocrystals hybrid hydrogels for wound dressing. *Polymers* 9 (4): 1–17. https://doi.org/10.3390/polym9040119.

10 Park, S.H., Shin, H.S., and Park, S.N. (2018). A novel pH-responsive hydrogel based on carboxymethyl cellulose/2-hydroxyethyl acrylate for transdermal delivery of naringenin. *Carbohydrate Polymers* 200: 341–352. https://doi.org/10.1016/j.carbpol.2018.08.011.

11 Chang, C., He, M., Zhou, J., and Zhang, L. (2011). Swelling behaviors of pH- and salt-responsive cellulose-based hydrogels. *Macromolecules* 44 (6): 1642–1648. https://doi.org/10.1021/ma102801f.

12 Biyani, M.V., Foster, E.J., and Weder, C. (2013). Light-healable supramolecular nanocomposites based on modified cellulose nanocrystals. *ACS Macro Letters* 2 (3): 236–240. https://doi.org/10.1021/mz400059w.

13 Reddy, N.N., Mohan, Y.M., Varaprasad, K. et al. (2010). Magnetic and electric responsive hydrogel–magnetic nanocomposites for drug-delivery application. *Journal of Applied Polymer Science* 122 (2011): 1364–1375. https://doi.org/10.1002/app.34016.

14 Bikram, M., and West, J.L. (2008). Thermo-responsive systems for controlled drug delivery. *Expert Opinion on Drug Delivery* 5 (10): 1077–1091. https://doi.org/10.1517/17425247.5.10.1077.

15 Zhang, K., Xue, K., and Loh, X.J. (2021). Thermo-responsive hydrogels: from recent progress to biomedical applications. *Gels* 7 (3): 77. https://doi.org/10.3390/gels7030077.

16 Mayba, J.N., and Gooderham, M.J. (2018). A guide to topical vehicle formulations. *Journal of Cutaneous Medicine and Surgery* 22 (2): 207–212. https://doi.org/10.1177/1203475417743234.

17 Weiss, S.C. (2011). Conventional topical delivery systems. *Dermatologic Therapy* 24 (5): 471–476. https://doi.org/10.1111/j.1529-8019.2012.01458.x.

18 Tan, X., Feldman, S.R., Chang, J., and Balkrishnan, R. (2012). Topical drug delivery systems in dermatology: a review of patient adherence issues. *Expert Opinion on Drug Delivery* 9 (10): 1263–1271. https://doi.org/10.1517/17425247.2012.711756.

19 Fumelli, C., Marconi, A., Salvioli, S. et al. (2000). Carboxyfullerenes protect human keratinocytes from ultraviolet-B-induced apoptosis. *Journal of Investigative Dermatology* 115 (5): 835–841. https://doi.org/10.1046/j.1523-1747.2000.00140.x.

20 Mishra, A., Panola, R., Vyas, B., Marothia, D., and Kansara, H. (2014). Topical antibiotics and semisolid dosage forms. *International Journal of Pharmaceutical Erudition* 4 (3): 33–54.

21 Rosen, J., Landriscina, A., and Friedman, A.J. (2014). Principles and approaches for optimizing therapy with unique topical vehicles. *Journal of Drugs in Dermatology* 13 (12): 1431–1435.

22 Ricciatti-Sibbald, D., and Sibbald, R.G. (1989). Dermatologic vehicles. *Clinics in Dermatology* 7 (3): 11–24. https://doi.org/10.1016/0738-081X(89)90003-5.

23 Lionelli, G.T., and Lawrence, W.T. (2003). Wound dressings. *Surgical Clinics of North America* 83 (3): 617–638. https://doi.org/10.1016/S0039-6109(02)00192-5.

24 Kathe, K., and Kathpalia, H. (2017). Film forming systems for topical and transdermal drug delivery. *Asian Journal of Pharmaceutical Sciences* 12 (6): 487–497. https://doi.org/10.1016/j.ajps.2017.07.004.

25 Chang, R., Raw, A., Lionberger, R., and Yu, L. (2013). Generic development of topical dermatologic products: formulation development, process development, and testing of topical dermatologic products. *AAPS Journal* 15 (1): 41–52. https://doi.org/10.1208/s12248-012-9411-0.

26 Boateng, J.S., Matthews, K.H., Stevens, H.N.E., and Eccleston, G.M. (2008). Wound healing dressings and drug delivery systems: a review. *Journal of Pharmaceutical Sciences* 97 (8): 2892–2923. https://doi.org/10.1002/jps.21210.

27 Escobar-Chávez, J.J., López-Cervantes, M., Naïk, A. et al. (2006). Applications of thermo-reversible Pluronic F-127 gels in pharmaceutical formulations. *Journal of Pharmacy and Pharmaceutical Sciences* 9 (3): 339–358.

28 Brown, T.L., Petrovski, S., Chan, H.T., Angove, M.J., and Tucci, J. (2018). Semi-solid and solid dosage forms for the delivery of phage therapy to epithelia. *Pharmaceuticals* 11 (1): 1–12. https://doi.org/10.3390/ph11010026.

29 Pershing, L.K., Silver, B.S., Krueger, G.G., Shah, V.P., and Skelley, J.P. (1992). Feasibility of measuring the bioavailability of topical betamethasone dipropionate in commercial formulations using drug content in skin and a skin blanching bioassay. *Pharmaceutical Research* 9: 45–51. https://doi.org/10.1023/A:1018975626210.

30 Hernández, A.C., Awad, M.E., Meléndez, W. et al. (2019). Colloidal and thermal behaviors of some Venezuelan kaolin pastes for therapeutic applications. *Minerals* 9 (12): 18–22. https://doi.org/10.3390/min9120756.

31 Londhe, A., and Patil, Y. (2021). Critical review of Malahara – a topical dosage form. *World Journal of Pharmaceutical Research* 10 (5): 15. https://doi.org/10.20959/wjpr20215-20269.

32 Lustig, A., and Gefen, A. (2021). Three-dimensional shape-conformation performances of wound dressings tested in a robotic sacral pressure ulcer phantom. *International Wound Journal* 18 (5): 670–680. https://doi.org/10.1111/iwj.13569.

33 Chai, Q., Jiao, Y., and Yu, X. (2017). Hydrogels for biomedical applications: their characteristics and the mechanisms behind them. *Gels* 3 (1): 6. https://doi.org/10.3390/gels3010006.

34 Chatterjee, S., and Hui, P.C. (2018). Stimuli-responsive hydrogels: an interdisciplinary overview. In: *Hydrogels: Smart Materials for Biomedical Applications*, ch. 2 (ed. L. Popa, M.V. Ghica, and C.-E. Dinu-Pîrvu) London: IntechOpen. http://dx.doi.org/10.5772/57353.

35 Ahmed, E.M. (2015). Hydrogel: preparation, characterization, and applications: a review. *Journal of Advanced Research* 6 (2): 105–121. https://doi.org/10.1016/j.jare.2013.07.006.

36 Akhtar, M.F., Hanif, M., and Ranjha, N.M. (2016b). Methods of synthesis of hydrogels ... A review. *Saudi Pharmaceutical Journal* 24: 554–559. https://doi.org/10.1016/j.jsps.2015.03.022.

37 Subramanian, K., and Vijayakumar, V. (2015). Hydrogels: classification, synthesis, characterization, and applications. In: *Concise Encyclopedia of Biomedical Polymers and*

Polymeric Biomaterials (ed. M. Mishra), 3879–3892. Boca Raton, FL: CRC Press. https://doi.org/10.1081/E-EBPP-120049894.

38 Ullah, F., Othman, M.B.H., Javed, F., Ahmad, Z., and Akil, H.M. (2015). Classification, processing and application of hydrogels: a review. *Materials Science & Engineering C* 57: 414–433. https://doi.org/10.1016/j.msec.2015.07.053.

39 Akther, F., Little, P., Li, Z., Nguyen, N.-T., and Ta, H.T. (2020). Hydrogels as artificial matrices for cell seeding in microfluidic devices. *RSC Advances* 10 (71): 43682–43703. https://doi.org/10.1039/d0ra08566a.

40 Chang, C., and Zhang, L. (2011). Cellulose-based hydrogels: present status and application prospects. *Carbohydrate Polymers* 84: 40–53. https://doi.org/10.1016/j.carbpol.2010.12.023.

41 Ciolacu, D.E., and Suflet, D.M. (2018). Cellulose-based hydrogels for medical/pharmaceutical applications. In: *Biomass as Renewable Raw Material to Obtain Bioproducts of High-Tech Value*(ed. V. Popa, and I. Volf), 401–439. Amsterdam: Elsevier. https://doi.org/10.1016/B978-0-444-63774-1.00011-9.

42 Maitra, J., and Shukla, V.K. (2014). Cross-linking in hydrogels – a review. *American Journal of Polymer Science* 4 (2): 25–31. https://doi.org/10.5923/j.ajps.20140402.01.

43 EUR-Lex (2008). *Regulation (EC) No 1272/2008 of the European Parliament and of the Council of 16 December 2008 on classification, labelling and packaging of substances and mixtures, amending and repealing Directives 67/548/EEC and 1999/45/EC, and amending Regulation (EC).* https://eur-lex.europa.eu/legal-content/EN/TXT/?uri=celex%3A32008R1272.

44 Groupe Veritas (2015). Material safety data sheet: Epichlorohydrin. https://groupeveritas.com/MSDS/Epoxy%20Resin.pdf.

45 Rimdusit, S., Somsaeng, K., Kewsuwan, P., Jubsilp, C., and Tiptipako, S. (2012). Comparison of gamma radiation crosslinking and chemical crosslinking on properties of methylcellulose hydrogel. *Engineering Journal* 16 (4): 15–28. https://doi.org/10.4186/ej.2012.16.4.15.

46 George, J., Hsu, C.C., Nguyen, L.T., Ye, H., and Cui, Z. (2020). Neural tissue engineering with structured hydrogels in CNS models and therapies. *Biotechnology Advances* 42: 1–17.

47 ChemWatch (2011) 1,2,3,4-Butanetetracarboxylic acid. Material Safety Data Sheet. https://www.szabo-scandic.com/pub/media/product_data/msds/SAC/SAC-MSDS-SACSC-251564.pdf.

48 Jubail Chemical Industries Company (2020). Epichlorohydrin. https://nama.com.sa.

49 LabChem (2017). Material Safety Data Sheet: Citric acid. https://www.labchem.com/tools/msds/msds/LC13140.pdf.

50 Sigma-Aldrich (2021). Divinyl sulfone. https://www.sigmaaldrich.com/FR/en/substance/divinylsulfone1181577770.

51 Spectrum (2006). Material Safety Data Sheet: Divinyl sulfone. https://www.spectrumchemical.com/media/sds/3135V.PDF.

52 TCI America (2010). Material safety data sheet: Ethylene glycol diglycidyl ether. https://www.tcichemicals.com/US/en/p/E0342.

53 PubChem (2021). Ethylene glycol diglycidyl ether. Material Safety Data Sheet. https://pubchem.ncbi.nlm.nih.gov/compound/Ethylene-glycol-diglycidyl-ether.

54 Central Drug House (2008). Material Safety Data Sheet: Succinic Anhydride. https://www.cdhfinechemical.com/images/product/msds/37_1475932756_SuccinicAnhydride-CASNO-108-30-5-MSDS.pdf.

55 Sigma-Aldrich (2021). Succinic anhydride. https://www.sigmaaldrich.com/FR/en/substance/succinicanhydride10007108305.

56 Chen, Y.W., Hassan, S.H.B., Yahya, M., and Lee, H.V. (2018). Novel superabsorbent cellulose-based hydrogels: present status, synthesis, characterization, and application prospects. In: *Cellulose-Based Superabsorbent Hydrogels* (ed. M.I.H. Mondal), 1–41. Cham: Springer. https://doi.org/10.1007/978-3-319-76573-0_9-1.

57 Gupta, A.K., and Siddiqui, A.W. (2012). Environmental responsive hydrogels: a novel approach in drug delivery system. *Journal of Drug Delivery & Therapeutics* 2 (1): 81–88.

58 Peppas, N.A., and Hoffman, A.S. (2020). Hydrogels. In: *Biomaterials Science: An Introduction to Materials in Medicine*, (ed. W.R. Wagner, S. Sakiyama-Ebert, G. Zhang, and M.J. Yaszemski) 153–166. London: Academic Press. https://doi.org/10.1016/B978-0-12-816137-1.00014-3.

59 Garg, S., and Garg, A. (2016). Hydrogel: classification, properties, preparation and technical features. *Asian Journal of Biomaterial Research* 2 (6): 163–170.

60 Hoffman, A.S. (2012). Hydrogels for biomedical applications. *Advanced Drug Delivery Reviews* 64: 18–23.

61 Ma, J., Li, X., and Bao, Y. (2015). Advances in cellulose-based superabsorbent hydrogels. *RSC Advances* 5: 59745–59757. https://doi.org/10.1039/C5RA08522E.

62 Harrison, I.P., and Spada, F. (2018). Hydrogels for atopic dermatitis and wound management: a superior drug delivery vehicle. *Pharmaceutics* 10 (2): 71. https://doi.org/10.3390/pharmaceutics10020071.

63 Ghasemiyeh, P., and Mohammadi-Samani, S. (2019). Hydrogels as drug delivery systems; pros and cons. *Trends in Pharmaceutical Sciences* 5 (1): 7–24. https://doi.org/10.30476/TIPS.2019.81604.1002.

64 Canal, T., and Peppas, N.A. (1989). Correlation between mesh size and equilibrium degree of swelling of polymeric networks. *Journal of Biomedical Materials Research* 23 (10): 1183–1193. https://doi.org/10.1002/jbm.820231007.

65 Huang, H., Qi, X., Chen, Y., and Wu, Z. (2019). Thermo-sensitive hydrogels for delivering biotherapeutic molecules: a review. *Saudi Pharmaceutical Journal* 27 (7): 990–999. https://doi.org/10.1016/j.jsps.2019.08.001.

66 Mohammed, M.A., Syeda, J.T.M., Wasan, K.M., and Wasan, E.K. (2017). An overview of chitosan nanoparticles and its application in non-parenteral drug delivery. *Pharmaceutics* 9 (4): 53. https://doi.org/10.3390/pharmaceutics9040053.

67 Mason, M.N., Metters, A.T., Bowman, C.N., and Anseth, K.S. (2001). Predicting controlled-release behavior of degradable PLA-b-PEG-b-PLA hydrogels. *Macromolecules* 34 (13): 4630–4635. https://doi.org/10.1021/ma010025y.

68 Moynihan, H.J., Honey, M.S., and Peppas, N.A. (1986). Solute diffusion in swollen membranes. Part V: solute diffusion in poly(2-hydroxyethyl methacrylate). *Polymer Engineering & Science* 26 (17): 1180–1185. https://doi.org/10.1002/pen.760261703.

69 Hamidi, M., Azadi, A., and Rafiei, P. (2008). Hydrogel nanoparticles in drug delivery. *Advanced Drug Delivery Reviews* 60 (15): 1638–1649. https://doi.org/10.1016/j.addr.2008.08.002.

70 Peng, L., Zhang, H., Feng, A. et al. (2015). Electrochemical redox responsive supramolecular self-healing hydrogels based on host-guest interaction. *Polymer Chemistry* 6 (19): 3652–3659. https://doi.org/10.1039/c5py00296f.

71 Chandrawati, R. (2016). Enzyme-responsive polymer hydrogels for therapeutic delivery. *Experimental Biology and Medicine* 241 (9): 972–979. https://doi.org/10.1177/1535370216647186.

72 AL-Rajabi, M.M., and Haan, T.Y. (2021). Green synthesis of thermo-responsive hydrogel from oil palm empty fruit bunches cellulose for sustained drug delivery. *Polymers* 13 (13): 2153. https://doi.org/10.3390/polym13132153.

73 Bustamante-Torres, M., Romero-Fierro, D., Arcentelas, B. et al. (2021). Hydrogels classification according to the physical or chemical interactions and as stimuli-sensitive materials. *Gels* 7 (4): 1–25. https://doi.org/10.3390/gels7040182.

74 Danby, S.G., and Cork, M.J. (2018). pH in atopic dermatitis. *Current Problems in Dermatology (Switzerland)* 54: 95–107. https://doi.org/10.1159/000489523.

75 Van Gheluwe, L., Chourpa, I., Gaigne, C., and Munnier, E. (2021). Polymer-based smart drug delivery systems for skin application and demonstration of stimuli-responsiveness. *Polymers* 13 (8): 1285. https://doi.org/10.3390/polym13081285.

76 Wang, F., Zhang, Q., Li, X. et al. (2019). Redox-responsive blend hydrogel films based on carboxymethyl cellulose/chitosan microspheres as dual delivery carrier. *International Journal of Biological Macromolecules* 134: 413–421. https://doi.org/10.1016/j.ijbiomac.2019.05.049.

77 Aimetti, A.A., Tibbitt, M.W., and Anseth, K.S. (2009). Human neutrophil elastase responsive delivery from poly(ethylene glycol) hydrogels. *Biomacromolecules* 10 (6): 1484–1489. https://doi.org/10.1021/bm9000926.

78 AL-Rajabi, M.M., and Teow, Y.H. (2023). Synthesis of thermoresponsive composite hydrogel from Pluronic F127 reinforced by oil palm empty fruit bunches-extracted cellulose for silver sulfadiazine drug delivery. *Sustainable Chemistry and Pharmacy* 31: 100939. https://doi.org/10.1016/j.scp.2022.100939.

79 Boustta, M., Colombo, P.-E., Lenglet, S., Poujol, S., and Vert, M. (2014). Versatile UCST-based thermoresponsive hydrogels for loco-regional sustained drug delivery. *Journal of Controlled Release* 174 (1): 1–6. https://doi.org/10.1016/j.jconrel.2013.10.040.

80 Willcock, H., Lu, A., Hansell, C.F. et al. (2014). One-pot synthesis of responsive sulfobetaine nanoparticles by RAFT polymerisation: the effect of branching on the UCST cloud point. *Polymer Chemistry* 5 (3): 1023–1030. https://doi.org/10.1039/c3py00998j.

81 Mary, P., Bendejacq, D.D., Labeau, M.-P., and Dupuis, P. (2007). Reconciling low- and high-salt solution behavior of sulfobetaine polyzwitterions. *Journal of Physical Chemistry B* 111 (27): 7767–7777. https://doi.org/10.1021/jp071995b.

82 Seuring, J., and Agarwal, S. (2012). First example of a universal and cost-effective approach: polymers with tunable upper critical solution temperature in water and electrolyte solution. *Macromolecules* 45 (9): 3910–3918. https://doi.org/10.1021/ma300355k.

83 Miao, L., Zhang, M., Tu, Y., Lin, S., and Hu, J. (2019). Stimuli-responsive cellulose-based hydrogels. In: *Cellulose-Based Superabsorbent Hydrogels* (ed. M. Mondal), 269–308. Cham: Springer. https://doi.org/10.1007/978-3-319-77830-3_12.

84 Kohno, Y., Saita, S., Men, Y., Yuan, J., and Ohno, H. (2015). Thermoresponsive polyelectrolytes derived from ionic liquids. *Polymer Chemistry* 6 (12): 2163–2178. https://doi.org/10.1039/c4py01665c.

85 Chatterjee, S., and Hui, P.C. (2019). Review of stimuli-responsive polymers in drug delivery and textile application. *Molecules* 24 (14): 2547. https://doi.org/10.3390/molecules24142547.

86 Sponchioni, M., Capasso, U., and Moscatelli, D. (2019). Thermo-responsive polymers: applications of smart materials in drug delivery and tissue engineering. *Materials Science & Engineering C* 102: 589–605. https://doi.org/10.1016/j.msec.2019.04.069.

87 Qiu, Y., Hamilton, S.K., and Temenoff, J. (2011). Improving mechanical properties of injectable polymers and composites. In: *Injectable Biomaterials Science and Applications* (ed. B. Vernon), 61–91. Oxford: Woodhead Publishing. https://doi.org/10.1533/9780857091376.1.61.

88 Hsu, S.H., Leu, Y.-L., Hu, J.-W., and Fang, J.-Y. (2009). Physicochemical characterization and drug release of thermosensitive hydrogels composed of a hyaluronic acid/Pluronic f127 graft. *Chemical and Pharmaceutical Bulletin* 57 (5): 453–458. https://doi.org/10.1248/cpb.57.453.

89 Wang, W., Wat, E., Hui, P.C.L. et al. (2016). Dual-functional transdermal drug delivery system with controllable drug loading based on thermosensitive poloxamer hydrogel for atopic dermatitis treatment. *Scientific Reports* 6 (1): 24112. https://doi.org/10.1038/srep24112.

90 Derakhshandeh, K., Fashi, M., and Seifoleslami, S. (2010). Thermosensitive Pluronic® hydrogel: prolonged injectable formulation for drug abuse. *Drug Design, Development and Therapy* 4: 255–262. https://doi.org/10.2147/DDDT.S13289.

91 Sarwan, T., Kumar, P., Choonara, Y.E., and Pillay, V. (2020). Hybrid thermo-responsive polymer systems and their biomedical applications. *Frontiers in Materials* 7: 73. https://doi.org/10.3389/fmats.2020.00073.

92 Hammouda, B., Ho, D., and Kline, S. (2002). SANS from poly(ethylene oxide)/water systems. *Macromolecules* 35 (22): 8578–8585. https://doi.org/10.1021/ma011657n.

93 Khimani, M., Patel, H., Patel, V., Parekh, P., and Vekariya, R.L. (2020). Self-assembly of stimuli-responsive block copolymers in aqueous solutions: an overview. *Polymer Bulletin* 77 (11): 5783–5810. https://doi.org/10.1007/s00289-019-03046-w.

94 Kasiński, A., Zielińska-Pisklak, M., Oledzka, E., and Sobczak, M. (2020). Smart hydrogels – synthetic stimuli-responsive antitumor drug release systems. *International Journal of Nanomedicine* 15: 4541–4572. https://doi.org/10.2147/IJN.S248987.

95 Schild, H.G., and Tirrell, D.A. (1990). Microcalorimetric detection of lower critical solution temperatures in aqueous polymer solutions. *Journal of Physical Chemistry* 94 (10): 4352–4356. https://doi.org/10.1021/j100373a088.

96 Jeong, B., Kim, S.W., and Bae, Y.H. (2012). Thermosensitive sol-gel reversible hydrogels. *Advanced Drug Delivery Reviews* 64 (Suppl.): 154–162. https://doi.org/10.1016/j.addr.2012.09.012.

97 Saad, A., Mills, R., Wan, H. et al. (2020). Thermo-responsive adsorption-desorption of perfluoroorganics from water using PNIPAm hydrogels and pore functionalized membranes. *Journal of Membrane Science* 599: 117821. https://doi.org/10.1016/j.memsci.2020.117821.

98 Crespy, D., and Rossi, R.M. (2007). Temperature-responsive polymers with LCST in the physiological range and their applications in textiles. *Polymer International* 56: 1461–1468. https://doi.org/10.1002/pi.

99 Mokhtarinia, K., and Masaeli, E. (2020). Transiently thermally responsive surfaces: concepts for cell sheet engineering. *European Polymer Journal* 141: 110076. https://doi.org/10.1016/j.eurpolymj.2020.110076.

100 Tager, A.A., Safronov, A.P., Berezyuk, E.A., and Galaev, I.Y. (1994). Lower critical solution temperature and hydrophobic hydration in aqueous polymer solutions. *Colloid & Polymer Science* 272 (10): 1234–1239. https://doi.org/10.1007/BF00657775.

101 Yu, Z., Yi, J., and Tang, D. (2020). Poly (N-vinyl caprolactam), a thermal responsive support with tunable phase transition temperature for catalyst. *Separation and Purification Technology* 249: 116888. https://doi.org/10.1016/j.seppur.2020.116888.

102 Bonetti, L., De Nardo, L., and Farè, S. (2020). Thermo-responsive methylcellulose hydrogels: from design to applications as smart biomaterials. *Tissue Engineering Part B: Reviews* 27 (5): 486–513. https://doi.org/10.1089/ten.teb.2020.0202.

103 Gao, J., Haidar, G., Lu, X., and Hu, Z. (2001). Self-association of hydroxypropylcellulose in water. *Macromolecules* 34 (7): 2242–2247. https://doi.org/10.1021/ma001631g.

104 Yoshida, K., Horii, K., Saito, A., Takashima, A., and Nishio, I. (2017). Confinement effects on polymer dynamics: thermo-responsive behaviours of hydroxypropyl cellulose polymers in phospholipid-coated droplets (water-in-oil emulsion). *Polymers* 9 (12): 680. https://doi.org/10.3390/polym9120680.

105 Versypt, A.F. (2015). Modeling of controlled-release drug delivery from autocatalytically degrading polymer microspheres. Doctoral dissertation, University of Illinois.

106 Turabee, M.H., Jeong, T.H., Ramalingam, P., Kang, J.H., and Ko, Y.T. (2019). N,N,N-trimethyl chitosan embedded in situ Pluronic F127 hydrogel for the treatment of brain tumor. *Carbohydrate Polymers* 203: 302–309. https://doi.org/10.1016/j.carbpol.2018.09.065.

107 Fang, J.Y., Hsu, S.-H., Leu, Y.-L., and Hu, J.-W. (2009). Delivery of cisplatin from Pluronic co-polymer systems: liposome inclusion and alginate coupling. *Journal of Biomaterials Science, Polymer Edition* 20 (7–8): 1031–1047. https://doi.org/10.1163/156856209×444493.

108 Chen, C.C., Fang, C.-L., Al-Suwayeh, S.A., Leu, Y.-L., and Fang, J.-Y. (2011). Transdermal delivery of selegiline from alginate-Pluronic composite thermogels. *International Journal of Pharmaceutics* 415 (1–2): 119–128. https://doi.org/10.1016/j.ijpharm.2011.05.060.

109 Qiao, P., Niu, Q., Wang, Z., and Cao, D. (2010). Synthesis of thermosensitive micelles based on poly(N-isopropylacrylamide) and poly(l-alanine) for controlled release of adriamycin. *Chemical Engineering Journal* 159 (1–3): 257–263. https://doi.org/10.1016/j.cej.2010.02.035.

110 Chatterjee, S., Hui, P.C.-L., Kan, C.-W., and Wang, W. (2019). Dual-responsive (pH/temperature) Pluronic F-127 hydrogel drug delivery system for textile-based transdermal therapy. *Scientific Reports* 9 (11658): 1–13. https://doi.org/10.1038/s41598-019-48254-6.

111 Rezazadeh, M., Akbari, V., Amuaghae, E., and Emami, J. (2018). Preparation and characterization of an injectable thermosensitive hydrogel for simultaneous delivery of paclitaxel and doxorubicin. *Research in Pharmaceutical Sciences* 13 (3): 181–191. https://doi.org/10.4103/1735-5362.228918.

112 AL-Rajabi, M.M., and Haan, T.Y. (2021). Influence of vertical diffusion cell set-up on in vitro silver sulfadiazine drug release from thermo-responsive cellulose hydrogel. *Materials Science Forum* 1030: 19–26.

113 Anastas, P., and Eghbali, N. (2010). Green chemistry: principles and practice. *Chemical Society Reviews* 39 (1): 301–312. https://doi.org/10.1039/b918763b.

114 Welton, T. (2015). Solvents and sustainable chemistry. *Proceedings of the Royal Society A: Mathematical, Physical and Engineering Sciences* 471 (2183): 20150502. https://doi.org/10.1098/rspa.2015.0502.

115 Mohanty, A.K., Vivekanandhan, S., Pin, J.-M., and Misra, M. (2018). Composites from renewable and sustainable resources: challenges and innovations. *Science* 362 (6414): 536–542. https://doi.org/10.1126/science.aat9072.

116 Ciolacu, D. (2021). Sustainable hydrogels from renewable resources. In: *Sustainability of Biomass through Bio-based Chemistry* (ed. V. Popa), 161–189. Boca Raton, FL: CRC Press. https://doi.org/10.1201/9780429347993-6.

117 Tuyet Phan, M.T., Pham, L.N., Nguyen, L.H., and To, L.P. (2021). Investigation on synthesis of hydrogel starting from Vietnamese pineapple leaf waste-derived carboxymethylcellulose. *Journal of Analytical Methods in Chemistry* 2021: 6639964. https://doi.org/10.1155/2021/6639964.

118 Teow, Y., Ming, K., and Mohammad, A. (2018). Synthesis of cellulose hydrogel for copper (II) ions adsorption. *Journal of Environmental Chemical Engineering* 6 (4): 4588–4597. https://doi.org/10.1016/j.jece.2018.07.010.

119 Khozemy, E.E., Nasef, S.M., and Mahmoud, G.A. (2018). Synthesis and characterization of antimicrobial nanocomposite hydrogel based on wheat flour and poly (vinyl alcohol) using γ-irradiation. *Advances in Polymer Technology* 37 (8): 3252–3261. https://doi.org/10.1002/adv.22094.

120 Gyles, D.A., Castro, L.D., Silva, J.O.C., Jr, and Ribeiro-Costa, R.M. (2017). A review of the designs and prominent biomedical advances of natural and synthetic hydrogel formulations. *European Polymer Journal* 88: 373–392. https://doi.org/10.1016/j.eurpolymj.2017.01.027.

121 Farag, R.K., and Farag, A.A. (2018). Cellulose-based hydrogels as smart corrosion inhibitors. In: *Cellulose-Based Superabsorbent Hydrogels* (ed. M.I.H. Mondal), 1–36. Cham: Springer.

122 Li, J., Osada, Y., and Cooper-White, J. (2018). *Functional Hydrogels as Biomaterials*. Berlin: Springer.

123 Sharma, K., Sharma, V., and Kumar, V. (2019). Synthesis of hydrogels by modification of natural polysaccharides through radiation cross-linking polymerization for use in drug delivery. In: *Recombinant Protein Production in Yeast* (ed. V. Kumar, B. Chaudhary, V. Sharma, and K. Verma) 269–292. Cham: Springer. https://doi.org/10.1007/978-3-030-05770-1_8.

124 Onofrei, M., and Filimon, A. (2012). Cellulose-based hydrogels: designing concepts, properties, and perspectives for biomedical and environmental applications. In: *Polymer Science: Research Advances, Practical Applications and Educational Aspects* (ed. A. Méndez-Vilas and A. Solano). 108–120. Norristown, PA: Formatex Research Center.

125 del Valle, L.J., Díaz, A. and Puiggalí, J. (2017). Hydrogels for biomedical applications: cellulose, chitosan, and protein/peptide derivatives. *Gels* 3 (27): 1–28. https://doi.org/10.3390/gels3030027.

126 Li, Q., and Renneckar, S. (2011). Supramolecular structure characterization of molecularly thin cellulose I nanoparticles. *Biomacromolecules* 12 (3): 650–659.

127 Xi, J., Du, W., and Zhong, L. (2013). Probing the interaction between cellulose and cellulase with a nanomechanical sensor. In: *Cellulose*, ch. 7. (ed. T.G.B. Van de Ven), London: IntechOpen. https://doi.org/10.5772/50285.

128 Demitri, C., Madaghiele, M., Raucci, M.G., Sannino, A., and Ambrosio, L. (2018). Investigating the structure-related properties of cellulose-based superabsorbent hydrogels. In: *Hydrogels: Smart Materials for Biomedical Applications*, (ed. L. Popa, M.V. Ghica, and C. Dinu-Pirvu), 1–27. London: IntechOpen. https://doi.org/10.5772/intechopen.80986.

129 Pinho, E., and Soares, G. (2018). Functionalization of cotton cellulose for improved wound healing. *Journal of Materials Chemistry B* 6: 1887–1898. https://doi.org/10.1039/C8TB00052B.

130 Vlaia, L., Coneac, G., Olariu, I., Vlaia, V., and Lupuleasa, D. (2016). Cellulose-derivatives-based hydrogels as vehicles for dermal and transdermal drug delivery. In: *Emerging Concepts in Analysis and Applications of Hydrogels*, ch. 7. (ed. Majee, S.B.), London: IntechOpen. https://doi.org/10.5772/63953.

131 Sannino, A., Demitri, C., and Madaghiele, M. (2009). Biodegradable cellulose-based hydrogels: design and applications. *Materials* 2 (2): 353–373. https://doi.org/10.3390/ma2020353.

132 Hiorth, M., Nilsen, S., and Tho, I. (2014). Bioadhesive mini-tablets for vaginal drug delivery. *Pharmaceutics* 6: 494–511. https://doi.org/10.3390/pharmaceutics6030494.

133 Karim, M.Z., Chowdhury, Z.Z., Hamid, S.B.A., and Ali, M.E. (2014). Statistical optimization for acid hydrolysis of microcrystalline cellulose and its physiochemical characterization by using metal ion catalyst. *Materials* 7 (10): 6982–6999. https://doi.org/10.3390/ma7106982.

134 AL-Rajabi, M., and Teow, Y.H. (2021). Effect of sodium hydroxide/urea/deionised water solution ratio on the solubility of oil palm empty fruit bunches extracted biocellulose. *ASM Science Journal* 16: 1–6. https://doi.org/10.32802/asmscj.

135 Thakur, V.K., Thakur, M.K., and Kessler, M.R. (2017). *Handbook of Composites from Renewable Materials, Volume 1: Structure and Chemistry*. Chichester: Wiley.

136 Athirah, W.N., Haan, T.Y., and Mohammad, A.W. (2018). Sustainable approach in palm oil industry-green synthesis of palm oil mill effluent based graphene sand composite (P-GSC) for aerobic palm oil mill effluent treatment. *Jurnal Kejuruteraan SI* 1 (7): 11–20. https://doi.org/10.17576/jkukm-2018-si1.

137 Dungani, R., Karina, M., Sulaeman, S.A., Hermawan, D., and Hadiyane, A. (2016). Agricultural waste fibers towards sustainability and advanced utilization: a review. *Asian Journal of Plant Sciences* 15 (1–2): 42–55. https://doi.org/10.3923/ajps.2016.42.55.

138 Trache, D., Hussin, M.H., Chuin, C.T.H. et al. (2016). Microcrystalline cellulose: isolation, characterization and bio-composites application – a review. *International Journal of Biological Macromolecules* 93: 789–804. https://doi.org/10.1016/j.ijbiomac.2016.09.056.

139 Ng, P., Chia, C.H., Zakaria, S. et al. (2015). Preparation of cellulose hydrogel from oil palm empty fruit bunch fibers cellulose. *Polymer Research Journal* 9 (4): 449–459.

140 Wong, L.C. (2020) Optimisation of biomass-based cellulose hydrogels for topical drug delivery. International Conference of Pharmacy and Health Sciences 2020, 27–28 October.

141 Salleh, K.M., Zakaria, S., Sajab, M.S., Gan, S., and Kaco, H. (2019). Superabsorbent hydrogel from oil palm empty fruit bunch cellulose and sodium carboxymethylcellulose. *International Journal of Biological Macromolecules* 131: 50–59. https://doi.org/10.1016/j.ijbiomac.2019.03.028.

142 Ibrahim, M.M., Abd-Eladl, M., and Abou-Baker, N.H. (2015). Lignocellulosic biomass for the preparation of cellulose-based hydrogel and its use for optimizing water resources in agriculture. *Journal of Applied Polymer Science* 42652: 1–12. https://doi.org/10.1002/app.42652.

143 Abou-Baker, N.H., Ouis, M., Abd-Eladi, M., and Ibrahim, M.M. (2020). Transformation of lignocellulosic biomass to cellulose-based hydrogel and agriglass to improve beans yield. *Waste and Biomass Valorization* 11 (7): 3537–3551. https://doi.org/10.1007/s12649-019-00699-6.

144 George, D., Sheriffa, K.M.M., and Uma, B.P. (2018). Sugarcane bagasse (SCB) based pristine cellulose hydrogel for delivery of grape pomace polyphenol drug. *Waste and Biomass Valorization* 11: 851–860. https://doi.org/10.1007/s12649-018-0487-3.

145 Selvakumaran, N., Azwani, M., and Lazim, M. (2016). Preparation and characterization of oil palm frond based cellulose hydrogel and its swelling properties. *AIP Conference Proceedings*, 1784: 030018. https://doi.org/10.1063/1.4966756.

146 Tovar-Carrillo, K.L., Tagaya, M., and Kobayashi, T. (2013). Bamboo fibers elaborating cellulose hydrogel films for medical applications. *Journal of Materials Science and Chemical Engineering* 2013: 7–12.

147 Zhou, H., Zhu, H., Yang, X., et al. (2015). Temperature/pH sensitive cellulose-based hydrogel: synthesis, characterization, loading, and release of model drugs for potential oral drug delivery. *BioResources* 10 (1): 760–771.

148 Li, J., Wan, C., Lu, Y., and Sun, Q. (2014). Fabrication of cellulose aerogel from wheat straw with strong absorptive capacity. *Frontiers of Agricultural Science and Engineering* 1 (1): 46–52. https://doi.org/10.15302/J-FASE-2014004.

149 Kaco, H., Zakaria, S., Razali, N.F. et al. (2014). Properties of cellulose hydrogel from kenaf core prepared via pre-cooled dissolving method. *Sains Malaysiana* 43 (8): 1221–1229.

150 Zhang, M., Yin, Q., Ji, X. et al. (2020). High and fast adsorption of Cd(II) and Pb(II) ions from aqueous solutions by a waste biomass based hydrogel. *Scientific Reports* 10 (1): 3285. https://doi.org/10.1038/s41598-020-60160-w.

151 Park, H., Kim, M.H., Yoon, Y.I., and Park, W.H. (2017). One-pot synthesis of injectable methylcellulose hydrogel containing calcium phosphate nanoparticles. *Carbohydrate Polymers* 157: 775–783. https://doi.org/10.1016/j.carbpol.2016.10.055.

152 Tomšič, M., Prossnigg, F., and Glatter, O. (2008). A thermoreversible double gel: characterization of a methylcellulose and κ-carrageenan mixed system in water by SAXS, DSC and rheology. *Journal of Colloid and Interface Science* 322 (1): 41–50. https://doi.org/10.1016/j.jcis.2008.03.013.

153 Tang, Y., Wang, X., Li, Y. et al. (2010). Production and characterisation of novel injectable chitosan/ methylcellulose/salt blend hydrogels with potential application as tissue engineering scaffolds. *Carbohydrate Polymers* 82 (3): 833–841. https://doi.org/10.1016/j.carbpol.2010.06.003.

154 Liu, Z., and Yao, P. (2015). Injectable thermo-responsive hydrogel composed of xanthan gum and methylcellulose double networks with shear-thinning property. *Carbohydrate Polymers* 132: 490–498. https://doi.org/10.1016/j.carbpol.2015.06.013.

155 Zhang, Y., Gao, C., Li, X. et al. (2014). Thermosensitive methyl cellulose-based injectable hydrogels for post-operation anti-adhesion. *Carbohydrate Polymers* 101 (1): 171–178. https://doi.org/10.1016/j.carbpol.2013.09.001.

156 Wang, T., Chen, L., Shen, T., and Wu, D. (2016). Preparation and properties of a novel thermo-sensitive hydrogel based on chitosan/hydroxypropyl methylcellulose/glycerol. *International Journal of Biological Macromolecules* 93: 775–782. https://doi.org/10.1016/j.ijbiomac.2016.09.038.

157 Mahmoudian, M., and Ganji, F. (2017). Vancomycin-loaded HPMC microparticles embedded within injectable thermosensitive chitosan hydrogels. *Progress in Biomaterials* 6 (1): 49–56. https://doi.org/10.1007/s40204-017-0066-x.

158 Nayak, A., Babla, H., Han, T., and Das, D.B. (2016). Lidocaine carboxymethylcellulose with gelatine co-polymer hydrogel delivery by combined microneedle and ultrasound. *Drug Delivery* 23 (2): 668–679. https://doi.org/10.3109/10717544.2014.935985.

159 Kim, J.K., Won, Y.-W., Lim, K.S., and Kim, Y.-H. (2012). Low-molecular-weight methylcellulose-based thermo-reversible gel/Pluronic micelle combination system for local and sustained docetaxel delivery. *Pharmaceutical Research* 29 (2): 525–534. https://doi.org/10.1007/s11095-011-0581-8.

160 Nasir, F., Iqbal, Z., Khan, A. et al. (2014). Development and evaluation of Pluronic- and methylcellulose-based thermoreversible drug delivery system for insulin. *Drug Development and Industrial Pharmacy* 40 (11): 1503–1508. https://doi.org/10.3109/03639045.2013.831441.

161 Orasugh, J.T., Sarkar, G., Saha, N.R. et al. (2019). Effect of cellulose nanocrystals on the performance of drug loaded in situ gelling thermo-responsive ophthalmic formulations. *International Journal of Biological Macromolecules* 124: 235–245. https://doi.org/10.1016/j.ijbiomac.2018.11.217.

162 Liu, W., Zhang, B., Lu, W.W. et al. (2004). A rapid temperature-responsive sol-gel reversible poly(N- isopropylacrylamide)-g-methylcellulose copolymer hydrogel. *Biomaterials* 25 (15): 3005–3012. https://doi.org/10.1016/j.biomaterials.2003.09.077.

163 Dutta, S., Samanta, P., and Dhara, D. (2016). Temperature, pH and redox responsive cellulose based hydrogels for protein delivery. *International Journal of Biological Macromolecules* 87: 92–100. https://doi.org/10.1016/j.ijbiomac.2016.02.042.

164 Wang, W.Y., Hui, P.C.L., Wat, E. et al. (2016). Enhanced transdermal permeability via constructing the porous structure of poloxamer-based hydrogel. *Polymers* 8 (11): 406. https://doi.org/10.3390/polym8110406.

165 Chatterjee, S., Hui, P.C.L., and Kan, C.W. (2018). Thermoresponsive hydrogels and their biomedical applications: special insight into their applications in textile based transdermal therapy. *Polymers* 10 (480): 1–25. https://doi.org/10.3390/polym10050480.

166 Qiu, X., and Hu, S. (2013). 'Smart' materials based on cellulose: a review of the preparations, properties, and applications. *Materials* 6: 738–781. https://doi.org/10.3390/ma6030738.

167 Sanna, R., Fortunati, E., Alzari, V. et al. (2013). Poly(N-vinylcaprolactam) nanocomposites containing nanocrystalline cellulose: a green approach to thermoresponsive hydrogels. *Cellulose* 20 (5): 2393–2402. https://doi.org/10.1007/s10570-013-9988-1.

168 Bodratti, A.M., and Alexandridis, P. (2018). Formulation of poloxamers for drug delivery. *Journal of Functional Biomaterials* 9 (1): 11. https://doi.org/10.3390/jfb9010011.

169 Schmolka, I.R. (1972). Artificial skin I. Preparation and properties of Pluronic F-127 gels for treatment of burns. *Journal of Biomedical Materials Research* 6: 571–582.

170 Zheng, Z., Zhang, L., Ling, Y., and Tang, H. (2019). Triblock copolymers containing UCST polypeptide and poly(propylene glycol): synthesis, thermoresponsive properties, and modification of PVA hydrogel. *European Polymer Journal* 115: 244–250. https://doi.org/10.1016/j.eurpolymj.2019.03.034.

8

Advanced Approaches in Green Univariate Spectrophotometric Methods

Hayam M. Lotfy[1], *Sarah S. Saleh*[2], *Yasmin Rostom*[3], *Reem H. Obaydo*[4], *and Dina A. Ahmed*[1]

[1] *Pharmaceutical Chemistry Department, Faculty of Pharmacy, Future University in Egypt, Street Teseen, New Cairo 1, Cairo Governorate, 11835, Egypt*
[2] *Analytical Chemistry Department, Faculty of Pharmacy, October University for modern sciences and Arts (MSA), 26 July Mehwar Road intersection with Wahat Road, 6th October City, Giza, 11787, Egypt*
[3] *Analytical Chemistry Department, Faculty of Pharmacy, Cairo University, Kasr El-Aini Street, Cairo 11562, Egypt*
[4] *Analytical and Food Chemistry Department, Faculty of Pharmacy, Ebla Private University, 22743, Idlib, Syria*

CONTENTS

8.1 Green Analytical Chemistry Overview

The birth of green analytical chemistry (GAC) was in 1999, when Anastasa published his paper about the rules for developing eco-friendly analytical methods instead of traditional ones depending on using benign solvents and reducing all steps, materials, and waste during analytical procedures that harm the environment [1]. In 2013, Gałuszka elaborated the principles of GAC, which include reducing the amount of solvent, energy, waste, analytical steps, and sample handling by using and developing new methods in all fields [2].

In the pharmaceutical field, many analytical processes must be carried out to ensure the quality of the final pharmaceutical preparations, such as the process of verifying the purity of raw material, analysis of active pharmaceutical ingredients, dissolution tests, purity determination, stability-indicating assays, impurities profiling, as well as analysing the trace amount of the drug in environmental and food studies. These analytical methods adopted during different pharmaceutical stages are either new analytical methods developed by researchers, after their efficiency and analytical ability have been validated according to the rules in the guidelines set by official organisations like the International Council for Harmonisation of Technical Requirements for Pharmaceuticals for Human Use (ICH)

Sustainable Approaches in Pharmaceutical Sciences, First Edition. Edited by Kamal Shah, Durgesh Nandini Chauhan, and Nagendra Singh Chauhan.

or the US Food and Drug Administration (FDA), or analytical ones mentioned in the different pharmacopoeias in Europe, the UK, and the United States.

8.2 Strategies for Greening Spectrophotometric Methods

Regarding the analytical apparatus used in the pharmaceutical field, we can consider some of it as green analytical equipment, because its analysis protocol agrees with the principles of GAC. Analysis with spectrophotometric equipment is considered a reasonable example here. However, during the development of advanced univariate spectrophotometric methods, having a balance between excellent performance parameters (analytical figures of merit) and the requirements of the GAC principles must be considered. The spectrophotometric analytical method is considered green because the strategy of this technique is fully compatible with the 12 principles of GAC, as shown in Table 8.1.

Table 8.1 Application of green analytical chemistry (GAC) principles in spectrophotometric pharmaceutical analysis.

No.	GAC principle	Univariate spectrophotometric analysis for pharmaceutical preparations
1)	Avoiding sample treatment using direct analytical techniques	Samples do not require any chemical treatment, only dissolving and diluting in appropriate solvents
2)	Minimum sample size and number	Less than 1 mL of the sample is enough to complete the analysis, and the scanned spectra samples can be stored for many analysis steps to be undertaken
3)	In situ measurements	Applications of in situ spectrophotometric analysis in the pharmaceutical field are still limited to extracting the dissolution profiles of pharmaceutical preparations [6]
4)	Combining analytical procedures to minimise energy and reagents	Spectrophotometric techniques can be combined with others such as high-performance liquid chromatography or programs like MATLAB to emphasise the capability of the analysis and save energy and solvent
5)	Miniaturisation [7]	Low consumption of reagents, solvents, and energy
6)	Derivatisation	No need for derivatisation
7)	Decreasing waste	The amount of waste for a single sample is less than 1 mL
8)	Multianalyte method [8]	Multicomponent analysis can be achieved, and each component can be analysed by a single measurement
9)	Energy consumption	Less than 0.1 kWh of energy consumption for a single analysis
10)	Using renewable solvent	Distilled water and ethanol derived from renewable resources are widely used [9]
11)	Replacing or eliminating toxic reagents	The most used solvents are considered safe
12)	Analyst safety	Ultraviolet-blocking safety glasses should be used and hazardous solvent should be avoided

From the point of view of GAC, the development of advanced spectrophotometric methods differs only in the type of solvent used to complete the analysis as well as the amount of waste generated by the method. Using meagre amounts of renewable and environmentally friendly solvents is the main key to increase the method's greenness. Fortunately, the criteria for selecting an appropriate solvent for spectroscopic analysis are its ability to dissolve the drug, stability, safety, availability, and low cost. Therefore, the use of distilled water and ethanol as solvents is very common, and both are green solvents, as well as green methanol or bio-methanol being produced during biological pathways [3, 4], making it a safe, biodegradable, and environmentally friendly solvent [5]. More than 90% of the solvents used are considered green (water, ethanol, and methanol), which increases the importance of spectrophotometric methods since they are safe, green, and used in very small quantities compared to other analytical methods such as chromatography. Several greenness metrics were developed for the assessment of analytical methods, as shown in Table 8.2.

Absorption spectroscopy is a commonly applied tool for quantitation of analytes of interest in different matrices. The basic principle of molecular spectroscopy is the interaction between light and molecules. In normal conditions, the molecule acquires the ground state, which is its lowest electronic energy state.

In the ultraviolet–visible (UV–VIS) region, the interaction of a molecule with photons leads to the displacement of the valence electrons due to absorbing energy. The transition of the molecule goes from its ground state energy level (Eg) to an excited state energy level (Es) [15]. The Beer–Lambert law can be expressed as A = abc, where A is absorbance, a is absorptivity, b is path length, and c is concentration. The law entails that absorbance will be equal to zero (A = 0) at zero concentration (c = 0) at path length = 1 [16]. Thus, the linear regression equation relating absorbance (y-axis) and concentration (x-axis) is expressed as y = mx + b, where m and b represent the slope and the intercept values, respectively. The Beer–Lambert law is valid for describing dilute solutions only. Deviations from the law occur at higher concentrations and linearity is lost. Spectrophotometric analysis transcends molecular spectroscopic techniques because of its simplicity, precision, accuracy, and low time consumption [17].

Spectrophotometric analysis of multicomponents should be applied where the components' spectra show partial or complete overlapping. Determination of the multicomponents can be done using simultaneous equations to calculate the concentration of each component; otherwise, resolution of the overlapped spectra into individual ones is carried out [18]. To resolve the spectrum of one component from a mixture, the spectrum of the second component should be subtracted from the total solution absorbance. The methods are classified according to the extent of overlapping into resolving either severely overlapped or partially overlapped spectra [19]. The spectrophotometric techniques developed in the last few decades for the analysis of multicomponent mixtures are classified based on manipulation steps into four windows [20]:

- Window 1: Spectrophotometric methods based on zero-order (D^0) absorption spectra.
- Window 2: Spectrophotometric methods based on derivative spectra.
- Window 3: Spectrophotometric methods based on ratio spectra.
- Window 4: Spectrophotometric methods manipulating ratio spectra.

Table 8.2 A summary of greenness metrics for assessment of analytical sample preparation.

Greenness metric	Merits	Demerits	Pictogram	References
AGREE (Analytical GREEnness) is an algorithmic green assessment tool that incorporates the 12 green analytical chemistry (GAC) principles	Covers all the principles of GAC Explainable Rich with green information Gives qualitative and quantitative assessment Comprehensive input Simplicity and clarity of output	Type of hazard is not clear Need special software to calculate Does not consider analytical efficiency	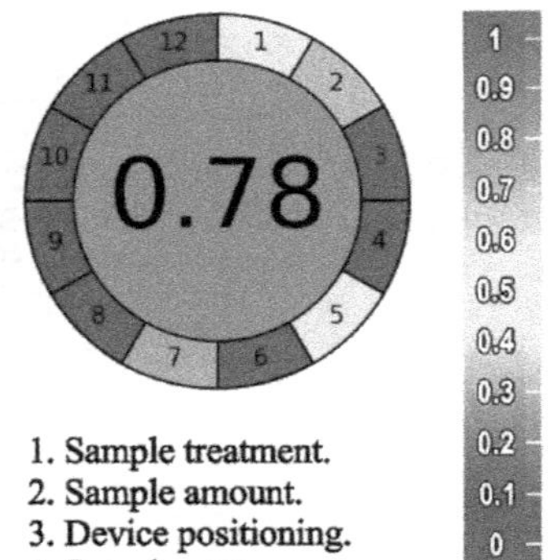 1. Sample treatment. 2. Sample amount. 3. Device positioning. 4. Sample prep. 5. Automated and miniaturized methods. 6. Derivatization. 7. Generation of a volume of waste. 9. Use of energy. 10. Renewable source of reagents. 11. Toxicity of reagents. 12. Safety of the Operator.	[10]

GAPI (Green Analytical Procedure Index) is based on the analytical methods and procedures used as well as providing the main information related to the prepared samples, solvents used, and instrumentation types	Semi-quantitative and qualitative tool Used to compare the greenness of two methods Does not need any special software to calculate the result Evaluates the analytical method in different steps	Information about hazards is not available Structure of the hazardous solvent is not clear Absence of sensitivity Analytical efficacy is not included	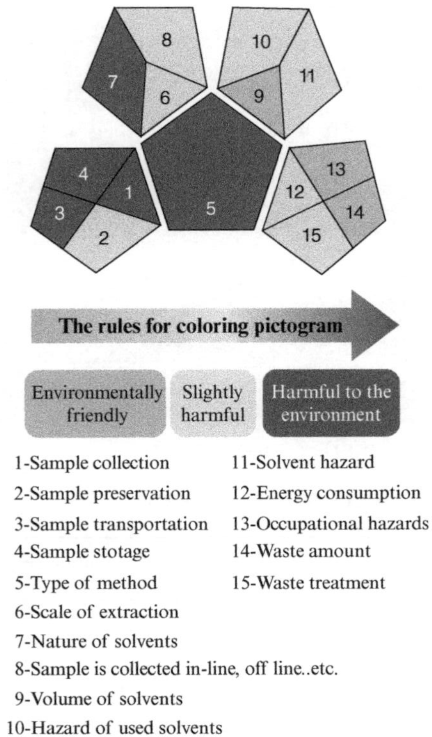	[11]

(Continued)

Table 8.2 (Continued)

Greenness metric	Merits	Demerits	Pictogram	References
AES (Analytical Eco-Scale) depends on calculating the penalty points (PPs) for reagents, hazards, energy, and waste, and then subtracting the total from 100 The outcome is graded on a scale and the greening of the analytical method is classified into four types	Semi-quantitative tool Easy to use Does not require any software to calculate the results Used to compare the greenness of two methods Gives information about the hazard and amount of the solvent used Evaluates the analytical method in different steps	No information provided in the final result (if the final score is 42, this does not reveal whether the waste is high or the solvent is hazardous) Not all of the GAC principles are relied on to calculate the final score Analytical efficacy is not ensured	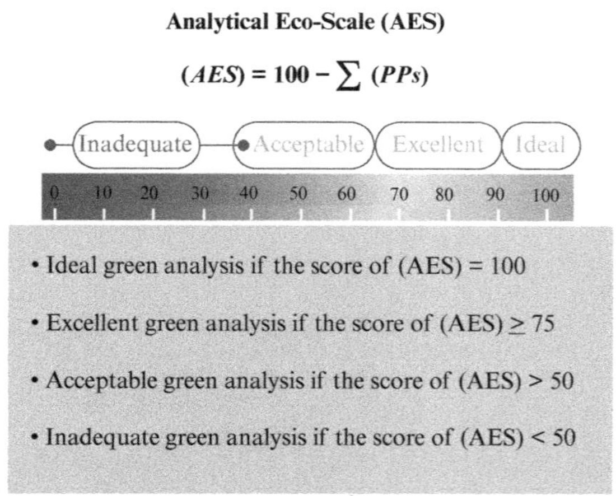	[12]

AGP (Assessment of Green Profile) is a semi-quantitative greenness tool depending on five risk potentials: health, safety, environmental, energy, and waste Outcomes are in pictogram form divided into five parts, each one coloured based on the sort of environmental effect	Semi-quantitative and qualitative tool Does not require any special software to calculate the result Easily compares two or more analytical greenness methods	Information about sample preparation is not available Structure of the hazardous solvent is not clear Absence of sensitivity Analytical efficacy is not ensured 12 principles of GAC are omitted	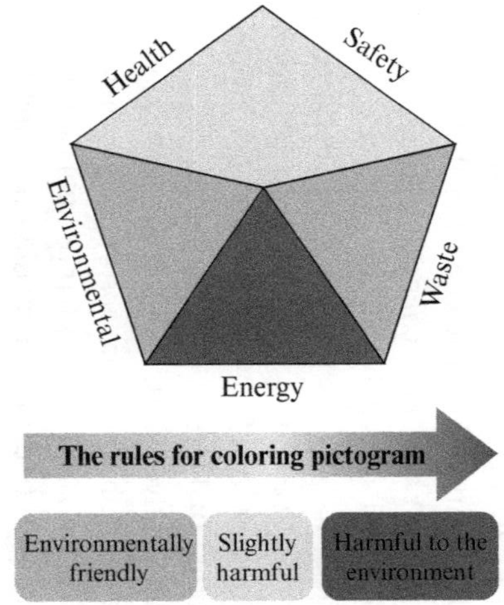	[13]
NEMI (National Environmental Methods Index) is considered as the first and oldest greenness tool and depends on getting information about where a sample fits in the following categories: • PBT (persistent, bio-cumulative, toxic) • Hazard • Corrosive • Waste amount	Easy to understand Qualitative tool Gives a general idea about the method's greenness in just one look No special software required	Does not cover all green analytical principles Not quantitative Little and general information Search for each chemical used in official lists is time consuming Energy use	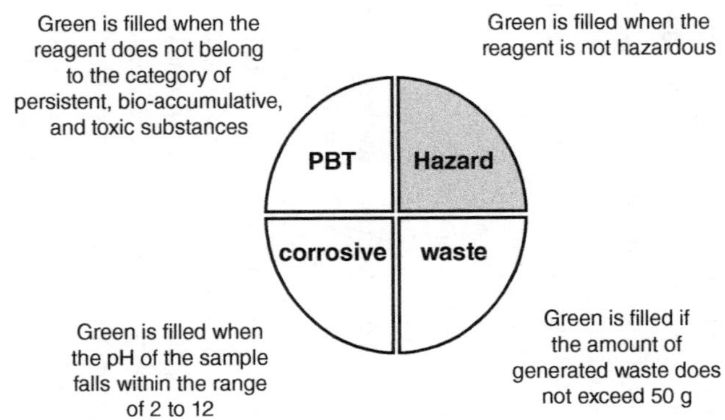	[14]

8.2.1 Window 1

Group A includes methods that depend on calculating the zero-order absorbance difference (ΔA) between two points (dual wavelength), which is in direct proportion to the concentration of the component of interest. This group includes dual wavelength (DW) [21–26] and induced dual wavelength (IDW) [23–25, 27, 28], where the interfering substance shown (ΔA) does not equal zero. Therefore, the absorbance of the interfering substance(s) will be equalised using a factor at the two selected wavelengths, while the component of interest will show different absorbance. The dual wavelength resolution technique (DWRT) is coupled with DW or IDW for solving the overlapping spectra [18, 23]. The absorption correction method (ACM) is applied for partial overlapped spectra where the absorbance of Y can be related at the two wavelengths using a factor and the X concentration can be estimated by subtracting the Y absorbance from the total absorbance [25, 29–31]. The H-point standard addition method (HPSAM) [32–34] is based on constructing a plot between the absorbance of mixed components at two assigned wavelengths against the concentration of X (the added analyte), where the difference in absorbance for Y (the interfering substance) equals zero, and thus two straight lines are plotted that have a common point.

Group B includes methods based on the isoabsorptive point, which is the point at which several components can act as a single one due to exhibiting equal absorptivity values, as in the conventional isoabsorptive point method [35–37]. The absorbance subtraction (AS) method is similar to the ACM, but using the isoabsorptive point regression equation for the calculation of each component concentration [38–41]. The advanced absorbance subtraction (AAS) method depends on calculating ΔA (the absorbance difference) between two selected wavelengths including the isoabsorptive point [22, 42–44]. The Q-absorbance ratio method [45–47] and the absorbance ratio method (ARM) [35, 48] apply an absorbance ratio at two selected wavelengths (isoabsorptive point and λ_{max} of one of the two components), followed by the application of mathematical equations. The absorptivity factor (a-factor) method is applied where there is a huge difference between the absorptivity of the components, so that the isoabsorptive point does not occur naturally but it is created by the a-factor [49–51].

Group C includes methods based on area under the curve (AUC-D^0) measurements instead of absorbance [52–54]. The AUC correction method (AUC-CM) was introduced to calculate the AUC of overlapped spectra instead of Cramer's rule [55, 56].

Group D includes methods that depend on mathematical calculation of an absorbance vector such as Vierordt's method, which uses two simultaneous equations and a bivariate procedure [57–59]. The spectrum subtraction method depends on the fact that the light absorption of a sample solution is additive [Mixture $(X + Y) - X = Y$]. It usually represents a complementary step to other methods [60–63].

8.2.2 Window 2

Derivative spectrophotometry follows the same laws as D^0 absorption, where the derivative amplitude is additive and dependent on the analyte concentration. The direct derivative method, in its four orders, has been performed for the quantitation of several drug mixtures and in the presence of impurities or degradation products. In spectroscopy software, numerous functions are utilised to achieve preliminary overlapped peak separation and noise filtering. The derivative function with different orders, such as the first derivative, second derivative, third derivative and fourth derivative, is commonly used for this purpose. On the other hand, Fourier self-deconvolution is not as widespread, but it serves as a simple mathematical technique to effectively eliminate broadening in the resulting spectra [37, 64–66]. Amplitude subtraction (PS) and its modification, modified amplitude subtraction (MPS), act by recording the mixture's peak of amplitude and then calculating the postulated value at the same wavelength. The drugs' maximum amplitude can be obtained after subtraction from the mixture's amplitude [24, 67, 68]. The amplitude correction (P-correction) method uses an experimentally tested factor [67–69]. The amplitude summation method (A-Sum) is similar to PS but shows an isoabsorptive point shift in derivative order rather than zero order [20, 36, 40, 62, 70]. The compensated area under the curve (CAUC) method involves calculating AUC for a mixture containing X + Y against different concentrations of pure drug positioned in the reference cell [71].

The coupling of successive derivative subtraction with constant multiplication (SDS-CM) is a resolution technique for mixtures showing severely overlapped D^0 spectra but partially overlapped derivative spectra [70, 72, 73]. Derivative transformation (DT) is applied by converting the derivative spectrum into its original zero-order spectrum using the normalised spectrum of the analyte [44, 61, 74, 75].

8.2.3 Window 3

Group A includes methods that depend on subtracting the ratio spectra amplitudes. The ratio subtraction method (RSM) deals with the extension of the D^0 spectrum of one component over the other(s) where the constant is measured [76–79]. The extended ratio subtraction method (EXRSM) is applied as a complementary step to RSM for quantitation of the less extended component, followed by the modified method to determine the extended one [78, 80–84]. Another modification to RSM is simultaneous ratio subtraction (SRS) [39, 85], where the two components (extended and less extended) can be recovered using their corresponding divisors.

Group B includes methods calculating the difference of ratio spectra amplitudes. The ratio difference spectrophotometric method (RDSM) [21, 78, 86–88] depends on calculating the difference in amplitudes at two selected wavelengths on the ratio spectra, which is directly proportional to the concentration of the component of interest, and not sensitive to the interfering component. The constant centre spectrophotometric method (CCSM) [89–93] includes two complementary steps, namely constant calculation via the amplitude difference method followed by constant multiplication where the components are determined via zero-order curves at λ_{max}. CCSM can be coupled with spectrum subtraction [43]. The amplitude centre method [94] is a progressive manipulating approach applied to a ternary mixture using a single divisor.

Group C includes methods that deal with modulation of ratio spectra amplitudes. Amplitude modulation method (AMM) [39, 40]. Differential amplitude modulation [75] uses the normalised spectrum of the divisor where one component is more extended than the other in the presence of the isoabsorptive point [41, 95–99]. Its extension, advanced amplitude modulation (AAM) [22, 23, 42], is appropriate for binary mixtures with severely overlapping spectra showing the isoabsorptive point either by merging the CCSM with the AMM or calculating the difference between the isosbestic point and another point in the wavelength. Induced amplitude modulation (IAM) [23, 27, 68] can be applied in case of a lack of isoabsorptive point or for an isoabsorptive point with low absorptivity, in addition to the concentration value method that modulates the amplitude to concentration [75].

Group D includes methods featuring a geometrical representation of ratio spectra amplitudes. The geometrical amplitude modulation method (GAM) [100, 101] offers a geometric representation of the standard addition effect of X on the binary mixture response of X + Y and shows it as a regression equation using a normalised divisor spectrum. A modification of this method, geometrically induced amplitude modulation (GIAM) [100, 101], was introduced for a binary mixture of X + Y showing absorptivities with large differences, and hence the zero spectrum exhibits no isoabsorptive point. The ratio H-point standard addition method (RHSAM) is an extension to the conventional HPSAM [100, 102, 103] using a normalised divisor spectrum.

8.2.4 Window 4

Ratio spectra are further manipulated using different approaches to estimate each component independently. Salinas et al. [21, 104, 105] introduced derivative ratio spectrophotometry (DR), which is done by calculating the derivative of the ratio spectrum of the mixture, which will be independent on the divisor. Double divisor-ratio spectra derivative spectrophotometry (DD-DR) is applied for ternary mixtures using a first derivative single divisor of two components [55, 106, 107]. Zero-crossing derivative spectrophotometry [66, 108] is applied for ternary mixtures where the derivative spectrum is measured at the zero crossing of the interferants. Simultaneous derivative ratio spectrophotometry (S^1DD) [103, 109] is transformed into simultaneous mode by adjusting with amplitude modulation. Mean centring [78, 110–112] involves data transformation of ratio spectra by calculating the geometric mean rather than the arithmetic mean to obtain a less biased central tendency. The pure component contribution algorithm (PCCA) is applied for extraction of components' signals [113–115] by coding a function that eliminates interfering components' signals using the tool of mean centring. Continuous wavelet transform (CWT) is a powerful signal processing tool close to Fourier transform in addition to trigonometric functions (sine and cosine) systems [116–120].

8.3 Advanced Ultraviolet Spectrophotometric Methods and Outcomes

8.3.1 Window 1

8.3.1.1 Absorptivity Centring [121

- *Spectral features*: D^0 spectra of binary mixture, X + Y, with partially (POS) or completely overlapped spectra (COS) intersecting in an isoabsorptive point (λ_{iso}).
- *Manipulation tools*: Preparation of a factorised spectrum employing the spectrophotometer's software via the division of the D_o spectrum of Y in its range of linearity by the recorded absorbance at the isoabsorptive point. The absorptivity factor between the two chosen wavelengths is calculated using the average of various concentrations of Y in its pure form (in POS) or via substitution in computing a statistical equation expressing the absorbance difference's relationship at two selected wavelengths $[\lambda_{iso}/\lambda_2]$, where X shows equal absorbance values versus the recorded absorbance at λ_{iso} for different concentrations of pure Y (in COS).

- *Mathematical resolution*: The actual absorbance of Y at λ_{iso} can be obtained either via multiplying the recorded absorbance by the absorptivity factor or via substituting in computing a regression equation expressing the absorbance difference's relationship at two selected wavelengths $[\lambda_{iso}/\lambda_2]$, where X shows equal absorbance values versus the recorded absorbance at λ_{iso} for different concentrations of pure Y (in COS). The calculated authentic absorbance of Y at λ_{iso} is multiplied by the previously prepared factorised spectrum of Y to obtain the D^0 of Y. Finally, subtracting the recovered D^0 spectrum of Y from the corresponding gross mixture's D^0 spectrum via the spectrum subtraction method will successfully recover the D^0 spectrum of X.
- *Quantification*: Applying the regression equations demonstrating the D^0 spectral absorbance of pure X and Y at their λ_{max} against the corresponding concentrations will enable the amount of each component in the mixture to be calculated.

8.3.1.2 Response Correlation [42]

- *Spectral features*: D^0 spectra of the binary mixture, X + Y, with POS or COS intersecting in an isoabsorptive point (λ_{iso}) as A_{iso} and retained as P_{iso} in the ratio spectra using pure X as the divisor.
- *Manipulation tools*: A statistical equation (SE_1) representing the relationship between the absorbance difference at two selected wavelengths $[\lambda_{iso}/\lambda_2]$, where X shows equal absorbance values versus the recorded absorbance at λ_{iso} for various amounts of pure Y. A second statistical equation (SE_2) expressing the relation between A_{iso} and P_{iso} (using X′ as a divisor) for various pure Y concentrations.
- *Mathematical resolution*: The actual Y absorbance at λ_{iso} could be obtained for analysing the mixture by substituting the recorded absorbance difference in SE_1. The mixture's amplitude corresponding to Y at λ_{iso} is calculated via SE_2. The noted amplitude at λ_{iso} of the mixture's ratio spectrum is subtracted from the calculated mixture's amplitude corresponding to Y to obtain the constant value of X in the mixture. For each mixture, multiplication of the calculated amplitude corresponding to X by the divisor (X′) will successfully obtain the D^0 spectrum of X, while subtraction of the D^0 spectrum X from the gross D^0 spectrum of the mixture will attain the D^0 spectrum of Y.
- *Quantification*: Exploiting the corresponding regression equation representing the absorbance values of pure X or Y in their D^0 spectra at their λ_{max} against their parallel amounts enables calculation of the X and Y concentrations in laboratory mixtures.

8.3.1.3 Advanced Balance Point-Spectrum Subtraction via Zero-Order Spectrum [42]

- *Spectral features*: D^0 spectra of the binary mixture, X + Y, with POS or COS where X is the minor component.
- *Manipulation tools*: A value for the pure Y response ratio (RR), which is the absorbance ratio (AR) at two maximum points. A statistical equation is representative of the direct relationship of the mixture's RR at the two selected wavelengths, λ_1, λ_2, of each different mixture's spectrum versus the corresponding pure X concentration, C_X.
- *Resolution*: Analysing a mix of two components, X and Y, the method observes the change in the AR of the mixture (on subtracting various concentrations of the pure minor component X above and below that expected to be in the mixture solution. The difference spectrum for each concentration of X is calculated using spectrum subtraction. As C_X

increases, the characteristic equilibrium point of the combination gradually approaches the pure drug (Y) and finally accords with the mixture's RR of the pure drug (Y). The balance point can be identified using the computed statistical equation as discussed previously, where C_X in the combination is equivalent to the subtracted C_X.
- *Quantification*: Calculating the minor component X's concentration in the combination is achieved by substituting the calculated value of RR for pure Y at the two selected wavelengths in the linear regression equation.

8.3.1.4 Induced Concentration Subtraction [27]

- *Spectral features*: D^0 spectra of the binary mixture, X + Y, with POS or COS where Y is more extended than X.
- *Manipulation tools*: Two absorptivity factors, the first ($F_{\lambda F}$) expressing the proportion of the absorptivity of X to the absorptivity of Y at λ_F. The second factor (F_Y) is calculated as the mean ratio between the two values of absorbance [abs (λ_F)/abs of various concentrations of pure Y].
- *Resolution*: For analysing the mixture comprising X and Y, multiplication of the formerly determined F_Y of Y by the recorded mixture's absorbance at λ_1 could successfully attain component Y's absorbance alone.
- *Quantification*: C_Y in the mixture is assessed by the unified regression equation (URE), expressing a direct relationship between the absorbance of pure Y at λ_F versus its corresponding concentrations, while the total mixture's concentration could be computed by the replacement of the recorded absorbance (A_m) in the URE at λ_F. Finally, the Y concentration is subtracted from the complete mixture, and the outcome will represent $F_{\lambda F}C_X$, which accordingly will be multiplied by $1/F_{\lambda F}$ to get the amount of component X in the mixture.

8.3.2 Window 2

8.3.2.1 Advanced Balance Point-Spectrum Subtraction via Derivative Spectrum [42]

- *Spectral features*: Two analytes, X and Y, in their binary mixture with POS or COS where X is a minor component in any derivative order, D^n.
- *Manipulation tools*: A value of the pure Y RR, which is the AR at the selected two amplitude maxima. A statistical equation is generated that demonstrates the linear relationship of the mixture's RR at the two selected wavelengths, λ_1, λ_2, of each different mixture's spectrum versus the corresponding pure X concentration, C_X.
- *Resolution*: To analyse a mixture of two components, X and Y, the method monitors the variation in AR for the mixture (on subtracting various concentrations of the pure minor component X above and below that expected to be in the mixture solution. The difference spectrum for each concentration of X is calculated using spectrum subtraction. As C_X increases, the characteristic equilibrium point gradually approaches the pure drug (Y) and finally accords with the mixture's RR of pure drug (Y). The equilibrium point can be identified using the computed statistical equation as discussed previously, where C_X in the combination is equivalent to the subtracted C_X.
- *Quantification*: Calculating the minor component X's concentration in the combination is achieved by substituting the calculated value of the RR of pure Y at the two wavelengths in the linear regression equation.

8.3.2.2 Relative Absorptivity Distribution via Amplitude at the Isosbestic Point [122]

- *Spectral features*: Derivative (D_n) of two analytes (X and Y) where n = 1 or 2 or 3 or 4 in their binary mixture with POS where D^0 intersects in an isoabsorptive point (λ_{iso}) as A_{iso} and is retained in the derivative spectra as P_{iso}.
- *Manipulation tools*: A factorised derivative spectrum is prepared by dividing the derivative spectrum of pure Y across the wavelengths (any concentration that fits into the Beer–Lambert law) by the recorded amplitude at the isosbestic point. The amplitude factor [$P_{\lambda iso}/P_{\lambda s}$] of pure Y is the mean of the proportion of the amplitude at the isosbestic point λ_{iso} to that at λ_s for all amounts of pure Y within the Beer–Lambert law. It should be computed where there is no impact of X at λ_s.
- *Resolution*: For analysing the mixture comprising X and Y in definite derivative mode D_n, the real amplitude of Y in the mixture at the isosbestic point is calculated via multiplying the computed amplitude factor of pure Y by its recorded amplitude at λ_s, followed by multiplying this real value by the factorised derivative that was previously prepared to obtain the YD_n spectrum in the combination. In order to extract the D_n of X (the co-formulated component), the extracted D_n of Y is subtracted from the D_n of the comparable mixture via the spectrophotometer software.
- *Quantification*: The concentrations of X and Y in the mixture can be successfully assessed by substituting the amplitude value of pure Y at the applied D_n in the regression equation.

8.3.3 Window 3

8.3.3.1 Ratio Difference-Isosbestic Points [44]

- *Spectral features*: Ratio spectra of Z component in a triplet mixture, X + Y + Z, with POS where D^0 intersects in two isoabsorptive points (λ_{iso}) as A_{iso} and is retained in the ratio spectra as P_{iso} using X′ in its normalised spectrum form as a divisor.
- *Manipulation tools*: None.
- *Resolution*: For analysing Z in the X + Y + Z mixture, amplitude differences P_1 and P_2 of the ratio spectrum at the two chosen wavelengths, λ_{iso1} and λ_{iso2}, of X and Y correspond to component Z alone where the amplitude values of X and Y are equal at these wavelengths.
- *Quantification*: Calculation of the Z concentration is achieved by means of the regression equation demonstrating the direct relationship of the ratio spectral amplitudes' differences using normalised X as a divisor at the two selected wavelengths versus the parallel concentration of drug Z.

8.3.3.2 Amplitude Modulation Coupled with Induced Ratio Difference [44]

- *Spectral features*: Ratio spectra of the X + Y + Z mixture with POS with an extension of Z over the other components using Z′ in its normalised spectral form as a divisor.
- *Manipulation tools*: Calculation of equality factor F_Y of pure Y/Z′ at the selected wavelengths which is the amplitude values' ratio of various pure Y concentrations at λ_1 and λ_2 wavelengths, where the interfering substance's amplitude is not equalised at those two wavelengths.
- *Resolution*: For analysing the X + Y + Z mixture, the constant of Z (corresponding to its concentration) is recorded at the extended region and deducted from the subsequent gross ratio spectrum to attain the ratio spectrum of the binary mixture. The proposed

method, induced ratio difference (IRD), can be performed for the extracted ratio spectrum of the binary mixture with severely overlapped spectra at λ_1 and λ_2 wavelengths, where the interfering substance's amplitudes at the selected wavelengths are equalised using the calculated F_Y of pure Y.

- *Quantification*: Calculation of the Z concentration is achieved by plotting the recorded amplitudes of the ratio spectra of Z at the extended region that represent their recorded concentration against their actual corresponding concentrations, and is represented by a regression equation. The concentration of X is obtained by substitution in the regression equation, found from the plot of the difference of amplitude values of the ratio spectra of X at the two selected wavelengths ($\Delta P = P_1 - F_Y P_2$) versus the corresponding concentrations of X. Meanwhile, the concentration of Y is achieved via similar steps using the pure equality factor of X at the two selected wavelengths (F_X).

8.3.3.3 Absorptivity Centring via Factorised Ratio Spectrum [101]

- *Spectral features*: Ratio spectra of binary analytes X and Y, with COS where no equalised interfering components' absorbance values all over the spectrum wavelength range are present in the D^0.
- *Manipulation tools*: The factorised ratio spectrum of Y′, $FSR_{\Delta P}$, is obtained by dividing the pure Y ratio spectrum (using X′ as a divisor) by the amplitude values' difference at the chosen wavelengths for component Y.
- *Mathematical resolution*: For analysing X and Y, by multiplying the difference of amplitudes at two chosen wavelengths by Y's factorised ratio spectrum, the Y/X ratio spectrum can be attained. By subtracting the extracted Y ratio spectrum from its parallel mixture's ratio spectrum, the ratio spectrum of the constant X can be regained and its value can be recorded.
- *Quantification*: Via substituting in subsequent regression equations demonstrating the Y amplitude at the maxima and the constant amplitude of X against their parallel amounts.

8.3.3.4 Ratio Subtraction Coupled with Unified Constant Subtraction [84]

- *Spectral features*: Ratio spectra of binary analytes, X and Y, with POS and Y extended over X.
- *Manipulation tools*: Standard analyte Y as a divisor (Y′).
- *Mathematical resolution*: For analysing the X + Y mixture, the method begins with the ratio subtraction method to get the spectrum of X then, using X′ as a divisor, subtract one value that represents the constant. The curve obtained is multiplied after subtraction of X′ (the divisor) to finally attain the original D^0 spectrum of Y.
- *Quantification*: The concentrations of X and Y are computed from the subsequent regression equations (attained by plotting X or Y's absorbance at its λ_{max} against the corresponding concentrations).

8.3.3.5 Constant Extraction [123]

- *Spectral features*: Ratio spectra of two components (X and Y) in a mixture with COS or POS with very poor extension.
- *Manipulation tools*: Using one of the standard analytes (X or Y) as a divisor, a statistical equation demonstrates the direct proportionality of the difference in amplitude values

(ΔP) for the ratio spectra of various amounts of pure Y using a definite amount of component X′ as a divisor at λ_1 and λ_2 versus their corresponding hypothesised amplitude summation ($P_{Postulated\ Sum}$).

- *Mathematical resolution*: For analysis of the binary mixture, X and Y, the amplitude difference for each mixture is substituted in the previously constructed statistical equation to get the postulated sum. The constant X/X′ is obtained using the difference between the recorded difference and the calculated postulated difference. The found constant will be multiplied by the divisor X′ to successfully attain the D^0 of X. The D^0 of Y can be obtained via subtracting the recovered X from the gross D^0 spectrum of the mixture.
- *Quantification*: The concentrations of X and Y are obtained via regression equations demonstrating the direct proportionality of the absorbance at their maxima versus their corresponding concentrations.

8.3.3.6 Advanced Amplitude Centring [124]

This novel approach can be used for analysing X, Y, and Z in their ternary mixture with POS or COS via a regression equation constructed at a single wavelength (λ_1).

8.3.3.3.1 Approach for Partially Overlapping Spectra

- *Spectral features*: Ratio spectra of ternary analytes, X, Y, and Z, with POS with an extension of Z over the other components, while X and Y are COS at λ_1 and λ_2 wavelengths.
- *Manipulation tools*: Standard analyte Z as a divisor (Z′). The equality factor of pure Y (F_Y) at λ_1 and λ_2 is calculated. The regression equation of X represents ΔP ($P_1 - F_YP_2$) against P_1 at λ_1 of pure component X (the amplitude difference of Y does not equal zero).
- *Mathematical resolution*: For analysing the X + Y + Z mixture at λ_1 and λ_2, first the Z component is quantified using the mixture's ratio spectrum by means of the divisor Z′. At the extended region, the Z/Z′ constant can be successfully determined, then subtracted via spectrum subtraction from the gross spectrum of the mixture to obtain the X + Y mixture at λ_1 and λ_2. The hypothesised amplitude value ($P_{postulated}$) of component X in the mixture of X + Y can be computed via the formerly calculated regression equation using the mixture's ΔP at λ_1 and λ_2. The recorded amplitude of the mixture's ratio spectrum ($P_{recorded}$) at λ_1 is subtracted from the $P_{postulated}$ of X at the same wavelength (λ_1) to attain the $P_{postulated}$ of component Y.
- *Quantification*: Calculation of the components' concentrations is achieved using the regression equation indicating the relation between the ratio spectra's amplitudes of X/Z′ or Y/Z′ or Z/Z′ at λ_1 and their corresponding concentrations.

8.3.3.3.2 Approach for Completely Overlapping Spectra

- *Spectral features*: Ratio spectra of ternary analytes, X, Y, and Z, with COS at two chosen wavelengths, λ_1 and λ_2.
- *Manipulation tools*: Standard analyte (Z) as a divisor. SE_1 represents the linear relationship between the ΔP of different concentrations of the pure Y ratio spectra at λ_1 and λ_2 using Z′ as a divisor versus the corresponding ratio amplitude at λ_1 where X shows equal amplitude at λ_1 and λ_2. SE_2 expresses the direct proportionality between the ΔP of the ratio spectra of various concentrations of pure X at λ_1 and λ_3 using Z′ as a divisor versus the corresponding amplitudes at λ_1 where Y shows equal amplitude at λ_1 and λ_3.

- *Mathematical resolution*: For the ratio spectrum of the X + Y + Z mixture, use Z as a divisor where Z/Z′ is constant while X/Z′ shows matched amplitudes at two selected wavelengths (λ_1 and λ_2). By amplitude difference calculation at λ_1 and λ_2 (for Y) or λ_1 and λ_3 (for X), the constant Z/Z′ will be eliminated together with any instrumental error or noise from an interfering analyte. The postulated amplitude value of Y/Z′ ($P_{postulated}$) and X/Z′ ($P_{postulated}$) at λ_1 is calculated via SE_1 and SE_2, respectively. Subtraction of the recorded amplitude of the mixture's ratio spectrum ($P_{recorded}$) at λ_1 and the calculated $P_{postulated}$ of X and Y at λ_1 will successfully attain the constant value, Z/Z′.
- *Quantification*: Calculation of the components' concentrations is performed using the regression equation demonstrating the relationship between X or Y or Z's centred amplitudes of ratio spectra using Z as a divisor at the single wavelength, λ_1, and the subsequent concentrations.

8.3.3.7 Dual Amplitude Difference [61]

- *Spectral features*: Ratio spectra of ternary analytes, X, Y, and Z, with COS at the selected λ_1 and λ_2 wavelengths.
- Manipulation tools: Standard analyte (Y) as a divisor. The factorised ratio spectrum (FRS_Z) of Z is formulated using the spectrophotometer software with Y′ as a divisor. The attained ratio spectrum is divided by the computed amplitude difference's numerical value where component X has equalised amplitudes at these wavelengths.
- *Mathematical resolution*: The ratio spectrum of X, Y, and Z is divided by the D^0 of Y′. Via calculating the difference in amplitude (ΔP) between λ_1 and λ_2 it will correspond to Z only, while Y is set off since it is a straight line; Y/Y′ and X/Y′ have an amplitude difference equal to zero. The ratio spectrum of Z is gained by multiplying the numerical value of the ΔP of the mixture and FRS_Z. Multiply the ratio spectrum $\left(\frac{Z}{Y'}\right)$ by Y′ (the divisor) so that the parent (D^0) of Z will be refurbished. Then determination of Z in the mixture can be accomplished through individual plotted regression equations linking the absorbance at λ_{max} to its concentrations. The D^0 of Z is subtracted from the mixture's gross D^0 to regain the binary mixture's D^0 spectrum composed of X and Y. These measures could be replicated to quantify X and Y in the mixture.
- *Quantification*: Then quantification of the analyte (X, Y, or Z) in the mixture could be accomplished through individual plotted regression equations linking the absorbance at λ_{max} to its corresponding concentrations.

8.3.3.8 Induced Dual Amplitude Difference Coupled with Spectrum Subtraction [125]

- *Spectral features*: Ratio spectra of the ternary mixture, X, Y, and Z, with POS where Z is extended using λ_1 and λ_2 and there is a significant amplitude difference for component X. Meanwhile for component Y the differences of amplitude at the two wavelengths are not equalised.
- *Manipulation tools*: Standard analyte Z as a divisor. For different concentrations of the pure ratio spectra of Y, the recorded amplitudes at λ_1 and λ_2 and the equality factor (F_Y) are calculated. F_Y is the mean of the amplitude ratios at λ_1 and λ_2 (where F $\geq$1 or $\leq$1). The factorised ratio spectrum of X (FRS_X) is prepared using the spectrophotometer software using Z′ as a divisor. The attained ratio spectrum is divided by the computed numerical value of the amplitude difference after multiplying by the calculated equality factor of pure Y.

- *Mathematical resolution*: For analysing the X + Y + Z mixture at λ_1 and λ_2, first the Z component is quantified utilising the mixture's ratio spectrum with Z as a divisor (Z′). At the extended region, the Z/Z′ constant can be successfully determined then subtracted via spectrum subtraction from the gross spectrum of the mixture to obtain the X + Y mixture at λ_1 and λ_2 and the amplitude difference (ΔP) between λ_1 and λ_2 is calculated. The ratio spectrum of X/Z′ is gained by multiplying the mixture's induced numerical value of ΔP (next to multiplication by pure Y's equality factor) and FRS_Z. The above ratio spectrum $\left(\frac{X}{Z'}\right)$ is multiplied by Z′ (the divisor) so that the parent (D^0) of X will be renovated. For resolving the component Y, the spectrum subtraction method is used to deduct the obtained ratio spectrum of X from the gross spectrum of the mixture.
- *Quantification*: The analyte (X, Y, or Z) could be accomplished through individual plotted regression equations linking the amplitude at maxima to its corresponding concentrations.

8.3.4 Window 4

8.3.4.1 Unlimited Derivative Ratio [126]

- *Spectral features*: The ternary mixture's derivative ratio spectra at any derivative order, first, second, third, or fourth, with COS using Z as a divisor. For determination of X in the mixture, two wavelengths are chosen, λ_1 and λ_2, where a significant amplitude difference is observed for X while an unequal amplitude difference is observed between those two wavelengths for Y.
- *Manipulation tools*: Standard analyte Z as a divisor. The equality factor (F_Y) of the recorded amplitudes of the pure ratio spectra of various amounts of Y at λ_1 and λ_2 is calculated, which is the average amplitude ratio at λ_1 and λ_2 (where F $\geq$1 or $\leq$1).
- *Mathematical resolution*: When analysing the X + Y + Z mixture, for X quantitation two wavelengths, λ_1 and λ_2, are selected in the ternary mixture's derivative ratio spectra using Z as a divisor. In the derivative ratio spectra of pure X, the amplitude difference between λ_1 and λ_2 is recorded and manipulated using the previously designed equality factor of Y. Thus, in the derivative ratio spectra of the mixture, the amplitude difference is reliant on X only and is independent of Y or Z.
- *Quantification*: The amounts of X are computed exploiting the regression equation, found by the derivative ratio spectra's amplitude difference (ΔP) of the X plot using Z as a divisor at two wavelengths (ΔP, after multiplying one of them by the designed equality factor of pure Y) against the corresponding concentrations of X. Calculation of the Y concentration exploits the same procedure after calculating pure X's equality factor, F_X, at the two selected wavelengths for Y.

8.3.4.2 Factorised Derivative Ratio Coupled with Spectrum Subtraction [127]

- *Spectral features*: Novelty method using the ternary mixture's derivative ratio spectra at any derivative order, first, second, third, or fourth, with COS using Z as a divisor.
- *Manipulation tools*: Standard analyte Z as a divisor. The factorisation of the derivative ratio of X ($FDDS_X$) is performed by the division of the X derivative of the ratio spectra (DD_1) by its measured peak amplitude value [$P_{X\,(\lambda\ \text{zero point})} = 1$].
- *Mathematical resolution*: For analysing the X + Y + Z mixture, for X determination two wavelengths, λ_1 and λ_2, are selected in the derivative ratio spectra of the X + Y + Z

mixture using the divisor Z′. Eliminating the Z contribution is achieved by applying a suitable order where the Z/Z′ constant is terminated by derivatisation. A suitable wavelength is chosen where the X/Z′ spectrum shows a positive or negative peak at the zero point of Y/Z′ (either by zero contribution point or zero crossing). The X/Z′ derivative ratio spectrum can be calculated by multiplying the previously calculated $FDDS_X$ for X by the recorded amplitude of the mixture at the selected wavelength ($\lambda_{zero\ point}$). The derivative ratio spectrum of Y (Y/Z′) is attained by its subtraction from the derivative ratio spectrum of the ternary mixture. Similarly, the derivative ratio spectrum of Z is attained via similar steps using X or Y as a divisor.

- *Quantification*: Calculation of X or Y or Z concentrations in the mixture is attained via regression equations showing the linear relation of the pure target component's amplitudes against the conforming concentrations using the quantified graphical illustration P_{maxima} to zero ($P_{max\text{-}zero}$), P_{minima} to zero ($P_{min\text{-}zero}$) or P_{maxima} to P_{minima} ($P_{max\text{-}min}$).

8.3.4.3 Factorised Derivative Ratio Null Contribution [125]

- *Spectral features*: A novelty method using the ternary mixture's derivative ratio spectra at any derivative order, first, second, third, or fourth, with COS using Y as a divisor.
- *Manipulation tools*: Standard analyte Y as a divisor. The factorisation of the derivative ratio of X ($FDDS_X$) is performed by dividing the X derivative of the ratio spectra (DD_1) by its calculated amplitude summation value [$P_{X\,(\lambda\ zero\ point)} = 1$] at specified wavelengths, λ_1 and λ_2, where the derivative spectrum of $\frac{X}{Y'}$ has a contribution with two amplitude values (either equal or unequal).
- *Mathematical resolution*: In the ternary mixture, component Z is determined in the derivative ratio spectra using the divisor Y′ via choosing two wavelengths at which the ratio spectrum of $\frac{Z}{Y'}$ displays the highest and lowest amplitudes while the spectrum of X has two minima of $\frac{X}{Y'}$ with equalised amplitudes. Thus, the maximum amplitude of $\frac{Z}{Y'}$ is reduced by the minima of $\frac{X}{Y'}$ at λ_1. On the other hand, the minimum amplitude of $\frac{Z}{Y'}$ is furnished by the minima of $\frac{X}{Y'}$ at λ_2. The reduced and furnished effects are equal since $PX1 = PX2$, maintaining the sum of the maximum and minimum amplitudes of similar Pz with null impact of P_X (no effect of X). Thus, the amplitudes when summed for Z / Y' at the chosen wavelengths will show dependence on the amounts of the Z component only, ignoring the sign. In general, this method could be employed if there are two minima of $\frac{X}{Y'}$ that acquire unequal amplitudes where the Fx equality factor is in the range $F \geq 1$ or ≤ 1 of pure X in case $Px1 \neq Px2$, where F_X is the ratio of peak amplitudes of different X concentrations at the specified minima and maxima. The computation of the Z/Y′ derivative ratio spectrum is done through multiplying the amplitude summation at the specified pair of wavelengths by the formerly prepared factorised derivative ratio spectrum of Z, $FDDS_Z$.
- *Quantification*: Computation of the Z concentration is attained via substituting in the regression equation indicating the direct proportionality of the amplitude summation values at the chosen wavelength pair against the corresponding concentrations of Z.

Requirements, advantages and limitations of the proposed advanced spectrophotometric methods are displayed in Table 8.3.

Applications of advanced univariate spectrophotometric applications in various matrices, including specifications for all the analytical methods discussed here, are listed in Table 8.4.

Table 8.3 Limitations and outcomes of advanced univariate spectrophotometric methods.

Methods and spectrum	Limitations and outcomes
Window 1	
Absorptivity centring 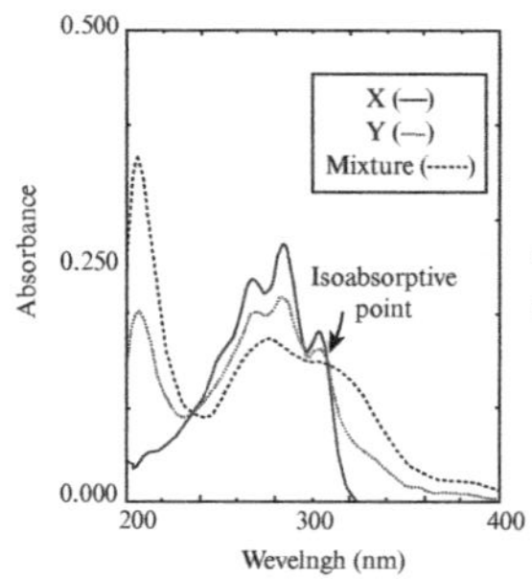 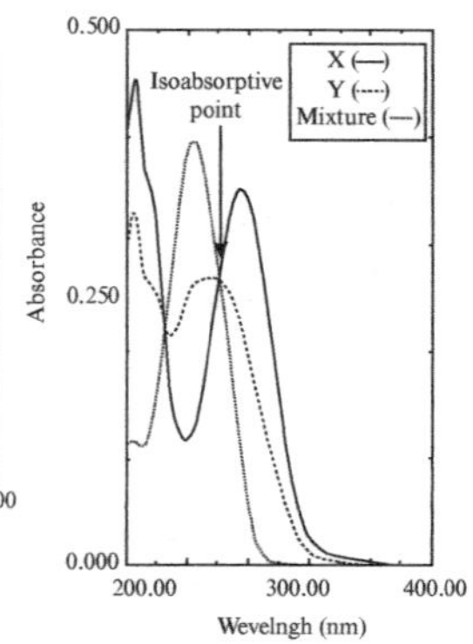	√ Could be applied in the presence of an extension region √ Could be applied in the absence of an extension region √ Recovery of parent spectra that confirm the spectral profile of the target component √ Concentrations are calculated at zero order √ Need a factorised spectrum × Need a divisor spectrum × Need special software
Response correlation 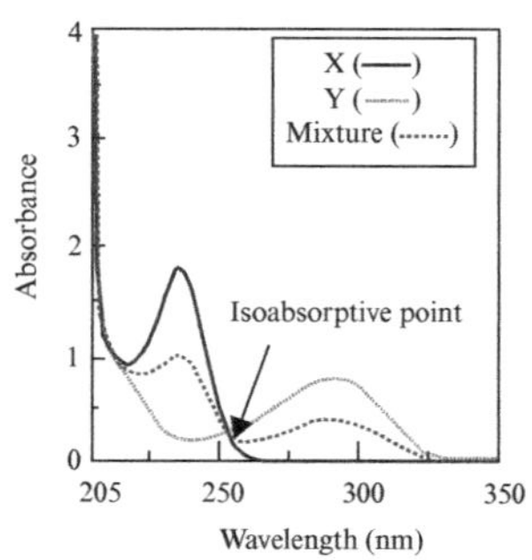 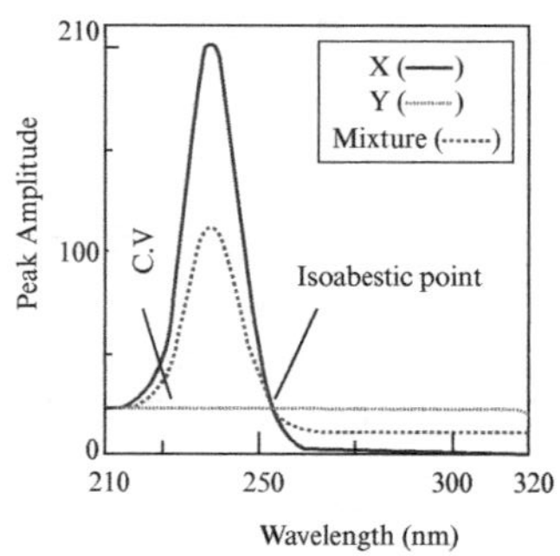	√ Could be applied in the presence of an extension region √ Could be applied in the absence of an extension region × Recovery of parent spectra that confirm the spectral profile of the target component √ Concentrations are calculated at zero order × Need a factorised spectrum √ Need a divisor spectrum × Could be used for minor components × Need special software

(Continued)

Table 8.3 (Continued)

Methods and spectrum	Limitations and outcomes
Advanced balance point-spectrum subtraction via zero-order spectrum 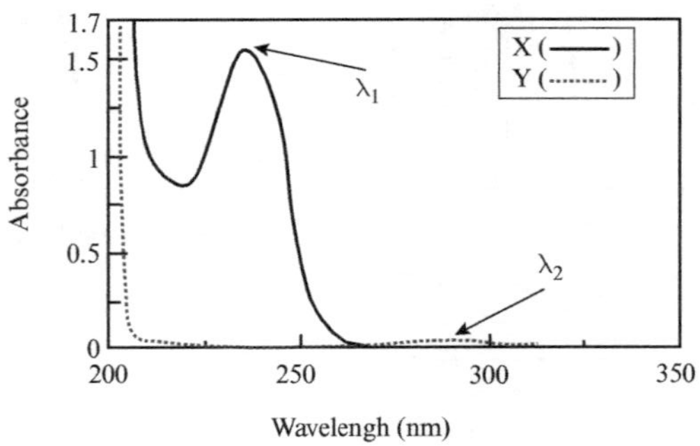 	√ Could be applied in the presence of an extension region √ Could be applied in the absence of an extension region × Recovery of parent spectra that confirm the spectral profile of the target component √ Concentrations are calculated at zero order × Need a factorised spectrum × Need a divisor spectrum √ Could be used for minor components × Need special software
Induced concentration subtraction 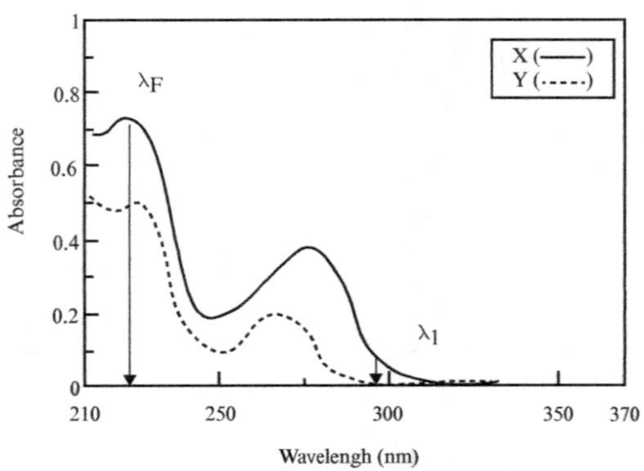 	√ Could be applied in the presence of an extension region √ Could be applied in the absence of an extension region × Recovery of parent spectra that confirm the spectral profile of the target component √ Concentrations are calculated at zero order × Need a factorised spectrum × Need a divisor spectrum √ Could be used for minor components × Need special software

Window 2

Advanced balance point-spectrum subtraction via derivative spectrum 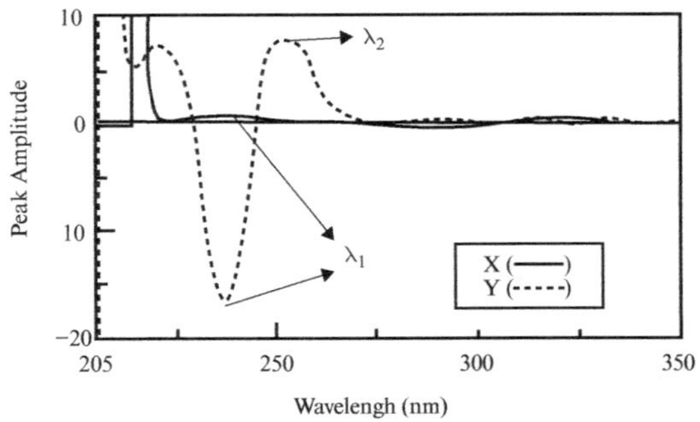	√ Could be applied in the presence of an extension region √ Could be applied in the absence of an extension region × Recovery of parent spectra that confirm the spectral profile of the target component √ Concentrations are calculated at zero order × Need a factorised spectrum × Need a divisor spectrum √ Could be used for minor components × Need special software
Relative absorptivity distribution via amplitude at the isosbestic point 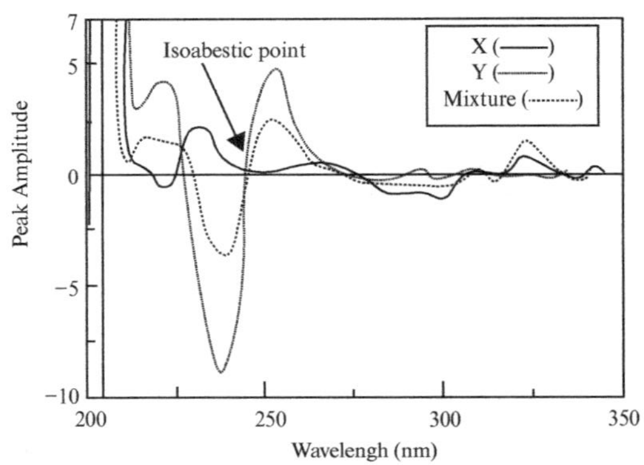	√ Could be applied in the presence of an extension region × Could be applied in the absence of an extension region × Recovery of parent spectra that confirm the spectral profile of the target component × Concentrations are calculated at zero order √ Need a factorised spectrum × Need a divisor spectrum × Could be used for minor components × Need special software

(Continued)

Table 8.3 (Continued)

Methods and spectrum	Limitations and outcomes
Window 3	
Ratio difference–isosbestic points 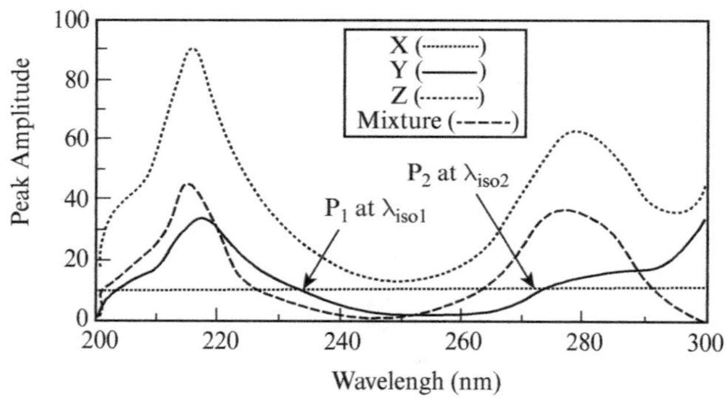	√ Could be applied in the presence of an extension region √ Could be applied in the absence of an extension region × Recovery of parent spectra that confirm the spectral profile of the target component × Concentrations are calculated at zero order × Need a factorised spectrum √ Need a divisor spectrum × Could be used for minor components × Need special software
Amplitude modulation coupled with induced ratio difference 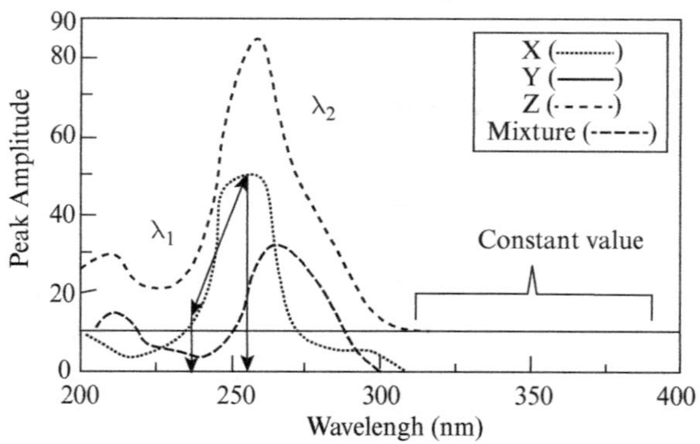	√ Could be applied in the presence of an extension region × Could be applied in the absence of an extension region × Recovery of parent spectra that confirm the spectral profile of the target component × Concentrations are calculated at zero order × Need a factorised spectrum √ Need a divisor spectrum × Could be used for minor components × Need special software

Absorptivity centring via factorised ratio spectrum 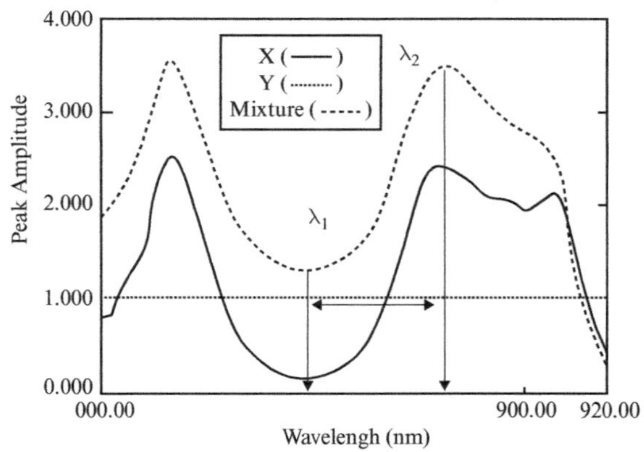	√ Could be applied in the presence of an extension region √ Could be applied in the absence of an extension region × Recovery of parent spectra that confirm the spectral profile of the target component × Concentrations are calculated at zero order √ Need a factorised spectrum √ Need a divisor spectrum × Could be used for minor components × Need special software
Ratio subtraction coupled with unified constant subtraction 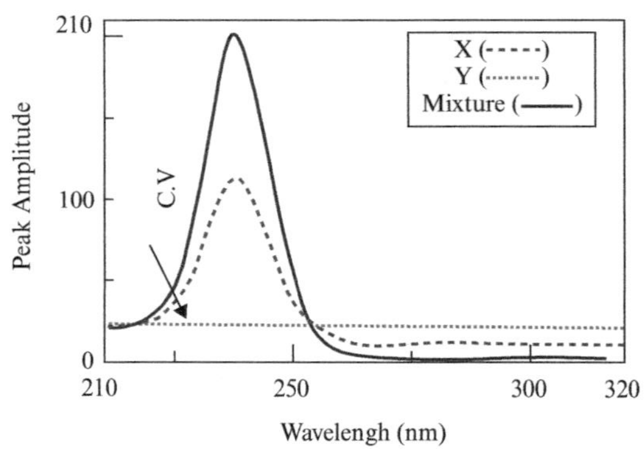	√ Could be applied in the presence of an extension region × Could be applied in the absence of an extension region √ Recovery of parent spectra that confirm the spectral profile of the target component √ Concentrations are calculated at zero order × Need a factorised spectrum √ Need a divisor spectrum × Could be used for minor components × Need special software

(Continued)

Table 8.3 (Continued)

Methods and spectrum	Limitations and outcomes
Constant extraction 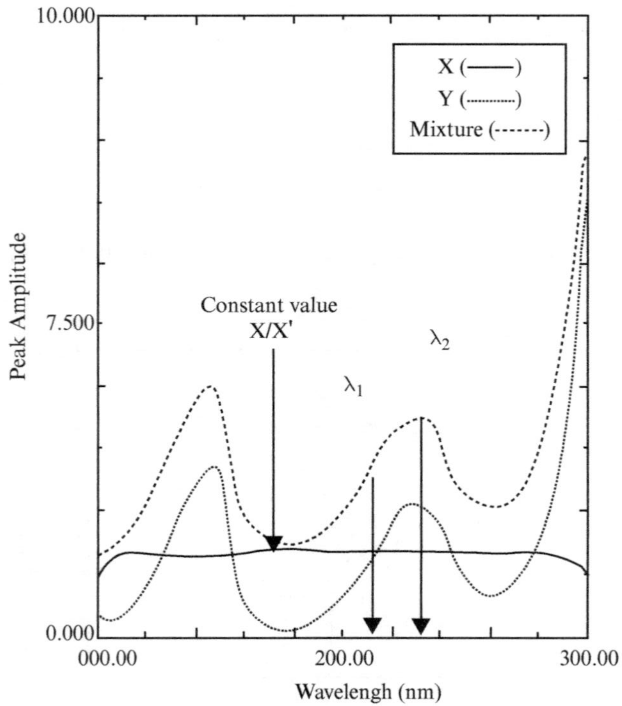 	√ Could be applied in the presence of an extension region √ Could be applied in the absence of an extension region √ Recovery of parent spectra that confirm the spectral profile of the target component √ Concentrations are calculated at zero order × Need a factorised spectrum √ Need a divisor spectrum × Could be used for minor components × Need special software

Advanced amplitude centring	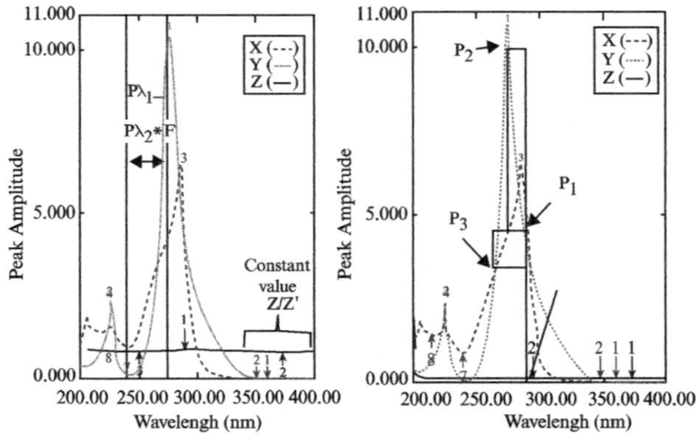	√ Could be applied in the presence of an extension region √ Could be applied in the absence of an extension region × Recovery of parent spectra that confirm the spectral profile of the target component × Concentrations are calculated at zero order × Need a factorised spectrum √ Need a divisor spectrum × Could be used for minor components × Need special software
Dual amplitude difference	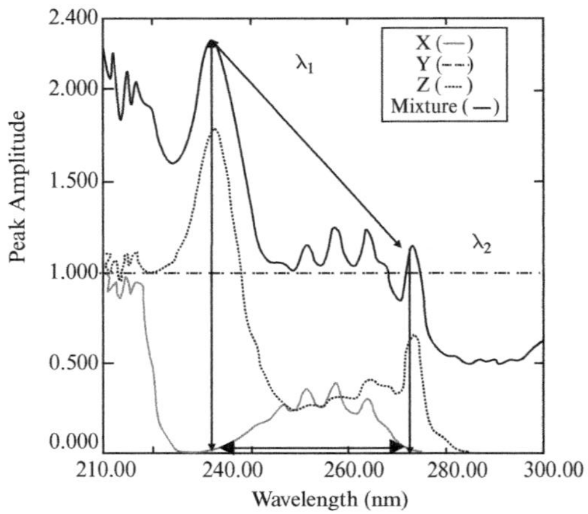	√ Could be applied in the presence of an extension region √ Could be applied in the absence of an extension region √ Recovery of parent spectra that confirm the spectral profile of the target component √ Concentrations are calculated at zero order √ Need a factorised spectrum √ Need a divisor spectrum × Could be used for minor components × Need special software

(Continued)

Table 8.3 (Continued)

Methods and spectrum	Limitations and outcomes
Induced dual amplitude difference coupled with spectrum subtraction 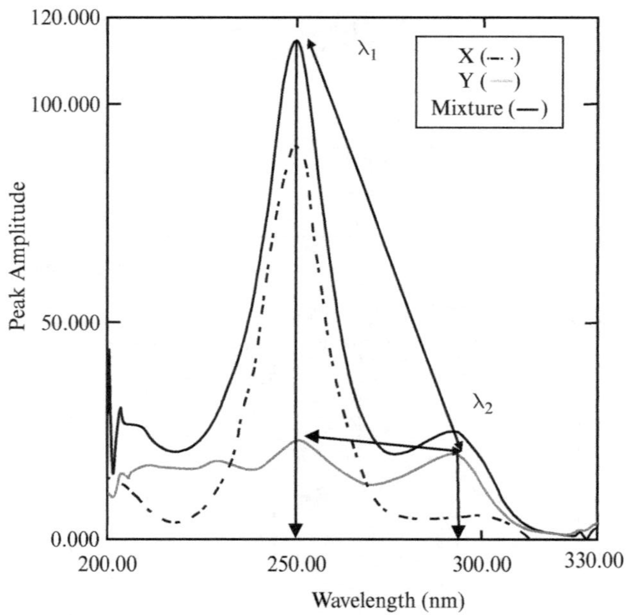 	√ Could be applied in the presence of an extension region √ Could be applied in the absence of an extension region √ Recovery of parent spectra that confirm the spectral profile of the target component √ Concentrations are calculated at zero order √ Need a factorised spectrum √ Need a divisor spectrum × Could be used for minor components × Need special software

Window 4

Unlimited derivative ratio

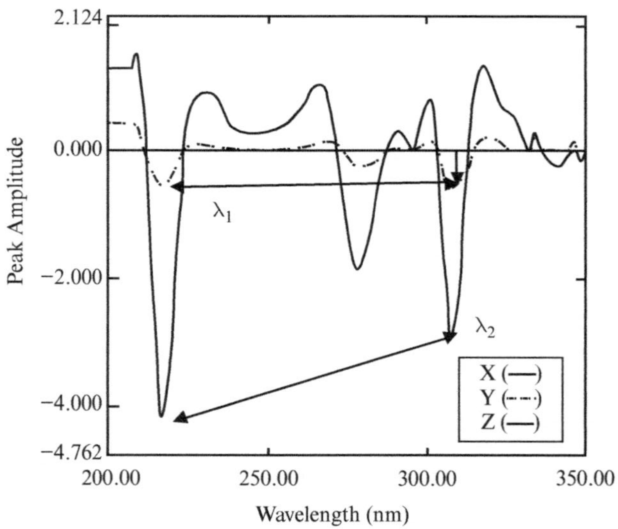

√ Could be applied in the presence of an extension region

√ Could be applied in the absence of an extension region

× Recovery of parent spectra that confirm the spectral profile of the target component

× Concentrations are calculated at zero order

× Need a factorised spectrum

√ Need a divisor spectrum

× Could be used for minor components

× Need special software

(Continued)

Table 8.3 (Continued)

Methods and spectrum	Limitations and outcomes
Factorised derivative ratio coupled with spectrum subtraction	√ Could be applied in the presence of an extension region √ Could be applied in the absence of an extension region × Recovery of parent spectra that confirm the spectral profile of the target component × Concentrations are calculated at zero order √ Need a factorised spectrum √ Need a divisor spectrum × Could be used for minor components × Need special software

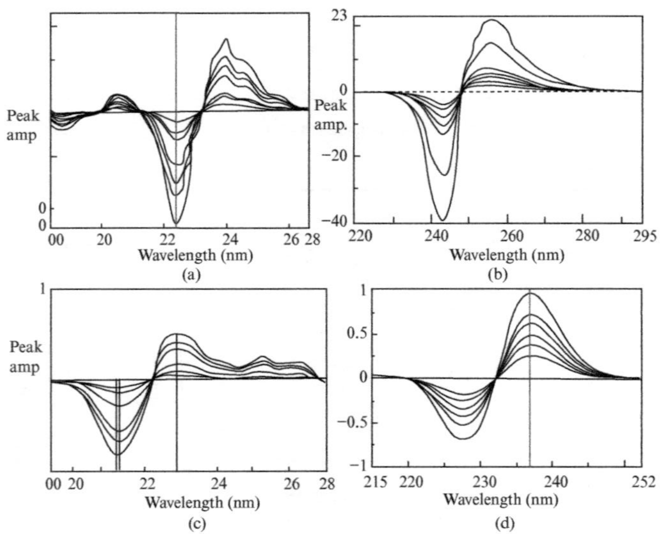

Factorised derivative ratio null contribution

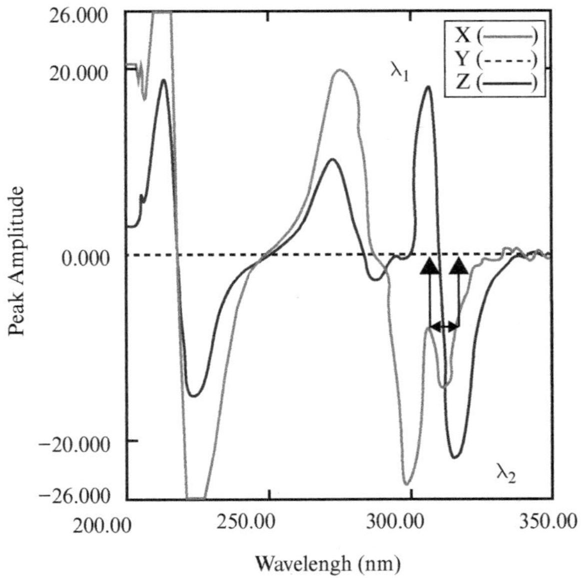

√ Could be applied in the presence of an extension region
√ Could be applied in the absence of an extension region
× Recovery of parent spectra that confirm the spectral profile of the target component
× Concentrations are calculated at zero order
√ Need a factorised spectrum
√ Need a divisor spectrum
× Could be used for minor components
× Need special software

Table 8.4 Advanced univariate spectrophotometric applications in different matrices since 2017.

Analytes	Methods	Matrix	Greenness assessment (GA)	Solvent	Year and window (W)	References
	Pharmaceutical applications					
Paracetamol, pseudoephedrine hydrochloride, and carbinoxamine maleate	Direct spectrophotometry Dual wavelength First derivative Derivative ratio Ratio difference Constant centre linked to spectrum subtraction Constant multiplication linked to spectrum subtraction	Michaelon® tablets	GA	Distilled water	2022 W1 W2 W3	[128]
Amlodipine and atorvastatin Amlodipine and candesartan	Constant extraction Ratio subtraction coupled with unified constant subtraction Constant centre	Caduet® and Tansifa® tablets	None	Methanol	2022 W3	[93]
Marbofloxacin	Modified ratio difference Mean centring	Marbofloxacin Veterinary tablets	None	Purified water + ethanol (80 : 20 v/v)	2022 W3	[129]
Dutasteride and silodosin	Amplitude modulation Absorptivity centring Constant extraction linked to spectrum subtraction Ratio subtraction linked to constant multiplication Absorbance subtraction	Maxvoid Plus-4 tablets	GA	Ethanol	2022 W3 W1	[[130]

Betrixaban on its own or mixed with lercanidipine	First derivative amplitudes Direct spectrophotometry	Laboratory-prepared capsules and Care-dipine tablets	GA	Methanol	2022 W1 W2	[131]
Aspirin and omeprazole	Dual wavelength Advanced absorbance subtraction First and second derivative Ratio difference Mean centring Derivative ratio	Yosprala 81/40 tablet	None	Methanol	2022 W1 W2 W3	[132]
Saxagliptin hydrochloride and dapagliflozin propanediol monohydrate	Ratio difference Ratio subtraction in conjunction with extended ratio subtraction Induced dual wavelength	Formigliptin® and Diglifloz® tablets	None	Methanol	2022 W3 W1	[133]
Amlodipine, telmisartan, hydrochlorothiazide, and chlorthalidone	Fourier self-deconvolution Amplitude factor First derivative	Telvas 3D and Telmikind-Ct tablets	None	Methanol	2022 W2 W3	[134]
Ibuprofen, pseudoephedrine hydrochloride, caffeine and chlorpheniramine maleate	Derivative ratio Constant multiplication in conjunction with spectrum subtraction Dual amplitude difference Factorised first derivative in conjunction with derivative transformation	Antiflu® capsules	None	Methanol	2021 W3 W4	[61]

(Continued)

Table 8.4 (Continued)

Analytes	Methods	Matrix	Greenness assessment (GA)	Solvent	Year and window (W)	References
Mix I: Olmesartan medoxomil and amlodipine besylate Mix II: Telmisartan and hydrochlorothiazide	Mix I: Induced dual wavelength Absorbance correction Ratio subtraction in conjunction with constant multiplication Mix II: Advanced absorbance subtraction Dual wavelength Constant centre in conjunction with spectrum subtraction	Excaliba® and Micardis® plus tablets	None	Methanol	2021 W1 W3 W4	[43]
Tenofovir alafenamide with its alkali degradation	Dual wavelength Ratio difference First derivative of ratio spectra	HEPBEST® tablets	GA	Methanol	2021 W1 W3 W4	[135]
Emogliflozin and metformin	First derivative First derivative of ratio spectra Amplitude difference	Mixers and tablets prepared in a laboratory	GA	Water	2021 W2 W3	[136]
Remogliflozin and vildagliptin	Ratio difference Derivative ratio spectrophotometry	Tablet formulation	GA	Water	2021 W3	[137]
Clotrimazole and tinidazole	Derivative spectrophotometry Area under the curve Absorptivity factor	Bulk and ointment	GA	10% v/v ethanol	2021 W1 W2	[138]

Paracetamol, aceclofenac, and thiocolchicoside	Simultaneous equation	Tablet formulation	GA	Phosphate buffer pH 7.8	2021 W1	[139]
Sofosbuvir and velpatasvir	Second derivative ratio spectra	Epclusa tablets	GA	Methanol	2021 W1 W2 W4	[140]
Dacarbazine and its related impurities	Double dual wavelength Dual ratio subtraction Successive ratio subtraction	Dacarbazine medac® powder for injection	None	Methanol for stock solution and water for working solution	2021 W1 W3	[141]
Sulfasalazine and its related compounds	Modified ratio difference Mean centring	Colosalazine-ECVR and Marsalaz VR tablets	GA	Acetone diluted with ethanol	2021 W3 W4	[142]
Flumethasone pivalate and clioquinol	Dual wavelength Fourier self-deconvolution First derivative ratio spectra Bivariate procedures Area under the curve	Combined formulation Viotic VR ear drops	None	Methanol	2021 W1 W4	[143]
Miconazole nitrate and nystatin	Dual wavelength Absorption correction Ratio difference First derivative ratio spectra Mean centring Ratio subtraction	Combined suppositories and dissolution testing	None	Methanol for working standard solution Bi-distilled water for inv itro dissolution	2021 W1 W2 W3	[144]

(Continued)

Table 8.4 (Continued)

Analytes	Methods	Matrix	Greenness assessment (GA)	Solvent	Year and window (W)	References
Azithromycin and levofloxacin	First derivative	Laboratory-prepared tablets	GA	Methanol	2020 W1 W2	[145]
Mebendazole and quinfamide	Extended ratio subtraction coupled with isoabsorptive point Dual wavelength Simultaneous ratio subtraction Absorbance subtraction	Vermox Plus® tablets	None	Methanol	2020 W1 W3	[146]
Acefylline piperazine and bromhexine hydrochloride	Dual wavelength within the ratio spectra Double divider-ratio spectra derivative	Mucophylline® syrup	None	Methanol	2020 W3 W4	[147]
Alfuzosin and solifenacin	Dual wavelength Determination in zero order First derivative ratio spectra Derivative ratio Ratio difference Mean centring	Solitral® capsules	GA	Water	2020 W1 W2 W3	[148]
Zofenopril calcium and hydrochlorothiazide	Absorbance subtraction Ratio subtraction linked to constant multiplication Advanced amplitude modulation Ratio difference	Zoprotec Plus® film-coated tablets	None	Methanol	2020 W3	[123]

Sulfadimidinesodium, sulfaquinoxaline sodium, diaveridine, and vitamin K_3	Amplitude modulation Successive ratio subtraction linked to constant multiplication Absorbance subtraction	Coccimix® powder veterinary formulation	None	Water	2020 W3	[149]
Ciprofloxacin hydrochloride and metronidazole	Continuous wavelet transform	Ciprodiazole tablets	None	Acidic pH monitoring solution (0,1 M) HCl with pH 1.2	2020 W3	[150]
Cetylpyridinium chloride and lidocaine hydrochloride with dimethylaniline	Ratio difference First derivative ratio spectra Dual wavelength linked to the isoabsorptive point	Dentinox® teething gel	None	Distilled water	2020 W4 W3 W1	[151]
Ranitidine hydrochloride and metronidazole	Response correlation Absorptivity centring	Flagyl® 500 mg and Zantac® 150 mg	None	Methanol	2020 W1 W3	[152]
Paracetamol, ibuprofen, and caffeine	Continuous wavelet transform	Bidi-Ipalvic capsules and Glotasic tablets Dissolution profiles	None	Phosphate buffer pH 7.8	2020 W4	[153]
Diphenhydramine, paracetamol, p-aminophenol and diphenofydramine degraded (N-oxide)	Dual wavelength Three divider ratio difference Double divider ratio difference	Quaternary mixtures prepared in a lab Panadol night® tablets for quantitative determination of diphenhydramine and paracetamol	None	Methanol	2020 W1 W3	[154]

(Continued)

Table 8.4 (Continued)

Analytes	Methods	Matrix	Greenness assessment (GA)	Solvent	Year and window (W)	References
Clioquinol, betamethasone tolnaftate, gentamicin and preservative chlorocresol	Constant value spectrum subtraction Constant multiplication Derivative ratio Concentration value Factorised derived ratio linked to spectrum subtraction	Quadriderm cream	None	Stock solutions in methanol, except for gentamicin in bi-distilled water	2020 W2 W3 W4	[127]
Alogliptin and pioglitazone	Induced amplitude modulation Induced concentration subtraction Induced dual wavelength	Oseni® tablets	None	Methanol	2020 W1 W3	[27]
Tylosin tartrate and doxycycline hydrochloride	Absorbance subtraction Amplitude summation Ratio subtraction linked to extended ratio subtraction Spectrum subtraction Successive derivative subtraction Concentration value Constant value Derivative transformation Direct spectrophotometry Successive derivative subtraction linked to spectrum subtraction Derivative subtraction linked to constant multiplication	Tydovet® powder veterinary medicine	None	Methanol	2020 W1 W3	[20, 70, 72, 73, 75, 84]

Cangliflozin and metformin	Absorbance difference Absorbance at isoabsorptive point Amplitude at isosbestic point	Vokanamet® tablets	GA	Methanol	2020 W2 W3	[122]
Tylosin tartrate and doxycycline hydrochloride	Induced dual wavelength Dual wavelength Absorption correction Absorbance subtraction Amplitude correction Derivative ratio Advanced amplitude modulation	Tydovet® powder veterinary medicine	None	Methanol	2020 W1 W3 W4	[24]
Ciprofloxacin and acidic degraded (chloro analogue)	Pure component contribution algorithm	CEPROZ® tablets	None	Methanol	2020 W4	[155]
Metoclopramide and aspirin (acetyl salicylic acid)	Ratio H-point standard addition Absorptivity centring Geometrically induced amplitude modulation	Migramax sachets	None	Water : methanol (50 : 50 v/v)	2020 W1 W3	[101]
Dapagliflozin and saxagliptin	Factorised zero order derivative Ratio difference	In-house formulation of Qtern® tablets	None	Methanol	2019 W1 W2 W3	[156]
Amlodipine besylate and rosuvastatin calcium	Induced dual wavelength Amplitude correction Absorbance subtraction Absorption correction Advanced amplitude subtraction	Rosucor® Plus film-coated tablets	None	Methanol	2019 W1 W3	[157]

(Continued)

Table 8.4 (Continued)

Analytes	Methods	Matrix	Greenness assessment (GA)	Solvent	Year and window (W)	References
Ofloxacin and dexamethasone	Absorptivity centring Absorbance subtraction Amplitude modulation Amplitude summation	Dexaflox® eye drops	None	Ethanol : water (50 : 50 v/v)	2019 W1	[121]
Pseudoephedrine sulfate and loratadine	Induced amplitude modulation Ratio difference Absorption correction Dual wavelength Direct analysis Constant multiplication Induced dual wavelength	Clarinase® tablets	None	0.1 M HCl	2019 W1 W3	[25]
Ciprofloxacin and fluocinolone acetonide	Absorptivity centring Extended ratio subtraction Constant multiplication Unified constant subtraction Spectrum subtraction Ratio subtraction	Otovel® otic solution	None	Methanol	2019 W1 W3	[82, 84]
Phenazone and benzocaine	Absorptivity centring Absorbance subtraction Amplitude modulation Concentration value	Tympanil® otic drops	None	Ethanol	2019 W1 W3	[75, 158]

Ciprofloxacin and fluocinolone acetonide	Isoabsorptive point coupled with direct spectrophotometry Isoabsorptive point linked to area under the curve Isoabsorptive point coupled with amplitude modulation	Otovel® otic solution	None	Methanol	2019 W1 W2 W3	[159]
Metformin hydrochloride, empagliflozine, linagliptin and pioglitazone hydrochloride	Mean centring Ratio derivative–zero crossing	Glucophage®, Jardiance®, Trajenta® and Actos® tablets	None	Methanol	2019 W4	[160]
Trimebutine maleate with degradation product (DEG) 1 (3,4,5-trimethoxy benzoic acid) and DEG 2 (2-dimethyl amino)-2 phenyl butanol	Dual wavelength Second derivative ratio spectra Ratio difference Constant centre linked to spectrum subtraction	Gast-reg® tablets, ampoules, and suspension	None	Methanol	2019 W1 W2 W3	[161]
Aceclofenac and paracetamol with degraded diclofenac sodium and 4-minophenol	Dual wavelength Induced dual wavelength Unlimited derivative Successive derivative subtraction linked to constant multiplication Ratio difference Constant centre	Hifenac-P® tablets	None	Methanol	2019 W1 W2 W3 W4	[126]
Daclatasvir, sofosbuvi and ribavirin	Pure component contribution algorithm	Daklanork® tablets	None	Methanol	2019 W4	[162]
Ciprofloxacin and metronidazole	Pure component contribution algorithm	Ciprodiazole® tablets	None	Distilled water	2019 W4	[115]

(Continued)

Table 8.4 (Continued)

Analytes	Methods	Matrix	Greenness assessment (GA)	Solvent	Year and window (W)	References
Thioctic acid, benfotiamine and cyanocobalamin	First derivative Ratio difference First derived ratio spectra Ratio subtraction	Thiotacid® compound capsules	None	Acetonitril : water (50 : 50 v/v)	2019 W3 W4	[163]
Hydrochlorothiazide and telmisartan	Q-absorbance ratio	Micardis Plus®	GA	Methanol	2019 W3	[164]
Pseudoephedrine hydrochloride and ibuprofen	Dual wavelength Ratio difference Constant multiplication linked to spectrum subtraction Absorption correction Constant centre linked to spectrum subtraction	Brufen-Flu® tablets	None	Methanol	2019 W1 W3	[31]
Salbutamol, theophylline, and ambroxol	Simultaneous equation (Vierordt's method)	Ambrolite-ST tablets	None	Methanol	2018 W1	[165]
Chloramphenicol and dexamethasone sodium phosphate	Ratio subtraction Unified constant subtraction Extended ratio subtraction Constant multiplication Spectrum subtraction	Spersadex® eye drops	None	Ethanol : water (50 : 50 v/v)	2018 W3	[84]
Ambroxol, fuaifenesin and theophylline	Direct spectrophotometry Dual wavelength First derivative ratio spectra Absorption correction	Trisolvin® capsules	None	Methanol	2018 W1 W4	[166]

Clotrimazole and dexamethasone acetate	Constant centre Constant value with amplitude difference Ratio difference Advanced concentration value Derived ratio spectra	Mycuten-D cream	None	Methanol	2018 W1 W3 W4	[75, 167]
Carbinoxamine maleate, pholcodine and ephedrine hydrochloride	Successive derived ratio spectra Successive derivative subtraction coupled with constant multiplication Ratio subtraction linked to ratio difference Amplitude summation Continuous wavelet transform	Cyrinol syrup	None	Distilled water	2018 W2 W3 W4	[70]
Paracetamol, chlorzoxazone and diclofenac potassium	Continuous wavelet transform	Myospazfort® tablet	None	Methanol	2018 W2 W4	[168]
Paracetamol, pseudoephedrine hydrochloride and cetirizine dihydrochloride	Ratio subtraction linked to ratio difference Derived ratio spectra linked to zero crossing Successive derivative ratio Pure component contribution algorithm	Allercet Cold® capsules	None	Distilled water	2018 W3 W4	[169]

(Continued)

Table 8.4 (Continued)

Analytes	Methods	Matrix	Greenness assessment (GA)	Solvent	Year and window (W)	References
Ketorolac tromethamine, phenylephrine hydrochloride and chlorpheniramine maleate	First derivative ratio spectra Derivative ratio Difference ratio Delta absorbance Convolution of derived data by discrete Fourier functions	MIDRIA® and KETO-PC® eye drops	None	Distilled water	2018 W1 W2 W3 W4	[170]
Furosemide spironolactone and canrenone	Successive ratio subtraction	Lasilactone® tablets	None	Methanol	2018 W3	[171]
Guaifenesin chlorpheniramine and pseudoephedrine	Continuous wavelet transform	Commercial cough syrup	None	Distilled water	2018 W4	[172]
Chlorzoxazone and ibuprofen	Amplitude modulation Amplitude summation Absorbance subtraction	Markfast® and Profenazone® capsules	None	Ethanol : water (50 : 50 v/v)	2018 W1 W2 W3	[95]
Mix 1: Simvastatin and ezetimibe Mix 2: Chloramphenicol and prednisolone acetate	Absorptivity centring	Inegy® tablets and Cortiphen® eye drops	None	Methanol for mix 1 Ethanol for mix 2	2018 W1	[173]
Clotrimazole and dexamethasone	Mean centring	Mycuten-D® cream	None	Methanol	2018 W4	[174]
Albendazole with alkaline degraded substance	Derivative ratio	Bendax® tablets	None	Methanol	2018 W4	[175]

Canagliflozin and metformin hydrochloride	Advanced balance point utilising spectrum subtraction Advanced amplitude modulation Advanced absorbance subtraction Response correlation	Vokanamet® tablets	None	Methanol	2018 W2 W3	[42]
Entacapone, levodopa and carbidopa	First derivative ratio spectra Double divider derivative ratio Continuous wavelet transform	Stalevo® tablets	None	Methanol : water (70 : 30, v/v))	2017 W4	[176]
Amlodipine, valsartan and hydrochlorothiazide	Advanced amplitude centring	Exforge HCT® film-coated tablets	None	Methanol : water (50 : 50 v/v,	2017 W3	[124]
Metronidazole, diloxanide, and mebeverine HCl	Absorption correction Modified amplitude centre Area under the curve	Dimetrol® tablets	None	Methanol	2017 W1 W3	[94, 177]
Drotaverine, caffeine, paracetamol, and para-aminophenol	Direct spectra linked to derivative transformation Dual wavelength Spectrum subtraction Advanced absorbance subtraction Advanced amplitude modulation Advanced ratio difference Simultaneous derived ratio Double divider ratio difference	Tablets of Panadol Extra®, Petro®, and Soumadril Compound®	None	Methanol	2017 W1 W2 W3 W4	[44]

(Continued)

Table 8.4 (Continued)

Analytes	Methods	Matrix	Greenness assessment (GA)	Solvent	Year and window (W)	References
Miconazole, mometasone furaoate and gentamicin	Successive derivative subtraction Spectrum subtraction linked to constant multiplication Differential amplitude modulation Constant value Successive derivative subtraction linked to constant multiplication	Momenta cream	None	Miconazol, mometasone in methanol, and gentamicin in bi-distilled water	2017 W2 W3	[75, 84]
Amlodipine, valsartan and hydrochlorothiazide	Pure component contribution algorithm	EXFORGE HCT® tablets	None	Methanol	2017 W4	[114]
Clotrimazole and dexamethasone	Absorbance subtraction Amplitude modulation	Mycuten-D cream	None	Methanol	2017 W1 W3	[178]
	Biological applications					
Vandetanib, dasatinib and sorafenib	Double divisor-ratio spectra derivative	Caprelsa®, Sprycel®, and Nexavar® tablets as well as spiked human plasma and urine samples	None	Acetonitrile	2022	[179]
Atenolol, paracetamol, hydrochlorothiazide and levofloxacin	Extended derivative ratio	Tenormin®, Panadrex®, HCT Georetic25® and Tavanic® tablets as well as spiked and real human urine samples	GA	Ethanol	2020 W4	[180]

Timolol maleate, rosuvastatin calcium and diclofenac sodium	First derivative ratio spectra Mean centring	Spiked human plasma	None	Methanol	2019 W4	[181]
Ribavirin, sofosbuvir, and daclatasvir	Direct spectrophotometry Ratio difference Constant centre Isoabsorptive point Mean centring	Copegus® tablets, spiked human urine and plasma Dissolution test	None	Methanol	2018 W1 W3 W4	[182]
Bromazepam, diazepam, and clonazepam	Mean centring Isoabsorptive point coupled with ratio subtraction	Calmepam®, Valinil®, Neuril®, Apetryl®, Amotril®, Lexotanil® tablets, Rivotril®drops, human urine samples	None	Methanol	2018 W3 W4	[183]
Imatinib, gemifloxacin, nalbuphine, and naproxen	Extended derivative ratio	Glivec®, Quinabiotic®, Naprofen® tablets, Nalufin® ampoules, human urine samples	None	Methanol	2018 W4	[184]
	Environmental analysis					
Tomato pesticides	Mean centring Three successive derivatisation steps on ratio spectra Modified ratio difference	Field tomato samples	None	Methanol	2020 W3 W4	[185]
Carboxin, chlorpyrifos, and tebuconazole	Successive derived ratio spectra Double divider Mean centring	Cabbage remains in the trial field	None	Methanol	2020 W4	[186]

References

1 Anastas, P.T. (1999). Green chemistry and the role of analytical methodology development. *Critical Reviews in Analytical Chemistry* 29: 167–175.

2 Gałuszka, A., Migaszewski, Z., and Namieśnik, J. (2013). The 12 principles of green analytical chemistry and the SIGNIFICANCE mnemonic of green analytical practices. *TrAC Trends in Analytical Chemistry* 50: 78–84.

3 Tekin, K., Hao, N., Karagoz, S., and Ragauskas, A.J. (2018). Ethanol: a promising green solvent for the deconstruction of lignocellulose. *ChemSusChem* 11: 3559–3575.

4 Lee, B., Choe, C., Kim, H. et al. (2021). Economic parity analysis of green methanol synthesis using water electrolysis based on renewable energy. *ACS Sustainable Chemistry & Engineering* 9: 15807–15818.

5 Sollai, S., Porcu, A., Tola, V. et al. (2023). Renewable methanol production from green hydrogen and captured CO_2: a techno-economic assessment. *Journal of CO_2 Utilization* 68: 102345. https://doi.org/10.1016/j.jcou.2022.102345.

6 Garrigues, S., and de la Guardia, S.M. (2020). Direct analysis by green spectroscopy and spectrometry. *Challenges in Green Analytical Chemistry* 66: 19–23.

7 Pena-Pereira, F., Costas-Mora, I., Romero, V. et al. (2011). Advances in miniaturized UV-Vis spectrometric systems. *TrAC Trends in Analytical Chemistry* 30: 1637–1648.

8 Abdulwahab, S., Ali, E.E., Hassan, W.S., and Azab, S.M. (2021). Mathematically assisted UV-spectrophotometry as a greener alternative to HPLC-UV for quality control analysis of free-drug combinations. *Microchemical Journal* 170: 106638–106645.

9 Prat, D., Hayler, J., and Wells, A. (2014). A survey of solvent selection guides. *Green Chemistry* 16 (10): 4546–4551.

10 Pena-Pereira, F., Wojnowski, W., and Tobiszewski, M. (2020). AGREE—Analytical GREEnness metric approach and software. *Analytical Chemistry* 92: 10076–10082.

11 Płotka-Wasylka, J. (2018). A new tool for the evaluation of the analytical procedure: Green Analytical Procedure Index. *Talanta* 181: 204–209.

12 Gałuszka, A., Migaszewski, Z.M., Konieczka, P., and Namieśnik, J. (2012). Analytical Eco-Scale for assessing the greenness of analytical procedures. *TrAC Trends in Analytical Chemistry* 37: 61–72.

13 Raynie, D., and Driver, J. (2009). Green assessment of chemical methods. 13th Annual Green Chemistry and Engineering Conference. https://www.researchgate.net/publication/267357856_Green_Assessment_of_Chemical_Methods.

14 National Environmental Methods Index https://www.nemi.gov/home.

15 Rodger, A. (2013). Absorption spectroscopy and transition polarizations: pictorial description. In: *Encyclopedia of Biophysics* (ed. Roberts, G.C.K.), 29. Berlin: Springer.

16 Wormell, P., and Rodger, A. (2013). Absorbance spectroscopy: overview. In: *Encyclopedia of Biophysics* (ed. Roberts, G.C.K.), 23. Berlin: Springer. https://doi.org/10.1007/978-3-642-16712-6_784.

17 Perkampus, H.-H. (2013). *UV-VIS Spectroscopy and Its Applications*. Berlin: Springer Science & Business Media.

18 Lotfy, H.M., and Saleh, S.S. (2016). Recent development in ultraviolet spectrophotometry through the last decade (2006–2016): a review. *International Journal of Pharmacy and Pharmaceutical Sciences* 8 (10): 40–56.

19 Obaydo, R.H., Al Zakri, D.J., Sakur, A.A., and Lotfy, H.M. (2021). Ultraviolet spectrophotometric methods for the determination of the minor component presented in fixed-dose pharmaceutical combinations through the last two decades (2000–2020). *Future Journal of Pharmaceutical Sciences* 7: 44.

20 Lotfy, H.M., Monir, H.H., Michael, A.M. et al. (2020). Impact study of mathematical manipulation on the resolution efficiency of the spectrophotometric technique—an application on veterinary binary mixture with overlapping absorption bands. *Journal of AOAC International* 103: 1412–1423.

21 Lotfy, H.M., Saleh, S.S., Hassan, N.Y., and Elgizawy, S.M. (2012). A comparative study of the novel ratio difference method versus conventional spectrophotometric techniques for the analysis of binary mixture with overlapped spectra. *American Journal of Analytical Chemistry* 3: 761–769.

22 Lotfy, H.M., Hegazy, M.A., Rezk, M.R., and Omran, Y.R. (2015). Comparative study of novel versus conventional two-wavelength spectrophotometric methods for analysis of spectrally overlapping binary mixture. *Spectrochimica Acta, Part A* 148: 328–337.

23 Lotfy, H.M., Saleh, S.S., Hassan, N.Y., and Salem, H. (2015). Novel two wavelength spectrophotometric methods for simultaneous determination of binary mixtures with severely overlapping spectra. *Spectrochimica Acta, Part A* 136: 1786–1796.

24 Lotfy, H.M., Fayez, Y.M., Michael, A.M. et al. (2020). Paired wavelength relevance as spectrophotometric strategy for evaluation the potency of medicine affecting human health. *Spectrochimica Acta, Part A* 239: 118461–118470.

25 Lotfy, H.M., El-Hanboushy, S., Fayez, Y.M., and Abdelkawy, M. (2019). Spectral analysis of overlapped absorption bands of binary mixtures—an application on combination of pseudoephedrine sulphate and loratadine mixture. *Future Journal of Pharmaceutical Sciences* 5: 1–14.

26 Lotfy, H.M., Fayez, Y.M., Michael, A.M., and Nessim, C.K. (2020). Evaluation of the efficiency of smart stability-indicating spectrophotometric methods based on mathematical and statistical processing of the obtained results via different manipulating pathways. *Current Pharmaceutical Analysis* 16: 186–200.

27 Lotfy, H.M., and Mohamed, E.H. (2020). Induced mathematical filtration as an innovative strategy for discrimination and estimation of glycemic control drugs in fixed dose combination. *Heliyon* 6: e05289–e05297.

28 Elsonbaty, A., Eissa, M.S., Hassan, W.S., and Abdulwahab, S. (2020). Separation-free spectrophotometric platforms for rapid assessment of combined antiplatelet therapy in complex matrices. *Bioanalysis* 12: 335–348.

29 Kavathia, A., Suchak, K., and Misra, M. (2013). Application of absorption correction method and first order derivative spectrophotometry for simultaneous determination of anti-hypertensive combination (amlodipine and benazepril). *International Journal of Pharmacy and Pharmaceutical Sciences* 5: 371–375.

30 Alves, E., Nazareth, C., and Pereira, S. (2020). Development and validation of a novel UV spectrophotometric method for simultaneous analysis of amlodipine, indapamide and perindopril. *Indian Journal of Pharmaceutical Sciences* 82: 843–850.

31 Lotfy, H.M., Ahmed, D.A., Abd El-Rahman, M.K., and Weshahy, S.A. (2019). Smart spectral processing of data for the estimation of commonly used over-the-counter (OTC) co-formulated drug; pseudoephedrine hydrochloride and ibuprofen. *Spectrochimica Acta, Part A* 223: 117322–117330.

32 Campins-Falco, P., Verdu-Andres, J., and Bosch-Reig, F. (1995). H-point standard additions method for resolution of binary mixtures with simultaneous addition of both analytes. *Analytica Chimica Acta* 315: 267–278.

33 Al-Sabha, T.A.N., Bunaciu, A.A., and Aboul-Enein, H.Y. (2011). H-point standard addition method (HPSAM) in simultaneous spectrophotometric determination of binary mixtures: an overview. *Applied Spectroscopy Reviews* 46: 607–623.

34 Abdollahi, H. (2001). Simultaneous spectrophotometric determination of chromium (VI) and iron (III) with chromogenic mixed reagents by H-point standard addition method and partial least squares regression. *Analytica Chimica Acta* 442: 327–336.

35 Lotfy, H.M., Hassan, N.Y., Elgizawy, S.M., and Saleh, S.S. (2013). Comparative study of new spectrophotometric methods; an application on pharmaceutical binary mixture of ciprofloxacin hydrochloride and hydrocortisone. *Journal of the Chilean Chemical Society* 58: 1651–1657.

36 Darwish, H.W., Bakheit, A.H., and Naguib, I.A. (2016). Comparative study of novel ratio spectra and isoabsorptive point based spectrophotometric methods: application on a binary mixture of ascorbic acid and rutin. *Journal of Analytical Methods in Chemistry* 2016: 2828647.

37 Hassan, N.Y., Elgizawy, S.M., Lotfy, H.M., and Saleh, S.S. (2013). Comparative study of spectrophotometric methods versus chemometric methods; an application on a pharmaceutical binary mixture of ofloxacin and dexamethasone. *International Research Journal of Pure & Applied Chemistry* 3: 90–110.

38 Lotfy, H.M. (2014). Absorbance subtraction and amplitude modulation as novel spectrophotometric methods for the analysis of binary mixtures. *International Journal of Pharmaceutical Sciences* 6: 735–741.

39 Lotfy, H.M., Hegazy, M.A., Rezk, M.R., and Omran, Y.R. (2014). Novel spectrophotometric methods for simultaneous determination of timolol and dorzolamide in their binary mixture. *Spectrochimica Acta, Part A* 126: 197–207.

40 Lotfy, H.M., Saleh, S.S., Hassan, N.Y., and Salem, H. (2014). A comparative study of novel spectrophotometric methods based on isosbestic points; application on a pharmaceutical ternary mixture. *Spectrochimica Acta, Part A* 126: 112–121.

41 El-Abasawy, N., Attia, K., Abouserie, A. et al. (2018). Different spectrophotometric methods applied for simultaneous analysis of binary mixture of formoterol and fluticasone: a comparative study. *Journal of Analytical & Pharmaceutical Research* 7: 160–165.

42 Lotfy, H.M., Mohamed, D., and Elshahed, M.S. (2018). Different mathematical processing of absorption, ratio and derivative spectra for quantification of mixtures containing minor component: an application to the analysis of the recently co-formulated antidiabetic drugs; canagliflozin and metformin. *Spectrochimica Acta, Part A* 189: 100–109.

43 Rostom, Y., Lotfy, H.M., Öztürk, M. et al. (2021). Trade-off efficacy and data processing strategy in the power of spectral resolution of co-formulated antihypertensive pharmaceuticals. *Spectrochimica Acta, Part A* 247: 119080–119087.

44 Mohamed, E.H., Lotfy, H.M., Hegazy, M.A., and Mowaka, S. (2017). Different applications of isosbestic points, normalized spectra and dual wavelength as powerful tools for resolution of multicomponent mixtures with severely overlapping spectra. *Chemistry Central Journal* 11: 1–15.

45 Patel, N.V., and Prajapati, A.M. (2012). Q-absorbance ratio spectrophotometric method for the simultaneous estimation of ciprofloxacin and metronidazole in their combined dosage form. *Journal of Pharmaceutical Science and Bioscientific Research* 2: 118–122.

46 Kotecha, B., Zala, P., and Faldu, S. (2014). Q-Absorbance ratio spectrophotometric method for the simultaneous estimation of amlodipine besylate and candesartan cilexetil in synthetic mixture. *PharmaTutor* 2: 167–178.

47 Pandey, G., and Mishra, B. (2013). A new analytical Q-absorbance ratio method development and validation for simultaneous estimation of lamivudine and isoniazid. *International Scholarly Research Notices* 2013: 912376.

48 Erk, N. (2002). Simultaneous determination of fosinopril and hydrochlorothiazide in pharmaceutical formulations by spectrophotometric methods. *Journal of Pharmaceutical and Biomedical Analysis* 27: 901–912.

49 Samir, A., Salem, H., and Abdelkawy, M. (2012). New developed spectrophotometric method for simultaneous determination of salmeterol xinafoate and fluticasone propionate in bulk powder and Seritide® diskus inhalation. *Bulletin of Faculty of Pharmacy Cairo University* 50: 121–126.

50 Saleh, S.S., Lotfy, H.M., Hassan, N.Y., and Elgizawy, S.M. (2013). A comparative study of validated spectrophotometric and TLC-spectrodensitometric methods for the determination of sodium cromoglicate and fluorometholone in ophthalmic solution. *Saudi Pharmaceutical Journal* 21: 411–421.

51 Mohammed, F.F., Badr El-Din, K., and Derayea, S.M. (2019). Two smart spectrophotometric methods for simultaneous determination of lisinopril and hydrochlorothiazide in binary mixtures. *Journal of Advanced Biomedical and Pharmaceutical Sciences* 2: 47–53.

52 Abdel-Aziz, O., El-Kosasy, A.M., Magdy, N., and El Zahar, N.M. (2014). Novel spectroscopic methods for determination of cromolyn sodium and oxymetazoline hydrochloride in binary mixture. *Spectrochimica Acta, Part A* 131: 59–66.

53 Abdelrahman, M.M. (2013). Simultaneous determination of cinnarizine and domperidone by area under curve and dual wavelength spectrophotometric methods. *Spectrochimica Acta, Part A* 113: 291–296.

54 Farid, N.F., and Abdelwahab, N.S. (2015). Two different spectrophotometric determinations of potential anticancer drug and its toxic metabolite. *Spectrochimica Acta, Part A* 145: 360–367.

55 Salem, H., Lotfy, H.M., Hassan, N.Y. et al. (2015). A comparative study of different aspects of manipulating ratio spectra applied for ternary mixtures: derivative spectrophotometry versus wavelet transform. *Spectrochimica Acta, Part A* 135: 1002–1010.

56 Abdelwahab, N.S., and Farid, N.F. (2016). Innovative spectrophotometric methods for determination of newly discovered combination for hepatitis C treatment. *Analytical Chemistry Letters* 6: 783–794.

57 Mendham, J., Bassett, J., and Jeffery, G. (2021). *Vogel's Textbook of Quantitative Chemical Analysis*. Harlow: Longman Scientific & Technical.

58 El-Leithy, E.S., and Abdel-Rashid, R.S. (2016). Validation and application of Vierordt's spectrophotometric method for simultaneous estimation of tamoxifen/coenzyme Q10 in their binary mixture and pharmaceutical dosage forms. *Asian Journal of Pharmaceutical Sciences* 11: 318–325.

59 Al Alamein, A.M.A., Elwy, H.M., and El-Din, S.H.S. (2019). Univariate and multivariate spectrophotometric methods for simultaneous determination of avobenzone and octinoxate in pure form and in cosmetic formulations: a comparative study. *Spectrochimica Acta. Part A, Molecular and Biomolecular Spectroscopy* 206: 37–47.

60 Samir, A., Lotfy, H.M., Salem, H., and Abdelkawy, M. (2014). Development and validation of simultaneous spectrophotometric and TLC-spectrodensitometric methods for determination of beclomethasone dipropionate and salbutamol in combined dosage form. *Spectrochimica Acta, Part A* 128: 127–136.

61 Ahmed, D.A., and Lotfy, H.M. (2021). Evaluation of in silico and in lab sample enrichment techniques for the assessment of challengeable quaternary combination in critical ratio. *Spectrochimica Acta, Part A* 260: 119943–119956.

62 Lotfy, H.M., and Saleh, S.S. (2019). Investigating advanced approaches based on iso-absorptivity coefficient in unresolved spectral signals of binary mixtures. *Journal of Analytical Methods in Chemistry* 2019: 7924821–7924832.

63 Lotfy, H.M., Tawakkol, S.M., Fahmy, N.M., and Shehata, M.A. (2015). A comparative study of novel spectrophotometric resolution techniques applied for pharmaceutical mixtures with partially or severely overlapped spectra. *Spectrochimica Acta, Part A* 136: 937–952.

64 Mohamed, M.E. (1986). First-derivative spectrophotometric determination of a mixture of pirbuterol hydrochloride and butorphanol tartrate. *Analytical Letters* 11: 1323–1339.

65 Hassan, S.M., Amer, S.M., and Amer, M.M. (1987). Determination of fusidic acid and sodium fusidate in pharmaceutical dosage forms by first-derivative ultraviolet spectrophotometry. *Analyst* 112: 1459–1461.

66 Ouanes, S., Kallel, M., Trabelsi, H. et al. (1998). Zero-crossing derivative spectrophotometry for the determination of haloperidol in presence of parabens. *Journal of Pharmaceutical and Biomedical Analysis* 17: 361–364.

67 Lotfy, H.M., Tawakkol, S.M., Fahmy, N.M., and Shehata, M.A. (2013). Validated stability indicating spectrophotometric methods for the determination of lidocaine hydrochloride, calcium dobesilate, and dexamethasone acetate in their dosage forms. *Analytical Chemistry Letters* 3: 208–225.

68 Lotfy, H.M., Mohamed, D., and Mowaka, S. (2015). A comparative study of smart spectrophotometric methods for simultaneous determination of sitagliptin phosphate and metformin hydrochloride in their binary mixture. *Spectrochimica Acta. Part A, Molecular and Biomolecular Spectroscopy* 149: 441–451.

69 Lotfy, H.M., Erk, N., and Rostom, Y. (2019). Developing spectral numerical factor technique for the determination of amlodipine besylate and the latest generation of statins in their new pharmaceutical combination. *Spectrochimica Acta. Part A, Molecular and Biomolecular Spectroscopy* 218: 320–330.

70 Moustafa, A.A., Hegazy, M.A., Mohamed, D., and Ali, O. (2018). Novel approach for the simultaneous determination of carbinoxamine maleate, pholcodine, and ephedrine hydrochloride without interference from coloring matter in an antitussive preparation using smart spectrophotometric methods. *Journal of AOAC International* 101: 414–426.

71 Lotfy, H.M., Saleh, S.S., Hassan, N.Y., and Elgizawy, S.M. (2013). Spectrophotometric and chromatographic methods for the determination of a binary mixture of sodium cromoglicate and xylometazoline hydrochloride. *Analytical Chemistry* 13: 152–160.

72 Lotfy, H.M., Tawakkol, S.M., Fahmy, N.M., and Shehata, M.A. (2014). Successive spectrophotometric resolution as a novel technique for the analysis of ternary mixtures of pharmaceuticals. *Spectrochimica Acta, Part A* 121: 313–323.

73 Magdy, R., Hemdan, A., Fares, N.V., and Farouk, M. (2018). Simultaneous spectrophotometric determination of drugs lacking peak maxima in their zero-order profiles by graphical or statistical representation of data. *European Journal of Chemistry* 9: 194–201.

74 Lotfy, H.M., Fayez, Y.M., Michael, A.M., and Nessim, C.K. (2016). Simultaneous determination of mebeverine hydrochloride and chlordiazepoxide in their binary mixture using novel univariate spectrophotometric methods via different manipulation pathways. *Spectrochimica Acta, Part A* 155: 11–20.

75 Lotfy, H.M., Fayez, Y.M., Tawakkol, S.M. et al. (2017). Evaluation of graphical and statistical representation of analytical signals of spectrophotometric methods. *Spectrochimica Acta, Part A* 184: 61–70.

76 El-Bardicy, M.G., Lotfy, H.M., El-Sayed, M.A., and El-Tarras, M.F. (2008). Smart stability-indicating spectrophotometric methods for determination of binary mixtures without prior separation. *Journal of AOAC International* 91: 299–310.

77 Darwish, H., Metwally, F.H., and El Bayoumi, A. (2015). Novel ratio subtraction and isoabsorptive point methods for determination of ambroxol hydrochloride and doxycycline in their combined dosage form: development and validation. *Tropical Journal of Pharmaceutical Research* 14: 133–140.

78 Lotfy, H.M., and Hagazy, M.A. (2012). Comparative study of novel spectrophotometric methods manipulating ratio spectra; an application on pharmaceutical ternary mixture of omeprazole, tinidazole and clarithromycin. *Spectrochimica Acta, Part A* 96: 259–270.

79 Bachri, M., Masfria, M., Syahputra, S., and Hafid, H. (2019). Quantitative estimation of anti hypertension combination by ratio subtraction spectrophotometry method. *Open Access Macedonian Journal of Medical Sciences* 7: 2940–2946.

80 Lotfy, H.M., Saleh, S.S., Hassan, N.Y., and Elgizawy, S.M. (2013). Univariate versus multivariate spectrophotometric methods for simultaneous determination of complex binary mixtures with overlapped spectra: a comparative study. *Analytical Chemistry Letters* 3: 70–84.

81 Mohammad, M.-A.-A., Mahrouse, M.A., Amer, E.A.H., and Elharati, N.S. (2021). Simultaneous determination of enalapril maleate and nitrendipine in tablets using spectrophotometric methods manipulating ratio spectra. *Spectrochimica Acta, Part A* 244: 118894–118902.

82 Obaydo, R.H., and Alhaj Sakur, A. (2019). Fingerprint spectrophotometric methods for the determination of co-formulated otic solution of ciprofloxacin and fluocinolone acetonide in their challengeable ratio. *Journal of Analytical Methods in Chemistry* 2019: 8919345.

83 Bagherian, G., Salehi Mobarake, F., Arab Chamjangali, M. et al. (2020). Comparison between univariate and multivariate calibration methods for simultaneous spectrophotometric determination of catechol and hydroquinone in their binary mixture. *Frontiers in Chemical Research* 2: 1–9.

84 Lotfy, H.M., and Saleh, S.S. (2018). Testing the purity of spectral profiles: finger-print resolution of complex matrices and extraction of absorbance signals. *Spectrochimica Acta, Part A* 205: 160–169.

85 Lotfy, H.M., and Hegazy, M. (2013). Simultaneous determination of some cholesterol-lowering drugs in their binary mixture by novel spectrophotometric methods. *Spectrochimica Acta, Part A* 113: 107–114.

86 Fayez, Y.M., Elghobashy, M.R., Goda, Z.M., and Shehata, M.A. (2016). Comparative study on four spectrophotometric methods manipulating ratio spectra for the simultaneous determination of binary mixture of diflucortolone valerate and isoconazole nitrate. *Bulletin of Faculty of Pharmacy Cairo University* 54: 39–47.

87 Mohsen, A.M., Lotfy, H.M., Badawey, A.M. et al. (2013). Application of three novel spectrophotometric methods manipulating ratio spectra for resolving a pharmaceutical mixture of chlorphenoxamine hydrochloride and caffeine. *International Journal of Pharmacy and Pharmaceutical Sciences* 5: 478–487.

88 Victor, N., Elfiky, H., Badawey, A., and Abdelghany, M. (2021). Simultaneous determination of xipamide and triamterene by first derivative, ratio difference, and derivative ratio spectrophotometric methods. *Archives of Pharmaceutical Sciences Ain Shams University* 5: 52–62.

89 Lotfy, H.M. (2012). Determination of simvastatin and ezatimibe in combined tablet dosage forms by constant center spectrophotometric method. *International Journal of Pharmaceutical Sciences* 4: 673–679.

90 El-Maraghy, C.M., and Lamie, N.T. (2019). Three smart spectrophotometric methods for resolution of severely overlapped binary mixture of ibuprofen and paracetamol in pharmaceutical dosage form. *BMC Chemistry* 13: 1–8.

91 Attia, K.A.-S., Abdel-Aziz, O., Nasef, N., and Mohamed, G. (2018). Determination of flucloxacillin-sodium in binary mixture with ampicillin-trihydrate using univariate and multivariate spectrophotometric methods: a comparative study. *Journal of Advanced Pharmacy Research* 2: 180–190.

92 Mostafa, N.M., Fayez, Y.M., Farid, J.F., and Abd El-Alim, A.E.-A.B. (2017). Stability indicating spectrophotometric methods for determination of ivabradine hydrochloride in the presence of its degradation product. *Analytical Chemistry Letters* 7: 280–294.

93 Saleh, S.S., Lotfy, H.M., Tiris, G. et al. (2022). The power of high impact amplitude manipulation (HIAM) technique for extracting the basic spectra of two fixed-dose combinations (FDC)—spectrophotometric purity analysis via spectral contrast angle. *Spectrochimica Acta, Part A* 273: 121036–121041.

94 Saleh, S.S., Lotfy, H.M., Hassan, N.Y., and Salem, H. (2014). A comparative study of progressive versus successive spectrophotometric resolution techniques applied for pharmaceutical ternary mixtures. *Spectrochimica Acta, Part A* 132: 239–248.

95 Saleh, S.S., and Riad, S.M. (2018). Analytical investigation on green smart spectrophotometric methods utilizing unified regression equation. *Analytical Chemistry Letters* 8: 268–276.

96 Kelani, K.M., Shalaby, A.A., Elmaamly, M., and Halim, M. (2015). Spectrophotometric and chemometric methods for simultaneous determination of two anti-hypertensive drugs in their combined dosage form. *Pharmaceutica Analytica Acta* 6: 2.

97 Zaghary, W.A., Mowaka, S., and Hendy, M.S. (2020). Sample enrichment of canagliflozin prior to its spectrophotometric determination in presence of metformin: application to recently approved binary dosage form. *Journal of Analytical Chemistry* 75: 742–753.

98 Moussa, B.A., Mahrouse, M.A., and Fawzy, M.G. (2021). Smart spectrophotometric methods for the simultaneous determination of newly co-formulated hypoglycemic drugs in binary mixtures. *Spectrochimica Acta, Part A* 257: 119763–119771.

99 Rizk, M.S., Sultan, M., Mohamed, D., and Tony, R.M. (2017). Simultaneous determination of levonorgestrel and ethinyl estradiol in combined dosage form utilizing spectrophotometric methods and high performance thin layer chromatographic method on nanosilica gel plates. *European Journal of Chemistry* 8: 52–59.

100 Lotfy, H.M., Saleh, S.S., Hassan, N.Y., and Salem, H. (2015). Computation of geometric representation of novel spectrophotometric methods used for the analysis of minor components in pharmaceutical preparations. *Spectrochimica Acta, Part A* 151: 628–643.

101 Lotfy, H.M., Saleh, S.S., and El-Maraghy, C.M. (2020). Advanced approaches for the treatment and amplification of weak spectral signals produced by critical concentrations in white multicomponent systems. *Spectrochimica Acta, Part A* 224: 117339–117406.

102 Yehia, A.M. (2013). Development and validation of new spectrophotometric ratio H-point standard addition method and application to gastrointestinal acting drugs mixtures. *Spectrochimica Acta, Part A* 109: 193–200.

103 Yehia, A.M., and Abd El-Rahman, M.K. (2015). Application of normalized spectra in resolving a challenging orphenadrine and paracetamol binary mixture. *Spectrochimica Acta, Part A* 138: 21–30.

104 Salinas, F., Berzas Nevado, J.J., and Mansilla, A.E. (1990). A new spectrophotometric method for quantitative multicomponent analysis resolution of mixtures of salicylic and salicyluric acids. *Talanta* 37: 347–351.

105 Darwish, H.W., Hassan, S.A., Salem, M.Y., and El-Zeiny, B.A. (2011). Three different spectrophotometric methods manipulating ratio spectra for determination of binary mixture of amlodipine and atorvastatin. *Spectrochimica Acta, Part A* 83: 140–148.

106 Dinç, E., Baydan, E., Kanbur, M., and Onur, F. (2002). Spectrophotometric multicomponent determination of sunset yellow, tartrazine and allura red in soft drink powder by double divisor-ratio spectra derivative, inverse least-squares and principal component regression methods. *Talanta* 58: 579–594.

107 Ayman, A., Zeid, A.M., Wahba, M.E.K., and El-Shabrawy, Y. (2022). Simultaneous determination of ergotamine, caffeine and dipyrone in their ternary mixture by applying double divisor and first derivative ratio spectra methods. *Annales Pharmaceutiques Françaises* 80 (5): 718–729.

108 Dinç, E., Kökdil, G., and Onur, F. (2001). Derivative ratio spectra–zero crossing spectrophotometry and LC method applied to the quantitative determination of paracetamol, propyphenazone and caffeine in ternary mixtures. *Journal of Pharmaceutical and Biomedical Analysis* 26: 769–778.

109 Lamie, N.T., and Yehia, A.M. (2015). Development of normalized spectra manipulating spectrophotometric methods for simultaneous determination of dimenhydrinate and cinnarizine binary mixture. *Spectrochimica Acta, Part A* 150: 142–150.

110 Issa, M.M., Nejem, R.M., Stefan Van Staden R.I., and Aboul-Enein H.Y. (2015). New approach application of data transformation in mean centering of ratio spectra method. *Spectrochimica Acta, Part A* 142: 204–209.

111 Afkhami, A., and Bahram, M. (2005). Mean centering of ratio spectra as a new spectrophotometric method for the analysis of binary and ternary mixtures. *Talanta* 66: 712–720.

112 Gorji, S., and Bahram, M. (2010). Spectrophotometric determination of acidity constants by mean centering of ratio spectra. *Analytical Methods* 2: 1514–1521.

113 Hegazy, M.A. (2015). A novel pure component contribution algorithm (PCCA) for extracting components' contribution from severely overlapped signals; an application to UV-spectrophotometric data. *Spectrochimica Acta, Part A* 151: 405–414.

114 Mowaka, S., Hegazy, M.A., Lotfy, H.M., and Mohamed, E.H. (2017). Novel pure component contribution algorithm (PCCA) and UHPLC methods for separation and quantification of amlodipine, valsartan, and hydrochlorothiazide in ternary mixture. *Journal of AOAC International* 100: 692–699.

115 Obaydo, R.H., and Sakur, A.A. (2019). A green analytical method using algorithm (PCCA) for extracting components' contribution from severely overlapped spectral signals in pharmaceutical mixtures. *Research Journal of Pharmacy and Technology* 12: 4332–4338.

116 Afkhami, A., and Abbasi-Tarighat, M. (2009). Application of continuous wavelet transformation to the simultaneous kinetic determination of binary mixtures. *Talanta* 78: 424–431.

117 Afkhami, A., Nematollahi, D., Madrakian, T. et al. (2009). Simultaneous spectrophotometric determination of binary mixtures of surfactants using continuous wavelet transformation. *Journal of Hazardous Materials* 166: 770–775.

118 Dinc, E., Kaya, S., Doganay, T., and Baleanu, D. (2007). Continuous wavelet and derivative transforms for the simultaneous quantitative analysis and dissolution test of levodopa–benserazide tablets. *Journal of Pharmaceutical and Biomedical Analysis* 44: 991–995.

119 Dastaran, R., Sheibani, A., Shishehbore, M.R., and Saeedi-Sourck, H. (2022). Continuous wavelet transform for simultaneous determination of atorvastatin and rosuvastatin in combined pharmaceutical formulations. *Journal of Applied Spectroscopy* 88: 1195–1201.

120 Dinç, E., Üstündağ, Ö., Tilkan, G.Y. et al. (2017). Continuous wavelet transform methods for the simultaneous determinations and dissolution profiles of valsartan and hydrochlorothiazide in tablets. *Brazilian Journal of Pharmaceutical Sciences* 53 (1): e16050.

121 Lotfy, H.M., and Saleh, S.S. (2019). Investigating advanced approaches based on iso-absorptivity coefficient in unresolved spectral signals of binary mixtures. *Journal of Analytical Methods in Chemistry* 2019: 7924821.

122 Lotfy, H.M., Elshahed, M.S., and Mohamed, D. (2020). The concept of relative absorptivity distribution for enhancing disbanding power of spectrophotometric technique to resolve co-formulated tablets: a tool for purity index and uniformity assessment. *Spectrochimica Acta Part A* 239: 118551–118560.

123 Lotfy, H.M., Monir, H.H., Erk, N., and Rostom, Y. (2020). Novel feature extraction approach for achieving potential spectral resolution: green analytical application on zofenopril calcium and hydrochlorothiazide in their spectrally overlapping binary mixture. *Spectrochimica Acta Part A* 230: 117998–118112.

124 Saleh, S.S., and Lotfy, H.M. (2017). Advanced amplitude centering as an invigorating manipulation for unified wavelength spectral resolution of ternary mixtures. *International Journal of Pharmacy and Pharmaceutical Sciences* 9: 43–50.

125 Ahmed, D.A., and Lotfy, H.M. (2022). Sticking-pulling strategy for assessment of combined medicine for management of tough symptoms in COVID-19 pandemic using different windows of spectrophotometric platform-counterfeit products' detection. *Spectrochimica Acta Part A* 277: 121256–121273.

126 Lotfy, H.M., Ahmed, D.A., Abdel Rahman, M.K., and Weshahy, S.A. (2019). Study of efficiency and spectral resolution for mathematical filtration technique using novel unlimited derivative ratio and classical univariate spectrophotometric methods for the multicomponent determination-stability analysis. *Heliyon* 5 (5): e01669–e01712.

127 Lotfy, H.M., and Fahmy, N.M. (2020). Coupling of liquid-liquid extraction and mathematical filtration techniques for the separation and quantification of five components in semisolid dosage form with severely overlapped spectra. *Spectrochimica Acta Part A* 235: 118299–118310.

128 Soliman, R.M., Mostafa, N.M., Fayez, Y.M. et al. (2022). Novel spectrophotometric approaches for the simultaneous quantification of ternary common cold mixture containing paracetamol with a challenging formulation ratio: greenness profile evaluation. *Journal of AOAC International* 105 (5): 1268–1279.

129 da Silva, T.L.A., Lustosa, I.A., Torres, L.M., and Kogawa, A.C. (2022). Eco-friendly UV spectrophotometric method for evaluation of marbofloxacin in tablets: stability study. *Journal of AOAC International* 5: 30–42.

130 Rostom, Y., Wadie, M., Rezk, M.R. et al. (2022). Fingerprinting and iso-absorptive resolution techniques for the spectrally overlapping dutasteride and silodosin mixture: content uniformity testing along with greenness profile assessment. *Spectrochimica Acta Part A* 273: 121063–121070.

131 El-Masry, A.A., El-Wasseef, D.R., Eid, M. et al. (2022). Development of three ecological spectroscopic methods for analysis of betrixaban either alone or in mixture with lercanidipine: greenness assessment. *Royal Society Open Science* 9: 211457–211462.

132 Elmasry, M.S., Hassan, W.S., El-Mammli, M.Y., and Badrawy, M. (2022). Earth friendly spectrophotometric methods based on different manipulation approaches for simultaneous determination of aspirin and omeprazole in binary mixture and pharmaceutical dosage form: comparative statistical study. *Spectrochimica Acta Part A* 266: 120436–120441.

133 Fawzy, M.G. (2022). Different approaches for the assessment of greenness of spectrophotometric methodologies utilized for resolving the spectral overlap of newly approved binary hypoglycemic pharmaceutical mixture. *Spectrochimica Acta Part A* 272: 120998–121005.

134 Attala, K., and Elsonbaty, K.A. (2021). Advanced eco-friendly UV spectrophotometric approach for resolving overlapped spectral signals of antihypertensive agents in their binary and tertiary pharmaceutical dosage form. *Spectrochimica Acta Part A* 258: 119855–11992.

135 Said, N., Nasr, Z., and El Razeq, S.A. (2021). Green stability indicating UV-spectrophotometric techniques for estimation of tenofovir alafenamide in bulk form and dosage forms. *Azhar International Journal of Pharmaceutical and Medical Sciences* 1 (1): 97–105.

136 Attimarad, M., Nair, A.B., Sreeharsha, N. et al. (2021). Development and validation of green UV derivative spectrophotometric methods for simultaneous determination metformin and remogliflozin from formulation: evaluation of greenness. *International Journal of Environmental Research and Public Health* 18: 448–452.

137 Attimarad, M., Venugopala, K.N., Al-Dhubiab, B.E. et al. (2021). Development of ecofriendly derivative spectrophotometric methods for the simultaneous quantitative analysis of remogliflozin and vildagliptin from formulation. *Molecules* 26: 6160–6169.

138 Kannaiah, K., and Sugumaran, A. (2022). Eco-friendly ultraviolet spectrophotometric methods for the determination of clotrimazole and tinidazole in bulk and ointment dosage form. *Current Chemistry Letters* 11 (1): 11–22.

139 Kokilambigai, K., and Lakshmi, K. (2021). Utilization of green analytical chemistry principles for the simultaneous estimation of paracetamol, aceclofenac and thiocolchicoside by UV spectrophotometry. *Green Chemistry Letters and Reviews* 14: 99–107.

140 El-Yazbi, A.F. (2021). Eco-friendly analytical methods for the determination of compounds with disparate spectral overlapping: application to antiviral formulation of sofosbuvir and velpatasvir. *Journal of Analytical Science and Technology* 12: 7.

141 Naguib, I.A., Abdelaleem, E.A., Hassan, E.S., and Emam, A.A. (2021). Validated spectral manipulations for determination of an anti-neoplastic drug and its related impurities including its hazardous degradation product. *RSC Advances* 11: 21332–21342.

142 Abdelwhab, N.S., Habib, N.M., Abdelrahman, M.M. et al. (2022). Determination of sulphasalazine and its related compounds by simple, smart, validated, green spectrophotometric methods. *Journal of AOAC International* 105: 352–361.

143 Sayed, A., Mohamed, A.R., Hassan, W.S., and Elmasry, M.S. (2021). Comparative study of novel green UV-spectrophotometric platforms for simultaneous rapid analysis of flumethasone pivalate and clioquinol in their combined formulation. *Drug Development and Industrial Pharmacy* 47: 867–877.

144 Sayed, R.A., Mohamed, A.R., Hassan, W.S., and Elmasry, M.S. (2021). Smart UV-spectrophotometric platforms for rapid green analysis of miconazole nitrate and nystatin in their combined suppositories and in vitro dissolution testing. *Drug Development and Industrial Pharmacy* 47 (9): 1469–1480.

145 El-Yazbi, A.F., Khamis, E.F., Youssef, R.M. et al. (2020). Green analytical methods for simultaneous determination of compounds having relatively disparate absorbance; application to antibiotic formulation of azithromycin and levofloxacin. *Heliyon* 6: e04819–e04825.

146 Naguib, I.A., Abdelaleem, E.A., Hassan, E.S., and Emam, A.A. (2020). Comparative study of eco-friendly spectrophotometric methods for accurate quantification of mebendazole and quinfamide combination; content uniformity evaluation. *Spectrochimica Acta Part A* 235: 118271–118280.

147 Merey, H., El-Mosallamy, S.S., Hassan, N.Y., and El-Zeany, B.A. (2020). Validated eco-friendly spectrophotometric methods for the determination of acefylline piperazine and bromhexine hydrochloride in the presence of dosage form additives. *Journal of Applied Spectroscopy* 87: 159–168.

148 Tantawy, M.A., Weshahy, S.A., Wadie, M., and Rezk, M.R. (2021). Eco-friendly spectrophotometric methods for assessment of alfuzosin and solifenacin in their new pharmaceutical formulation; green profile evaluation via Eco-Scale and GAPI tools. *Current Pharmaceutical Analysis* 17: 1093–1103.

149 Fayez, Y.M., Michael, A.M., Monir, H.H. et al. (2020). Comprehensive comparative study of eco-friendly univariate and multivariate methodological approaches on processing multi-component formulation quality. *Spectrochimica Acta Part A* 243: 118816–118825.

150 Lotfy, H., Obaydo, R., and Sakur, A. (2021). Evaluation of assay and in-vitro dissolution profile of certain fixed-dose combination using green analytical method. *Annales Pharmaceutiques Françaises* 79 (1): 3–15.

151 Merey, H.A., Ramadan, N.K., Diab, S.S., and Moustafa, A.A. (2020). Green spectrophotometric methods for the determination of a binary mixture of lidocaine hydrochloride and cetylpyridinium chloride in the presence of dimethylaniline. *Spectrochimica Acta Part A* 242: 118743–118750.

152 Mohamed, E.H., and El-Maraghy, C.M. (2020). Eco-friendly-assessed TLC-densitometry and absorptivity coefficient based spectrophotometric methods for resolution and simultaneous analysis of two gastrointestinal acting drugs with superimposed spectra. *Microchemical Journal* 158: 105161–105170.

153 Vu Dang, H., Truong, H., Dong, L., and Nguyen, H. (2020). RP-HPLC and UV spectrophotometric analysis of paracetamol, ibuprofen, and caffeine in solid pharmaceutical dosage forms by derivative, Fourier, and wavelet transforms: a comparison study. *Journal of Analytical Methods in Chemistry* 2020: 8107571.

154 Abdelhamid, N.S. (2020). A comparative study of two novel validated spectrophotometric techniques for resolution of four-component mixtures with severely overlapping spectra. *Spectrochimica Acta Part A* 233: 118213–118220.

155 Sakur, A.A., and Obaydo, R.H. (2020). PCCA algorithm as a fingerprint resolution technique for the analysis of ciprofloxacin in the presence of its acid induced degradation product. *Research Journal of Pharmacy and Technology* 13: 5999–6006.

156 Lotfy, H.M., Mohamed, D., and Elshahed, M.S. (2019). Novel univariate spectrophotometric determination of the recently released solid dosage form comprising dapagliflozin and saxagliptin via factorized response spectra: assessment of the average content and dosage unit uniformity of tablets. *Spectrochimica Acta Part A* 222: 117120–117130.

157 Lotfy, H.M., Erk, N., and Rostom, Y. (2019). Developing spectral numerical factor technique for the determination of amlodipine besylate and the latest generation of statins in their new pharmaceutical combination. *Spectrochimica Acta Part A* 218: 320–330.

158 Al Zakri, D.J., Obaydo, R.H., and Sakur, A.A. (2019). New spectral resolution techniques for resolving and determining the components in binary fixed-dose combinations. *Heliyon* 5: e02637–e02642.

159 Obaydo, R.H., and Sakur, A.A. (2019). Spectrophotometric strategies for the analysis of binary combinations with minor component based on isoabsorptive point's leveling effect: an application on ciprofloxacin and fluocinolone acetonide in their recently delivered co-formulation. *Spectrochimica Acta Part A* 219: 186–194.

160 Amin, K.F., Abdullah, A.M., and Fakhre, N.A. (2019). Mean centering-triple divisor and ratio derivative-zero crossing for simultaneous determination of some diabetes drugs in their quaternary mixture with severely overlapping spectra. *Spectrochimica Acta Part A* 222: 117261–117270.

161 Lotfy, H.M., Morgan, E.M., Fayez, Y.M., and Abdelkawy, M. (2019). Different aspects in manipulating overlapped spectra used for the analysis of trimebutine maleate and structure elucidation of its degradation products. *Future Journal of Pharmaceutical Sciences* 5: 7.

162 El-Alamin, M.M.A., Sultan, M.A., Hegazy, M. et al. (2019). Pure component contribution (PCCA) and synergy interval partial least squares (siPLS) algorithms for efficient resolution and quantification of overlapped signals; an application to novel antiviral tablets of daclatasvir, sofosbuvir and ribavirin. *European Journal of Chemistry* 10: 350–357.

163 Hegazy, M.A., Badawey, A.M., Bakr, M.A., and Abbas, S.S. (2019). Spectrophotometric resolution and quantification of ternary co-formulated mixture of thioctic acid, benfotiamine and cyanocobalamin. *Research Journal of Pharmacy and Technology* 12: 2648–2656.

164 Ibrahim, F.A., El-Brashy, A.M., El-Awady, M.I., and Abdallah, N.A. (2019). Assessment of the greenness of spectrophotometric and micellar liquid chromatographic methods using two approaches: application to pharmaceutical analysis of hydrochlorothiazide and telmisartan. *Microchemical Journal* 148: 197–205.

165 Kalyani, L., and Rao, C.V. (2018). Simultaneous spectrophotometric estimation of salbutamol, theophylline and ambroxol three component tablet formulation using simultaneous equation methods. *Karbala International Journal of Modern Science* 4: 171–179.

166 Boltia, S.A., Fayed, A.S., Hegazy, M.A., and Musaed, A. (2018). Four validated spectrophotometric methods for determination of ambroxol, guaifenesin, and theophylline in their ternary mixture in bulk powder and dosage form. *Journal of Pharmacy Research* 12: 7–16.

167 Lotfy, H.M., Fayez, Y.M., Tawakkol, S.M. et al. (2018). Spectrophotometric resolution of the severely overlapped spectra of clotrimazole with dexamethasone in cream dosage form by mathematical manipulation steps. *Spectrochimica Acta Part A* 202: 115–122.

168 Hegazy, M., Elshahed, M., Toubar, S., and Helmy, M. (2018). Efficient processing of single and multiple spectral variables for resolution and quantitation of paracetamol, chlorzoxazone and diclofenac. *Journal of Advanced Pharmacy Research* 2: 269–282.

169 Youssef, S.H., Hegazy, M.A., Mohamed, D., and Badawey, A.M. (2018). Analysis of paracetamol, pseudoephedrine and cetirizine in Allercet Cold® capsules using spectrophotometric techniques. *Chemistry Central Journal* 12: 67.

170 Ragab, M.A., El Yazbi, F.A., Hassan, E. et al. (2018). Spectrophotometric analysis of two eye preparations, vial and drops, containing ketorolac tromethamine and phenylephrine hydrochloride binary mixture and their ternary mixture with chlorphenirmaine maleate. *Bulletin of Faculty of Pharmacy, Cairo University* 56: 91–100.

171 Emam, A.A., Abdelaleem, E.A., Naguib, I.A. et al. (2018). Successive ratio subtraction as a novel manipulation of ratio spectra for quantitative determination of a mixture of furosemide, spironolactone and canrenone. *Spectrochimica Acta Part A* 192: 427–436.

172 Sohrabi, M.R., Mirzabeygi, V., and Davallo, M. (2018). Use of continuous wavelet transform approach for simultaneous quantitative determination of multicomponent mixture by UV–Vis spectrophotometry. *Spectrochimica Acta Part A* 201: 306–314.

173 Lotfy, H.M., and Omran, Y.R. (2018). Novel absorptivity centering method utilizing normalized and factorized spectra for analysis of mixtures with overlapping spectra in different matrices using built-in spectrophotometer software. *Spectrochimica Acta Part A* 200: 167–178.

174 Fayez, Y.M., Tawakkol, S.M., Fahmy, N.M. et al. (2018). Comparative study of the efficiency of computed univariate and multivariate methods for the estimation of the binary mixture of clotrimazole and dexamethasone using two different spectral regions. *Spectrochimica Acta Part A* 194: 126–135.

175 Ahmed, D.A., Abdel-Aziz, O., Abdel-Ghany, M., and Weshahy, S.A. (2018). Stability indicating determination of albendazole in bulk drug and pharmaceutical dosage form by chromatographic and spectrophotometric methods. *Future Journal of Pharmaceutical Sciences* 4: 161–165.

176 Abdel-Ghany, M.F., Hussein, L.A., and Ayad, M.F. Youssef, M.M. (2017). Investigation of different spectrophotometric and chemometric methods for determination of entacapone, levodopa and carbidopa in ternary mixture. *Spectrochimica Acta Part A* 171: 236–245.

177 Abdelwahab, N.S. and Mohamed, M.A. (2017). Three new methods for resolving ternary mixture with overlapping spectra: comparative study. *Chemical and Pharmaceutical Bulletin* 65: 558–565.

178 Lotfy, H.M., Fayez, Y.M., Tawakkol, S.M. et al. (2017). Spectrophotometric determination for the binary mixture of clotrimazole and dexamethasone in pharmaceutical dosage form. *Analytical Chemistry Letters* 7: 30–42.

179 Abdelhameed, A.S., Attwa, M.W., Attia, M.I. et al. (2022). Development of novel univariate and multivariate validated chemometric methods for the analysis of dasatinib, sorafenib, and vandetanib in pure form, dosage forms and biological fluids. *Spectrochimica Acta Part A* 264: 120336–120342.

180 Haque, S.M. (2022). Box–Behnken experimental design for optimizing the HPLC method to determine hydrochlorothiazide in pharmaceutical formulations and biological fluid. *Journal of Molecular Liquids* 352: 118708–118718.

181 Hassouna, M.E. and Salem, H.O. (2019). Novel spectrophotometric methods for simultaneous determination of rosuvastatin calcium, timolol maleate and diclofenac sodium in pharmaceutical ternary mixture and spiked human plasma. *Journal of Pharmaceutical Research International* 31: 1–21.

182 Hassan, W.S., Elmasry, M.S., Elsayed, H.M., and Zidan, D.W. (2018). Comparative study of six sequential spectrophotometric methods for quantification and separation of ribavirin, sofosbuvir and daclatasvir: an application on laboratory prepared mixture, pharmaceutical preparations, spiked human urine, spiked human plasma, and dissolution test. *Spectrochimica Acta Part A* 202: 159–173.

183 Belal, F., Ibrahim, F., Sheribah, Z.A., and Alaa, H. (2018). Novel univariate and multivariate regression methods for the simultaneous analysis of ternary mixture of 1,4-benzodiazepines in dosage forms and human urine. *Clinica Chimica Acta* 482: 108–119.

184 Belal, F., Ibrahim, F., Sheriah, Z.A., and Alaa, H. (2018). New spectrophotometric/ chemometric assisted methods for the simultaneous determination of imatinib, gemifloxacin, nalbuphine and naproxen in pharmaceutical formulations and human urine. *Spectrochimica Acta Part A* 198: 51–60.

185 Abdelfatah, R.M., Mahmoud, H.M., Elsayed, M.A., and Hegazy, A.M. (2020). Green spectrophotometric approaches for simultaneous analysis of tomato pesticides in commercial formulations and environmental samples. *Microchemical Journal* 152: 104305–104315.

186 Omer, S.A., and Fakhre, N.A. (2020). Simultaneous determination of ternary mixture of carboxin, chlorpyrifos, and tebuconazole residues in cabbage samples using three spectrophotometric methods. *Journal of Analytical Methods in Chemistry* 2020: 4912762.

9

Cyclodextrin-Based Molecular Inclusion by Grinding

Quality by Design in Green Chemistry

Sanyam Sharma, Subh Naman and Ashish Baldi

Pharma Innovation Lab, Department of Pharmaceutical Sciences and Technology, Maharaja Ranjit Singh Punjab Technical University, Bathinda, Punjab, India

CONTENTS

9.1 Introduction

In the chemical sector, where there is a requirement for more eco-friendly methods, and particularly in the pharmaceutical field, where methods for assessing the greenness of processes and solvents are utilised in the manufacture of fine chemicals and pharmaceuticals, the total reduction of solvent utilisation by using green chemistry approaches is a key objective. Green chemistry must be used due to increasing environmental limitations [1, 2]. One of the most challenging problems in pharmaceutical technology is increasing the physicochemical characteristics of less soluble drugs. The Biopharmaceutical Classification System (BCS) divides active pharmaceutical ingredients (APIs) into four classifications depending on their solubility and permeability. Drugs in Classes II and IV have poor water solubility, which can be enhanced by CD complexes [3]. Numerous industries, including the food, pharmaceutical, and cosmetics industries, utilise cyclodextrins (CDs) extensively [4]. As members of the cyclic oligosaccharide family, CDs have a conical or truncated cone shape because of the chair conformation of the glucopyranoside units. The secondary hydroxyl functions of the sugar residues are found in the larger end of the torus, whereas the primary hydroxyl functions are found near the smaller lower edge. The skeletal carbons and ethereal oxygen of the glucose residue are covered in the core cavity of the molecule. This structure allows CDs to interact with a wide range of hydrophobic guest molecules to generate host–guest interactions [5]. The ability of CDs to combine multiple active substances into inclusion complexes, which enhance their physicochemical characteristics (solubility, stability, bioavailability, etc.), is the reason for their prevalence [6]. The development of non-covalent dynamic inclusion complexes is the basis for the mechanism of complexation [7]. In an aqueous solution, energetically unfavourable water molecules

Sustainable Approaches in Pharmaceutical Sciences, First Edition. Edited by Kamal Shah, Durgesh Nandini Chauhan, and Nagendra Singh Chauhan.

occupy the slightly apolar CD cavity, making it simple for compatible guest compounds that are less polar than water to occupy their place. The complex is produced as a result of the substitution of the high-enthalpy water molecules with a suitable guest component. The host molecule is the dispersed CD. One or more guest molecules are trapped within one, two, or three CD molecules. The host : guest ratio is typically 1 : 1, which is what molecular encapsulation is all about [8].

CDs can be utilised to achieve a variety of goals, including improving solubility, bioavailability, and stability, converting liquids and oils into amorphous powder, limiting evaporation, preserving flavour, reducing tastes and odours, preventing admixture incompatibilities, and haemolysis [7]. The structures of some of the different derivatives of CD are shown in Figure 9.1.

Widely viable varieties of CDs include the naturally occurring α-CD, β-CD, and γ-CD, as well as their numerous chemically modified variants [2]. The hydrophilic CD derivatives with pharmaceutical relevance include hydroxypropyl α cyclodextrin (HPαCD), hydroxypropyl–cyclodextrin (HPγCD), hydroxypropyl β cyclodextrin (HPβCD), crystalline dimethyl β cyclodextrin (DIMEB), randomly methylated β cyclodextrin (RAMEB), hydroxyethyl β cyclodextrin (HEβCD), sulfobutyl ether β cyclodextrin sodium salt (SBEβCD), and triacetyl-cyclodextrin (TAγCD). There are also other hydrophobic CD derivatives [2].

9.2 Cyclodextrin Inclusion Complex Formation by Grinding

For the combination with methyl-cyclodextrin, a greater stability constant value and a greater enhancement in terbinafine solubility up to 200-fold were discovered by Uzqueda and co-workers. Fourier transform infrared spectroscopy (FTIR), X-ray diffraction, and thermal analysis were used to create and characterise solid systems with a 1 : 1 drug : CD molar ratio [9–11]. They suggested that the co-evaporation approach was probably the most effective way to make these solid compounds. With the exception of the CD, the complexes of terbinafine with native CD were crystalline, but the methyl and hydroxypropyl derivatives produced amorphous phases.

Studies on the dissolution rate of terbinafine : CD and other complexes demonstrated the beneficial effects of complexation on drug dissolution [12]. The dry co-grinding

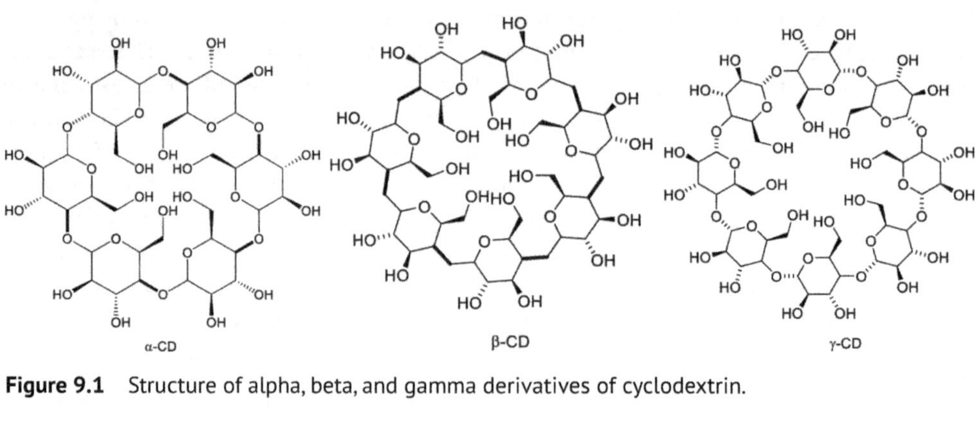

Figure 9.1 Structure of alpha, beta, and gamma derivatives of cyclodextrin.

technique was used by Arias and colleagues to create binary systems of triamterene and CD [13]. Scanning electron microscopy (SEM) and FTIR were used to characterise them. The key finding from this research was a strong drug–carrier interaction, which was clearly correlated with an increase in the amorphous nature of the drug. The dissolution rate was increased up to fivefold, with dissolving efficiency over the first 60 minutes of free drug. This might be explained by the increase in wettability of the drug in its amorphous state, inclusion complex development in the liquid state, and the amorphous state itself.

Aigner and his core group developed an inclusion complex of gemfibrozil and dimethyl cyclodextrin by the co-grinding method. Differential scanning calorimetry (DSC), X-ray powder diffractometry, and FTIR with curve-fitting analysis were used for evaluation of the complexes [14]. After 35 minutes of co-grinding, the authors judged that the sample's crystallinity had dropped too slowly and that the final product was totally amorphous. By using X-ray powder diffractometry and FTIR, a linear relationship was found between CD complex formation and co-grinding duration. The ratio of complex formation remained the same after co-grinding for 30 minutes. These investigations showed that complexing gem fibrozil with dimethyl β cyclodextrin can be accomplished through co-grinding. The result showed that the gem fibrozil–dimethyl β cyclodextrin product was amorphous.

The structure of different inclusion complexes of various ratios of CD is shown in Figure 9.2. Table 9.1 covers all the previously published research related to inclusion complex formation through grinding techniques involving various mills.

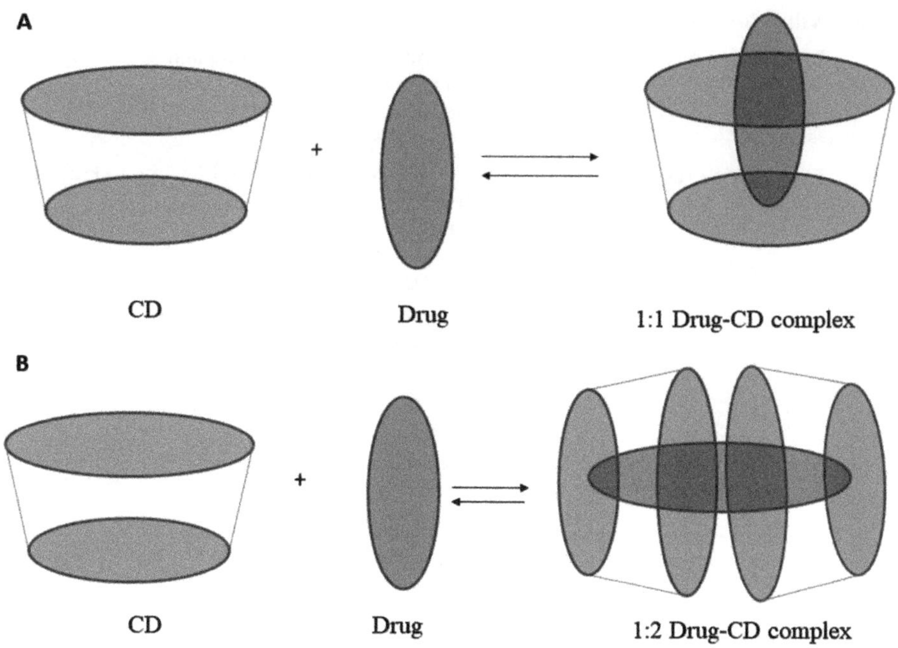

Figure 9.2 Different structures of inclusion complexes of cyclodextrin (CD) with different ratios of CD.

Table 9.1 Preparation of inclusion complexes of various drugs with cyclodextrin (CD) by grinding.

Type of CD used	Drug	Drug/CD ratio	Strategies and outcome	References
Mortar and pestle				
α-CD, β-CD, γ-CD, DIMEB, RAMEB	Trimetoprim, sulfadiazine, sulfamethoxazole	1 : 1	The grinding time was 15 min and results concluded that amorphous product was formed with RAMEB	[47]
HPβCD	Rifampicin	1 : 1	After 3 min of trituration and 30 min of grinding, the complex was created, yielding an amorphous product with 2.5× higher solubility	[49]
β-CD	Rifaldazine	1 : 1	After 3 min of trituration and 30 min of grinding, the complex was synthesised, yielding an amorphous product with 4.4× solubility	[50]
β-CD-EPI, β-CD-EPS	Naproxen	–	The amorphous product was formed by 40 min of grinding with enhanced dissolution	[48]
DIMEB	Gemifibrozil	1 : 1	The grinding time was 35 min and amorphous product was formed	[14]
α-CD	Naproxen	–	Pseudo inclusion was formed after 30 min grinding	[46]
α-CD	Chloramphenicol	1 : 1	Partial inclusion was formed after 120 min grinding	[45]
High-energy vibrational mills				
β-CD	Indomethacin nicotinamide cocrystals	1 : 1	The grinding time was 15 min and results showed a significant increase in dissolution rate with an amorphous system	[51]
HEβCD, HPβCD, SBEβCD, β-CD-EPI	Econazole nitrate	1 : 1	20 Hz and 15–60 min of grinding were done in normal surroundings. The result was an amorphous product with both HPβCD and SBEβCD.	[52]
α-CD	Econazole	1 : 1	The parameters for grinding were 60 min at 24 Hz yielding an amorphous product	[53]
HPβCD, SBEβCD	Daidzein, genistein	1 : 1	The product was prepared at ambient conditions for 30 min. Partially crystalline product was formed and SBEβCD was more efficient as the amorphising agent	[54]

Table 9.1 (Continued)

Type of CD used	Drug	Drug/ CD ratio	Strategies and outcome	References
β-CD-EPI, CMβCD-EPI	Ketoprofen	10 : 90	The grinding time was 10-120 min at 24 Hz, and the required temperature was used for preparation of the drug–CD complex. The results concluded that amorphisation occurred in moist conditions after 30 min and 120 min for β-CD-EPI and CMβCD-EPI, respectively	[28]
HPβCD	Loratadine	1 : 1 and 1 : 2	Stainless steel jar (25 mL) with two 15 mm balls at 15 Hz for up to 30 min After 7 min with HPβCD at a ratio of 1 : 1, the amorphisation was finished, and after 15 min an inclusion complex with a ratio of 1 : 2 was created, which was confirmed by FTIR	[55]
TAβCD	Metformin HCl	1 : 1	Grinding time was 30 min at 20 Hz with ambient conditions. The authors concluded that amorphous product was obtained by spray drying, which was characterised by a sustained release profile	[56]
β-CD, DIMEB, RAMEB	Oxaprozin	1 : 1	Grinding was carried out for 30 min at 24 Hz. The study's findings showed that partly crystalline products containing CD, DIMEB, and RAMEB enhanced medication dissolving rates 1.9×, 4.4×, and 7.2×, respectively	[25]
β-CD	Telmisartan	1 : 2 and 1 : 3	Results concluded that after 30 min of grinding new solid phases were formed, with the dissolution rate increased 19×. Animal studies on a rat model showed very effective and rapid action of the drug as an antihypertensive agent	[57]
β-CD, β-CD-EPI	Zaleplon	1 : 1	Grinding time was 10–90 min at 24 Hz in ambient conditions. The study concluded that the residual drug crystallinity of β-CD-EPI was 51.10%, which has a 25% faster dissolution rate	[34]
β-CD	Pranlukast hemihydrate	1 : 2	Grinding time was 10 min and the authors reported that by inclusion complex formation using grinding, a fine suspension was formed when resultant product was poured into water	[29]

(Continued)

Table 9.1 (Continued)

Type of CD used	Drug	Drug/ CD ratio	Strategies and outcome	References
TAβCD	Prilocaine HCl	1 : 1	Grinding time was 30 min at 24 Hz in ambient conditions. The results revealed that residual drug crystallinity was 28%, i.e. a partially crystalline product by grinding	[40]
β-CD, β-CD-EPI	Triclosan	1 : 1	Grinding period ranged between 10 and 90 min, at a frequency of 24 Hz. After 60 and 80 min of grinding, complete amorphisation was attained with β-CD-EPI and β-CD, respectively. Increased drug dissolution and antimicrobial properties were found after complexation with β-CD-EPI.	[58]
β-CD	Telmisartan	1 : 2 and 1 : 3	Grinding was done with a stainless steel jar and steel balls and milling times of 7, 15, and 30 min. The desired product quality was achieved after 30 min of grinding.	[57]
β-CD	Zaltoprofen	1 : 1	Grinding was done for 5 h at room temperature and the results revealed that the dissolution rate was increased but no improvement in solubility was observed	[59]
β-CD, HPβCD	Thiadiazole	1 : 1	Grinding was done for 60 min at room temperature and inclusion complex formed with an increase in bioavailability	[34]

CMβCD, carboxymethyl-β-cyclodextrin; DIMEB, crystalline dimethyl β cyclodextrin; EPI, epichlorohydrin; EPS, epichlorohydrin soluble; FTIR, Fourier transform infrared spectroscopy; HeβCD, hydroxyethyl β cyclodextrin; HPβCD, hydroxypropyl β cyclodextrin; RAMEB, randomly methylated β cyclodextrin; SBEβCD, sulfobutyl ether β cyclodextrin sodium salt; TaβCD, triacetyl-β-cyclodextrin.

9.3 Mechanisms of Inclusion Complex Formation by Grinding

Mechanochemistry describes processes that are typically driven by mechanical energy and take place in solids [15]. It is an effective technology with a variety of applications, including material engineering and nanoscience. Traditional grinding with a mortar and pestle and more efficient mechanical crushing with vibratory mills, ball mills, or oscillating are the commonly used techniques to produce mechanochemical modifications [16]. Grinding has evolved into a constantly growing toolset for the synthesis and screening of various supramolecular and covalent components, completing conventional approaches based on solvent-based synthesis. Grinding is now used for more than just basic particle size reduction [17, 18]. The remarkable performance of grinding-based mechanochemical production is due to its capacity to produce metal–ligand coordination bonds in addition to non-covalent bonding including stacking, hydrogen bonds, halogen bonds, and so on. This success allows not only for the activation of otherwise inactive reactants, but also for the incorporation and systematic study of supramolecular structure-templating effects in a synthesis that is solvent free. As a result, grinding is used to produce inclusion complexes, polymeric dispersions, permeable meta-organic structures, polymorphs, and co-crystals, all of which are crucial to the pharmaceutical sector [16, 18, 19].

Based on the typical three-step method for mechanochemical reactions, we propose a plausible scenario, illustrated in Figure 9.3 [20], that accounts for additional procedures taking place during mechanochemical drug stimulation through grinding [21]. The precise process of the synthesis of inclusion complex through grinding consisting of a drug–CD combination has not been thoroughly studied to date [16].

Every time a substance becomes stuck between grinding media that are clashing with each other or between the mill wall and the grinding medium while being ground into powder, it experiences a mechanical power pulse that leads to the creation of a meta-stable configuration [16]. The vast majority of the energy provided is converted into heat on a macroscopic scale, which may facilitate interactions between the medication and CD in the solid form. While performing a DSC evaluation of drug–CD systems, it is usual practice to look at the thermally induced drug–CD interaction [22, 23].

Additionally, the equilibrium among the aggregation and combination processes results in crystal breaking, when the strain field is concentrated in specific crystal zones, which

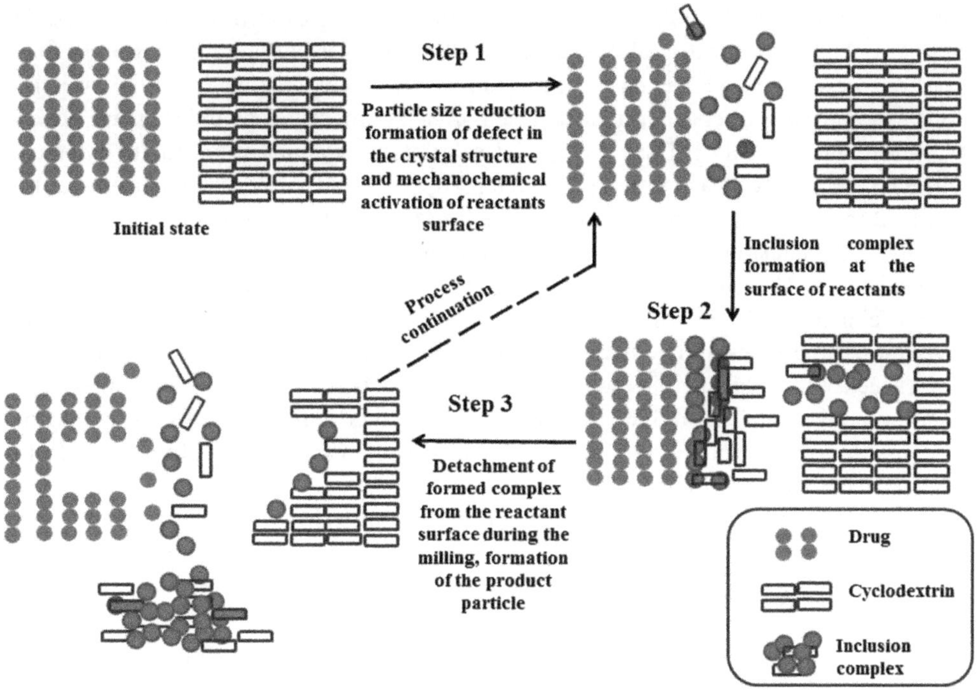

Figure 9.3 Inclusion complex formation by grinding.

results in a reduction in particle size up to a critical threshold. In the solid form, this raises the total surface that is open to the drug–CD interaction. Furthermore, energy delivery causes the crystalline minerals in the treated mixture to amorphise. This process often begins on a narrow surface layer and spreads into the bulk, resulting in a rise in the development of active materials [16]. It is reasonable to suppose that the surface particles of drug and CD react to form inclusion complexes. This process may involve a number of intermediate phases, such as the formation of solid dispersions, which can gradually transform into actual inclusion complexes in the solid state through molecular diffusion [24–27]. The inclusion complex could dissociate from the drug–CD particulates as the grinding procedure goes on, freeing the drug–CD particle interfaces again for the reaction to continue. More importantly, grinding also offers vigorous homogenisation and mixing of the reactants, which enhances the drug–CD interaction in the solid form.

Depending on the length and amount of grinding, as well as the physicochemical characteristics of the drug and CD that are being ground, a drug–CD mixture is frequently ground into an amorphous product or one that contains only traces of the crystalline drug [24–28]. Instances from the research include the creation of solid complexes of 1,2,4-thiadiazole derivatives with CDs by grinding and freeze-drying for the treatment of Alzheimer's based on thiadiazole. The existence of complexes in the solid state was demonstrated using DSC, microscopy, powder X-ray diffractometry, and FTIR spectroscopy [29–32]. The resultant solubility was also tested. The complex of thiadiazole and hydroxypropyl-CD showed better solubility in a phosphate buffer than free thiadiazole and its combinations with CD [33]. For enhancing the solubility of thiadiazole in water, formulations containing hydroxypropyl and CDs were created by grinding the compound. The results of the in vitro and in vivo testing were uniform, and they showed that the thiadiazole and hydroxypropyl-CD freeze-dried complexes had the highest solubility, bioavailability, and dissolution rates. For oral administration, these complexes can be suggested to be more efficient dosage formulations [34].

Ogawa and co-workers investigated a fentanyl–CD inclusion complex using powder X-ray diffraction (PXRD), DSC, FTIR, and solid state ^{13}C nuclear magnetic resonance (NMR) spectroscopy measurements after a fentanyl base and β-CD were co-ground at 1 : 1 and 1 : 2 molar ratios in order to look at the interactions between fentanyl and β-CD. A fentanyl–CD inclusion complex was generated in the humidified mixture, according to solid-state ^{13}C NMR data [35]. Co-crystallization, co-evaporation, and co-grinding were all successful methods for creating bisacodyl-CD inclusion complexes in the solid state by co-evaporation and co-grinding, as demonstrated by Li and co-workers [36]. By using ^{13}C NMR spectroscopy, Jablan and co-authors showed that the actual inclusion complexation in amorphous drug–CD products obtained through co-grinding still consists of a significant amount of remaining crystalline drug, which could easily convert into an inclusion complex when dissolved in aqueous solutions [37].

The different types of mills for inclusion complex formation by grinding are discussed next.

9.3.1 High-Energy Vibrational Mills

A mixer mill, often called a high-energy vibrational mill, consists of metal discs or toroidal-shaped bowls that carry individual cylindrical grating jars coupled to an engine. The grating jars oscillate radially in a horizontal position as the engine runs, and the grinding balls strike the sample material at the circular edges of the jars with great force due to their inertia. Furthermore, ball sliding and particle matter strike add to the mechanical energy source, resulting in sample pulverisation and subsequent mechanochemical activation. Additionally, the material is vigorously mixed as a result of the motions of the balls and the crushing jars. By combining multiple smaller balls, the degree of mixing can be enhanced even more [16]. Polycarbonate, zirconia ceramic, methacrylate, Teflon®, alumina ceramic, stainless steel, silicon nitride, polystyrene, tungsten carbide, hardened steel, and agate are the materials utilised to make the jars and balls. While continuous vibrating mills are appropriate for small-scale processes and manufacturing uses, batch-operated vibrational mills are best suited to laboratory manufacturing of goods on a gram scale [16, 38].

9.3.2 Planetary Mills

In planetary mills, one or more grating vials are positioned eccentrically inside a round basement that rotates around its primary symmetry axis. The rotation with relation to the basement causes the grinding balls in the grating jars to experience superimposed rotational motions. The interplay of frictional and impact forces induced by the difference in speeds between the grating jars and the balls releases high dynamic energy. The interaction of these forces results in the treated sample being activated mechanochemically and a significant reduction in particle size. Planetary mills come in laboratory and pilot plant sizes, and the grinding jars and balls can be manufactured from various materials [16, 39]. To prevent the sample from excessive heat, the mill is generally run with alternate milling and rest periods, with a total grinding time of 1–5 hours and a rotational speed of 400–600 rpm. This method allowed for the efficient manufacture of different 1-, 2-, and 4-thiadiazole anti-Alzheimer's medication candidates in the solid-state complex [40, 41].

9.3.3 Ball Mills

A desktop tumble ball mill is used to create CD inclusion complexes in solid form, although this is uncommon. The sample to be treated and several milling balls are put into a spinning cylinder (drum). Here, the applied speed and the drum diameter have a significant impact on the total energy transmitted to the treated material [16]. Due to the comparatively small drum diameters of desktop tumble ball mills, longer milling times are required to induce mechanochemical stimulation of the sample and perhaps inclusion complex formation in the solid form. Milling normally takes between 12 and 48 hours, with rotating rates ranging from 120 to 150 rpm [35, 42, 43]. For example, when fentanyl was crushed with β-CD, solid-state ^{13}C NMR spectroscopy was utilised to verify genuine inclusion complexation using 40 glass balls, 20 of which had an 8 mm diameter and the other 20 had a 12 mm diameter. The end products were amorphous [35].

9.3.4 Mortar and Pestle Grinding

Since the stone age, the mortar and pestle has been the primary tool for grinding science, and it is still beneficial in mechanochemical preparation today [44]. Mortar and pestle grinding has been successfully used as a CD complex synthesis method in the solid form, despite the minimal energy input and difficulty in quantifying it. Some examples from the literature show that hand grinding only results in partial drug complexation, particularly when crystalline natural CDs are used as the complexing agents [45–47]. Amorphous products were produced when amorphous CD derivatives were employed [14, 47, 48]. RAMEB seems to be particularly effective at drug amorphisation in grinding through the manual method, even in the case of drugs that generally have higher melting temperatures such as sulfadiazine, sulfamethoxazole, and trimethoprim, where after just 15 minutes of grinding full amorphisation and likely inclusion complex development happen [47]. Interestingly, FTIR analyses showed that in the instance of gemfibrozil, a medication with a comparatively low melting point, a longer grinding time was required to accomplish full drug complex formation with RAMEB (thus a less tabular crystal structure) [14].

9.4 Implementation of Quality by Design in Inclusion Complex Formation by Grinding

Using multiple statistical and experimental development tools, quality by design (QbD) is a important technique that is combined with quality risk management (QRM) to create a high-quality product [60]. To build an extremely effective and high-quality final product, development scientists have already begun applying the QbD principles. The QbD approach for green chemistry (Figure 9.4) begins by defining the quality target product profile (QTPP) and critical material attributes (CMAs), choosing an appropriate preparation technique, determining critical process parameters (CPPs) through the use of QRM, developing a control strategy, and then ensuring continued improvement with regular performance monitoring.

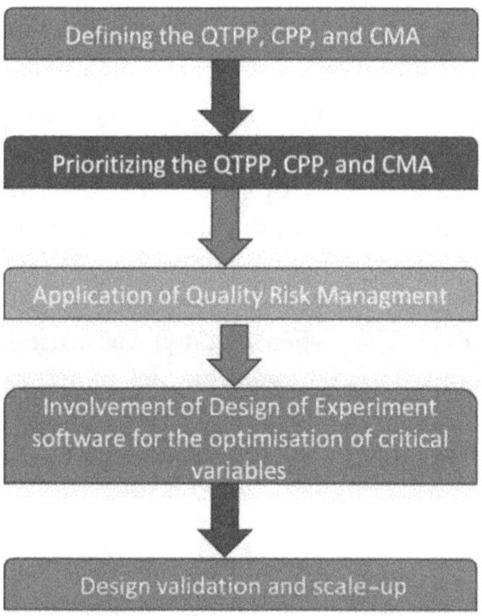

Figure 9.4 Five steps involved in quality by design during the formulation of inclusion complex. CMA, critical material attribute; CPP, critical process parameter; QTPP, quality target product profile.

Comparing QbD to traditional formulation development and optimisation, there are several benefits. These include creating a controlled and reliable grinding technology for use throughout a pharmaceutical product's lifespan [61]. QRM is a planned technique for assessing, controlling, communicating, and reviewing the risks to a product's quality in a grinding process, according to the ICH Q9 guideline. The scientific evaluation of various hazards and the efforts taken to control them through the necessary formalities and documentation methods constitute the basis of QRM. The most vital information for producing a quality product may be provided by QRM, which is an essential part of QbD [62].

9.4.1 Step I: Defining the Quality Attributes, Material Attributes, and Process Parameters/Process Variables

In the formulation of inclusion complex, the only process parameter that has been used is grinding, so instead it is important to find the process variables (PVs) involved in the grinding process [63]. The quality attributes (QAs), PVs, and material attributes (MAs) involved in the formulation of inclusion complex through grinding are shown in Table 9.2.

9.4.2 Step II: Prioritizing the Defined Quality Attributes, Process Variables, and Material Attributes as Critical Quality Attributes, Critical Process Variables, and Critical Material Attributes

After determination or identification of all possible variables, it is important to prioritize the identified variables into critical ones. For prioritizing the identified variables in the grinding process, each of the identified variables is analysed by two questions [64]:

- *Severity analysis*: Can failure to reach the quality variables affect the quality of the final formulation?
- *Impact analysis*: If any of the variables selected are quantitative, is there an impact on the quality of the final formulation?

After analysing all the identified PVs, QAs, and MAs for the grinding process for the formation of inclusion complexes, the results are shown in Table 9.3.

Table 9.2 List of different critical process variables, material attributes, and quality attributes involved in the formulation of inclusion complex.

Process variables	Material attributes	Quality attributes
Energy input in grinding Grinding time Grinding temperature Grinding volume Filling degree of grinding jars Cleaning of jars	Amount of active ingredients Amount of correct derivative of cyclodextrin	Inclusion efficiency Thermal behaviour Physicochemical behaviour

In the study outlined in Table 9.3, all the manufacturing variables excluding the filling degree of grinding jars and cleaning of jars were found to be critical for the desired quality of inclusion complex formed by using the grinding technique.

Table 9.3 Identification of critical quality attributes, critical material attributes, and critical process variables.

Identified manufacturing variables	Question 1 (severity analysis)	Question 2 (impact Analysis)	Criticality of manufacturing variables	Justification
Process variables				
Energy input in grinding	Y	Y	C	Energy input has a linear impact on the formation of the inclusion complex
Grinding time	Y	Y	C	Grinding time has an impact on the quality of the inclusion complex
Grinding temperature	Y	Y	C	Grinding temperature has an impact on the stability of the inclusion complex
Grinding volume	Y	Y	C	Grinding volume has a positive impact on the efficiency of inclusion complex formation
Filling degree of grinding jars	N	Y	NC	Filling degree of grinding jars does not have a major impact on the process of inclusion complex formation and hence can be ignored in the optimisation process
Cleaning of jars	N	N	NC	Cleaning of jars can be ignored in the optimisation process by maintaining hygiene and avoiding cross-contamination during manufacturing of the inclusion complex
Material attributes				
Amount of cyclodextrin	Y	Y	C	The amount of cyclodextrin should be in the optimum range for the formulation of inclusion complex of the desired quality
Amount of active ingredient	Y	Y	C	The amount of active ingredient has always been critical as it affects the final amount in the inclusion complex in stochiometric ratios
Quality attributes				
Inclusion efficiency	Y	Y	C	Inclusion efficiency determines the amount of active ingredients present in the inclusion complex

Table 9.3 (Continued)

Identified manufacturing variables	Question 1 (severity analysis)	Question 2 (impact Analysis)	Criticality of manufacturing variables	Justification
Thermal behaviour	Y	Y	C	Thermal characterisation is utilised to determine the stability of the inclusion complex
Physicochemical behaviour	Y	Y	C	Physicochemical characterisation has also been utilised for the stability of the inclusion complex and its physicochemical properties

C, Critical; N, No; NC, Not critical; Y, Yes.

9.4.3 Step III: Application of Quality Risk Management

Understanding the causal relationship among the prospective method variables and CQAs is the first step in QRM. To do this, a standard fishbone schematic can be created for the grinding process, as shown in Figure 9.5. Control–Noise–Experimental (CNX) analysis and Failure Mode and Effect Analysis (FMEA) were used in this investigation to identify the riskiest factors influencing the CQAs of CD-based molecular inclusion complexes [65–68]. The QRM advice and a QbD-based life-cycle strategy may both be adhered to by combining the FMEA and CNX approaches. Doing so expands the manufacturer's knowledge base and gives it a greater awareness of how potential technique factors might influence the

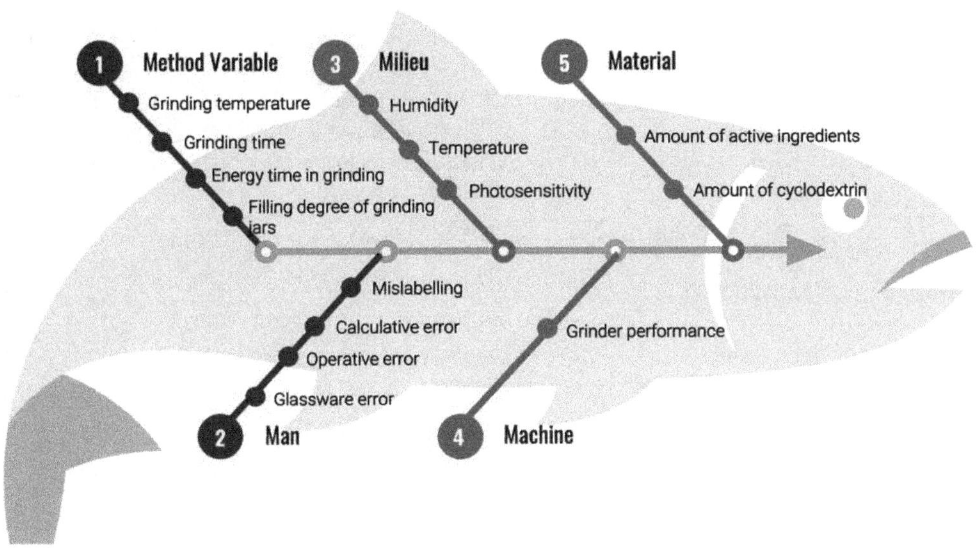

Figure 9.5 Ishikawa fishbone diagram depicting the possible risks involved in the formulation of inclusion complex using grinding techniques.

effectiveness of their analysis. Additionally, obtaining an appropriate score, termed the risk priority number (RPN), through an FMEA analysis depends on the CNX categorisation. Any manufacturing variables obtaining an RPN more than 100 are considered critical and require further investigation and optimisation by the application of response surface methodology. The RPN can be calculated by Equation 9.1:

$$RPN = S * O * D \tag{9.1}$$

where S is severity, O is occurrence, and D is Detectability.

In this scenario of grinding-based inclusion complex formation, all the manufacturing variables have been analysed through the FMEA with CNX approach and are shown in Table 9.4.

With the analysis of different risk factors, energy input in grinding, grinding time, and grinding temperature can be considered the most critical risk factors that can affect the final desired quality of the inclusion complex, as the RPN of all three factors is more than 100. All three identified factors should be further investigated through response surface methodology with the help of Design Expert software.

Table 9.4 Failure Mode and Effect Analysis (FMEA) and Control–Noise–Experimental (CNX) analysis combined.

Source	Cause of failure	CNX	Effect	S	O	D	RPN
Method	Energy input in grinding	X	Multiple	7	7	7	343
	Grinding time	X	Multiple	6	5	6	180
	Grinding temperature	X	Multiple	5	5	6	150
	Filling degree of grinding jars	C	Varied ratio, inclusion efficiency, and yield	5	3	5	75
Material	Amount of cyclodextrin	C	Varied ratio, inclusion efficiency, and yield	4	3	5	60
	Amount of active ingredient	C	Varied action	3	3	5	45
Milieu	Humidity	C	Wrong weighing of samples	4	3	2	24
	Temperature	C	Varying resolution	3	3	3	27
	Photosensitivity	C	Instability of sample	2	2	2	8
Machine	Grinder	C	Decreased performance	4	4	4	64
Man	Mislabelling	C	Faulty identification	2	2	2	8
	Calculative error	C	Incorrect purity	3	4	2	24
	Glassware error	C	Faulty preparation	2	2	2	8
	Operative error	N	Incorrect procedure	2	2	2	8

D, Detectability; O, Occurrence; RPN, Risk priority number; S, Severity.
The scores for S, O, and D are given on a scale of 1 (low risk) to 10 (high risk).

9.4.4 Step IV: Involvement of Design of Experiment for Optimisation of Critical Process Variables

After selection of the CPVs, it is important to optimise them by a design of experiment (DoE) approach through response surface methodology. Generally, software is available for performing DoE, such as Design Expert or Mini Tab. There are two types of response surface methodology available, screening design and optimisation design. Screening design is design that is utilised for screening different critical variables. If there are more than three critical variables, it is important to screen out the most important one for optimisation. If an attempt is made to optimise more critical factors, the software suggests an extremely large number of experiments that will be harder and costlier to perform. So a screening design such as Taguchi design or factorial design is applied to reduce the number of critical factors. After screening of the critical factors, the two or three most important critical variables should be further subjected to optimisation through a central composite design, Box-Behnken design, or Plackett-Burman design, for determining the optimum amount/concentration/range of the variable to obtain the desired quality profile of the formulation. Various features of the optimisation design such as point prediction and sample equation have been utilised for finding the optimum value. These designs also give a 2D contour plot and a 3D response surface plot to depict the relationship between the selected independent (manufacturing/critical variable) variable and dependent variable (selected CQA for characterisation of the final formulation). Design space is one of the important features that has also been generated through this kind of software, which also determines the working range of all the selected critical variables for obtaining the desired output from the grinding process.

9.4.5 Step V: Model Validation and Scale-Up for Commercial Production

The last step in QbD during formulation of a product is the validation of the digital model developed for optimisation. The model developed through the DoE software needs to be validated by comparing the result obtained from the digital model and the result obtained by performing the same experiment in the lab. Any error less than 2% makes the model acceptable for optimisation of the selected critical variables.

Pilot plant scale-up is a process that increases the manufacturing scale of the formulation. By obtaining a deeper understanding through QbD, effective control can be achieved of all the risk factors that can affect the quality of the inclusion complex formed by grinding. By keeping all the risk factors constant or at the lowest level, the batch size of CD-based product can be scaled up by precisely optimising the critical variables associated with the methodology [61–63, 66, 69].

9.5 Conclusion

For the synthesis of CD inclusion complex in solid form, grinding has proven to be a flexible, user-friendly, extremely effective, and environmentally safe and hence green methodology. The operating parameters must be properly optimised taking into consideration the type of mill used in addition to the physiochemical characteristics of each of the therapeutic agents and CDs exposed to grinding in order to accomplish a productive solid-state interaction among the components, continuing to improve the biopharmaceutical characteristics of the drug, and increasing its bioavailability and therapeutic characteristics. Despite the method's widespread use, very limited knowledge is available comparing grinding with other methods of drug–CD inclusion complex formation. In order to become the foundation for further scientific research that will result in a deeper knowledge of the fundamental mechanisms of this valid and beneficial methodology, this chapter presents a structured overview of the information currently available. With its detailed overview of the concept of QbD during the formation of inclusion complex by grinding, the deeper insights into this green chemistry approach will surely offer readers a platform for optimisation of this high-energy process by keeping in view the process of scaling up at an industrial level using cost-efficient methodologies.

References

1 Carlier, L., Baron, M., Chamayou, A., and Couarraze, G. (2011). Use of co-grinding as a solvent-free solid state method to synthesize dibenzophenazines. *Tetrahedron Letters* 52 (36): 4686–4689.

2 Jansook, P., Ogawa, N., and Loftsson, T. (2018). Cyclodextrins: structure, physicochemical properties and pharmaceutical applications. *International Journal of Pharmaceutics* 535 (1–2): 272–284.

3 Kondoros, B.A., Jójárt-Laczkovich, O., Berkesi, O. et al. (2022). Development of solvent-free co-ground method to produce terbinafine hydrochloride cyclodextrin binary systems; structural and *in vitro* characterizations. *Pharmaceutics* 14 (4): 744(1–19).

4 Szejtli, J. (1997). Utilization of cyclodextrins in industrial products and processes. *Journal of Materials Chemistry* 7 (4): 575–587.

5 Rasheed, A. (2008). Cyclodextrins as drug carrier molecule: a review. *Scientia Pharmaceutica* 76 (4): 567–598.

6 Loftsson, T., and Duchêne, D. (2007). Cyclodextrins and their pharmaceutical applications. *International Journal of Pharmaceutics* 329 (1–2): 1–11.

7 Davis, M.E., and Brewster, M.E. (2004). Cyclodextrin-based pharmaceutics: past, present and future. *Nature Reviews: Drug Discovery* 3 (12): 1023–1035.

8 Szejtli, J. (1998). Introduction and general overview of cyclodextrin chemistry. *Chemical Reviews* 98 (5): 1743–1754.

9 Sharma, N., and Baldi, A. (2016). Exploring versatile applications of cyclodextrins: an overview. *Drug Delivery* 23 (3): 729–747.

10 Gupta, R., Behera, C., Paudwal, G. et al. (2019). Recent advances in formulation strategies for efficient delivery of vitamin D. *AAPS Pharmscitech* 20 (1): 1–12.

11 Sethi, S., Choudhary, S., Sharma, D. et al. (2021). Armamentarium of anticancer analogues of curcumin: portray of structural insight, bioavailability, drug-target interaction and therapeutic efficacy. *Journal of Molecular Structure* 1231: 129691.

12 Uzqueda, M., Martín, C., Zornoza, A. et al. (2010). Physicochemical characterization of terbinafine-cyclodextrin complexes in solution and in the solid state. *Journal of Inclusion Phenomena and Macrocyclic Chemistry* 66 (3): 393–402.

13 Arias, M.J., Moyano, J.R., and Gines, J.M. (1997). Investigation of the triamterene–β-cyclodextrin system prepared by co-grinding. *International Journal of Pharmaceutics* 153 (2): 181–189.

14 Aigner, Z., Berkesi, O., Farkas, G., and Szabó-Révész, P. (2012). DSC, X-ray and FTIR studies of a gemfibrozil/dimethyl-β-cyclodextrin inclusion complex produced by co-grinding. *Journal of Pharmaceutical and Biomedical Analysis* 57: 62–67.

15 Jones, W., and Eddleston, M.D. (2014). Introductory lecture: mechanochemistry, a versatile synthesis strategy for new materials. *Faraday Discuss* 170: 9–34.

16 Colombo, I., Grassi, G., and Grassi, M. (2009). Drug mechanochemical activation. *Journal of Pharmaceutical Sciences* 98 (11): 3961–3986.

17 Hernández, J.G., and Bolm, C. (2017). Altering product selectivity by mechanochemistry. *Journal of Organic Chemistry* 82 (8): 4007–4019.

18 Friščić, T. (2012). Supramolecular concepts and new techniques in mechanochemistry: cocrystals, cages, rotaxanes, open metal–organic frameworks. *Chemical Society Reviews* 41 (9): 3493–3510.

19 Bikiaris, D.N. (2011). Solid dispersions, part I: recent evolutions and future opportunities in manufacturing methods for dissolution rate enhancement of poorly water-soluble drugs. *Expert Opinion on Drug Delivery* 8 (11): 1501–1519.

20 Friscic, T., and Jones, W. (2009). Recent advances in understanding the mechanism of cocrystal formation via grinding. *Crystal Growth & Design* 9 (3): 1621–1637.

21 Popielec, A., and Loftsson, T. (2017). Effects of cyclodextrins on the chemical stability of drugs. *International Journal of Pharmaceutics* 531 (2): 532–542.

22 Jablan, J., Szalontai, G., and Jug, M. (2012). Comparative analysis of zaleplon complexation with cyclodextrins and hydrophilic polymers in solution and in solid state. *Journal of Pharmaceutical and Biomedical Analysis* 71: 35–44.

23 Aigner, Z., Hassan, H.B., Berkesi, O. et al. (2005). FTIR and X-ray studies of gemfibrozil-cyclodextrin complexes. *Journal of Thermal Analysis and Calorimetry* 81 (2): 267–272.

24 Lin, H.-L., Lin, S.-Y., Lin, -C.-C. et al. (2012). Mechanical grinding effect on thermodynamics and inclusion efficiency of loratadine–cyclodextrin inclusion complex formation. *Carbohydrate Polymers* 87 (1): 512–517.

25 Mennini, N., Bragagni, M., Maestrelli, F., and Mura, P. (2014). Physico-chemical characterization in solution and in the solid state of clonazepam complexes with native and chemically-modified cyclodextrins. *Journal of Pharmaceutical and Biomedical Analysis* 18 (15): 142–149.

26 Cirri, M., Maestrelli, F., Mennini, N., and Mura, P. (2009). Influence of the preparation method on the physical–chemical properties of ketoprofen–cyclodextrin–phosphatidylcholine ternary systems. *Journal of Pharmaceutical and Biomedical Analysis* 50 (5): 690–694.

27 Maestrelli, F., Cecchi, M., Cirri, M. et al. (2009). Comparative study of oxaprozin complexation with natural and chemically-modified cyclodextrins in solution and in the solid state. *Journal of Inclusion Phenomena and Macrocyclic Chemistry* 63 (1): 17–25.

28 Cirri, M., Bragagni, M., Mennini, N., and Mura, P. (2012). Development of a new delivery system consisting in 'drug–in cyclodextrin–in nanostructured lipid carriers' for ketoprofen topical delivery. *European Journal of Pharmaceutics and Biopharmaceutics* 80 (1): 46–53.

29 Wongmekiat, A., Tozuka, Y., Oguchi, T., and Yamamoto, K. (2002). Formation of fine drug particles by cogrinding with cyclodextrins. I. The use of β-cyclodextrin anhydrate and hydrate. *Pharmaceutical Research* 19 (12): 1867–1872.

30 Wongmekiat, A., Tozuka, Y., Oguchi, T., and Yamamoto, K. (2003). Formation of fine drug particle by cogrinding with cyclodextrins: part II. The influence of moisture condition during cogrinding process on fine particle formation. *International Journal of Pharmaceutics* 265 (1–2): 85–93.

31 Sun, Y., Zhang, Y., Xu, K. et al. (2015). Thermal, mechanical properties, and low-temperature performance of fibrous nanoclay-reinforced epoxy asphalt composites and their concretes. *Journal of Applied Polymer Science* 132 (12): 41694.

32 Gu, F.G., Wang, Y., Meng, G.D.L. et al. (2012). Investigation of a fenofibrate-hydroxypropyl-β-cyclodextrin system prepared by a co-grinding method. *Die Pharmazie International Journal of Pharmaceutical Sciences* 67 (2): 143–146.

33 Brusnikina, M., Silyukov, O., Chislov, M. et al. (2017). Effect of cyclodextrin complexation on solubility of novel anti-Alzheimer 1, 2, 4-thiadiazole derivative. *Journal of Thermal Analysis and Calorimetry* 130 (1): 443–450.

34 Promzeleva, M., Volkova, T., Proshin, A. et al. (2018). Improved biopharmaceutical properties of oral formulations of 1, 2, 4-thiadiazole derivative with cyclodextrins: *in vitro* and *in vivo* evaluation. *ACS Biomaterials Science and Engineering* 4 (2): 491–501.

35 Ogawa, N., Higashi, K., Nagase, H. et al. (2010). Effects of cogrinding with β-cyclodextrin on the solid state fentanyl. *Journal of Pharmaceutical Sciences* 99 (12): 5019–5029.

36 Li, S., Zhai, Y., Yan, J. et al. (2016). Effect of preparation processes and structural insight into the supermolecular system: bisacodyl and β-cyclodextrin inclusion complex. *Materials Science and Engineering C* 58: 224–232.

37 Jablan, J., Bačić, I., Kujundžić, N., and Jug, M. (2013). Zaleplon co-ground complexes with natural and polymeric β-cyclodextrin. *Journal of Inclusion Phenomena and Macrocyclic Chemistry* 76 (3): 353–362.

38 Howard, J.L., Cao, Q., and Browne, D.L. (2018). Mechanochemistry as an emerging tool for molecular synthesis: what can it offer? *Chemical Sciences* 9 (12): 3080–3094.

39 Jug, M., and Mura, P.A. (2018). Grinding as solvent-free green chemistry approach for cyclodextrin inclusion complex preparation in the solid state. *Pharmaceutics* 10 (4): 189.

40 Bragagni, M., Maestrelli, F., and Mura, P. (2010). Physical chemical characterization of binary systems of prilocaine hydrochloride with triacetyl-β-cyclodextrin. *Journal of Inclusion Phenomena and Macrocyclic Chemistry* 68 (3): 437–445.

41 Higashi, K., Tozuka, Y., Moribe, K., and Yamamoto, K. (2010). Salicylic acid/γ-cydodextrin 2: 1 and 4: 1 complex formation by sealed-heating method. *Journal of Pharmaceutical Sciences* 99 (10): 4192–4200.

42 Mitrevej, A., Sinchaipanid, N., and Junyaprasert, V. (2008). Effect of grinding of β-cyclodextrin and glibenclamide on tablet properties. Part I. *In vitro. Drug Development and Industrial Pharmacy* 22 (12): 1237–1241.

43 Iwata, M., Fukami, T., Kawashima, D. et al. (2009). Effectiveness of mechanochemical treatment with cyclodextrins on increasing solubility of glimepiride. *Die Pharmazie International Journal of Pharmaceutical Sciences* 64 (6): 390–394.

44 Takacs, L. (2013). The historical development of mechanochemistry. *Chemical Society Reviews* 42 (18): 7649–7659.

45 Ramos, A.I., Braga, T.M., Silva, P. et al. (2013). Chloramphenicol cyclodextrin inclusion compounds: co-dissolution and mechanochemical preparations and antibacterial action. *Crystal Engineering Communications* 15 (15): 2822–2834.

46 Bettinetti, G., Sorrenti, M., Negri, A. et al. (1999). Interaction of naproxen with alpha-cyclodextrin and its noncyclic analog maltohexaose. *Pharmaceutical Research* 16 (5): 689–694.

47 Veiga, M.-D., Ahsan, F., and Merino, M. (1999). Differential scanning calorimetry as an analytical tool in determining the interaction between drug and cyclodextrin. In: *Proceedings of the Ninth International Symposium on Cyclodextrins* (eds. J.J.T. Labandeira, and J.L. Vila-Jato), 329–332. Dordrecht: Springer.

48 Mura, P., Faucci, M.T., Maestrelli, F. et al. (2002). Characterization of physicochemical properties of naproxen systems with amorphous β-cyclodextrin-epichlorohydrin polymers. *Journal of Pharmaceutical and Biomedical Analysis* 29 (6): 1015–1024.

49 Tan, Q., He, D., Wu, M. et al. (2013). Characterization, activity, and computer modeling of a molecular inclusion complex containing rifaldazine. *International Journal of Nanomedicine* 8: 477–484.

50 He, D., Deng, P., Yang, L. et al. (2013). Molecular encapsulation of rifampicin as an inclusion complex of hydroxypropyl-β-cyclodextrin: design; characterization and *in vitro* dissolution. *Colloids Surfaces B Biointerfaces* 103: 580–585.

51 Ali, H.R.H., Saleem, I.Y., and Tawfeek, H.M. (2016). Insight into inclusion complexation of indomethacin nicotinamide cocrystals. *Journal of Inclusion Phenomena and Macrocyclic Chemistry* 84 (3): 179–188.

52 Jug, M., Mennini, N., Kövér, K.E., and Mura, P. (2014). Comparative analysis of binary and ternary cyclodextrin complexes with econazole nitrate in solution and in solid state. *Journal of Pharmaceutical and Biomedical Analysis* 91: 81–91.

53 Mura, P., Faucci, M.T., Manderioli, A., and Bramanti, G. (2001). Multicomponent systems of econazole with hydroxyacids and cyclodextrins. *Journal of Inclusion Phenomena and Macrocyclic Chemistry* 39 (1): 131–138.

54 Fumić, B., Jablan, J., Cinčić, D. et al. (2018). Cyclodextrin encapsulation of daidzein and genistein by grinding: implication on the glycosaminoglycan accumulation in mucopolysaccharidosis type II and III fibroblasts. *Journal of Microencapsulation* 35 (1): 1–12.

55 Lin, S.-Y., Hsu, C.-H., and Sheu, M.-T. (2010). Curve-fitting FTIR studies of loratadine/hydroxypropyl-β-cyclodextrin inclusion complex induced by co-grinding process. *Journal of Pharmaceutical and Biomedical Analysis* 53 (3): 799–803.

56 Corti, G., Capasso, G., Maestrelli, F. et al. (2007). Physical–chemical characterization of binary systems of metformin hydrochloride with triacetyl-β-cyclodextrin. *Journal of Pharmaceutical and Biomedical Analysis* 45 (3): 480–486.

57 Borba, P.A., Pinotti, M., Andrade, G.R. et al. (2015). The effect of mechanical grinding on the formation, crystalline changes and dissolution behaviour of the inclusion complex of telmisartan and β-cyclodextrins. *Carbohydrate Polymers* 133: 373–383.

58 Jug, M., Kosalec, I., Maestrelli, F., and Mura, P. (2011). Analysis of triclosan inclusion complexes with β-cyclodextrin and its water-soluble polymeric derivative. *Journal of Pharmaceutical and Biomedical Analysis* 54 (5): 1030–1039.

59 Li, S., Lin, X., Xu, K. et al. (2017). Co-grinding effect on crystalline zaltoprofen with β-cyclodextrin/cucurbit [7] uril in tablet formulation. *Scientific Reports* 7 (1): 1–10.

60 Naman, S., Madhavi, N., Singh, B. et al. (2021). Implementing risk-based quality by design for development and optimization of flavored oral disintegrating mini tablets. *Journal of Drug Delivery Science and Technology* 66: 102799.

61 Sumit, K., Shikha, T., Deepika, T., and Ashish, B. (2012). A quantitative approach for pharmaceutical quality by design patterns. *Inventi Rapid: Pharm Analysis and Quality Assurance* 4: 1–8.

62 Naman, S., Madhavi, N., Singh, M. et al. (2019). Formulation design and pharmaceutical considerations for paediatric patients: current status and future dimensions. *Journal of Drug Delivery and Therapeutics* 9 (4): 601–606.

63 Bajwa, N., Naryal, S., Mahal, S. et al. (2022). Quality-by-design strategy for the development of arteether loaded solid self-micro emulsifying drug delivery systems. *Journal of Drug Delivery Science and Technology* 77: 103707.

64 Naman, S., Naryal, S., Palliwal, R. et al. (2022). Combating atherosclerosis with nanodrug delivery approaches: from bench side to commercialization. In: *Drug Delivery Systems for Metabolic Disorders*, (eds. H. Dureja, S.N. Murthy, P.R. Wich, and K. Dua), 97–136. London: Academic Press.

65 Kumar, D., Arora, M., and Baldi, A. (2015). Understanding industrial practices for pharmaceutical quality management—I, existing approaches and guidelines. *Advanced Research Pharmaceutical Biology* 5 (1): 802–811.

66 Bhandari, S.B.B., and Baldi, A. (2014). Total quality management of pharmaceuticals: recent approaches and advancements total quality management of pharmaceuticals: recent approaches and advancements. *Advanced Research Pharmaceutical Biology* 4 (2): 655–663.

67 Kumar, B., and Baldi, A. (2015). Understanding industrial practices for pharmaceutical quality management—II, process validation. *Advanced Research Pharmaceutical Biology* 5: 812–824.

68 Kumar, S., and Ashish, B. (2015). Formulation by design approach for fizzy granules using statistical optimization methodologies. *Asian Journal of Pharmaceutical* 9 (4): S59–67.

69 Bajwa, N., Mahal, S., Naryal, S. et al. (2022). Development of novel solid nanostructured lipid carriers for bioavailability enhancement using a quality by design approach. *AAPS PharmSciTech* 23 (7): 1–14.

10

Synthesis of Graphitic Carbon Nitride Quantum Dots from Bulk Graphitic Carbon Nitride

Jegam Noel Joseph and Selvaraj Mohana Roopan

Chemistry of Heterocycles and Natural Product Research Laboratory, Department of Chemistry, School of Advanced Sciences, Vellore Institute of Technology, Vellore, Tamil Nadu, India

CONTENTS

10.1 Introduction

Carbon nitrides are compounds that belong to the group of polymeric materials that mostly contain carbon and nitrogen. Carbon nitrides Includes azafullerenes, cyanofullerenes, percyanoalkynes, dicyanopolyynes, percyanoheterocycles, aromatic cyanocarbons, and the cyanogen family (Figure 10.1) [1–3]. Carbon nitrides are said to be next-generation materials because of their excellent optoelectronic properties and wide range of applications in energy conversion, storage, and catalysis [4]. Among all these types of carbon nitriles, graphitic carbon nitride (g-C_3N_4) is by far the most robust pattern. Studies state that its stability might be due to its hexagonal structure, which contains AB-stacked graphene sheets that are constructed ideally from tri-s-triazine units bound by planar amino groups [5]. g-C_3N_4 was first discovered by Berzelius and was named 'melon' according to reports by Leibig [6]. It was not until a few decades ago that the actual potential of the material, such as its chemical stability and insolubility in acidic, neutral, or basic solvents, was recognised. It has been trending for the past few decades because of its various time-saving methods of synthesis and its wide range of applications. It has been reported that reactions such as CO_2 activation, transesterification, oxygen reduction, hydrogen production, and photodegradation of dyes show better results when g-C_3N_4 is used as the catalyst [6]. Although g-C_3N_4 has numerous applications, there are a few limitations too. One

Sustainable Approaches in Pharmaceutical Sciences, First Edition. Edited by Kamal Shah, Durgesh Nandini Chauhan, and Nagendra Singh Chauhan.

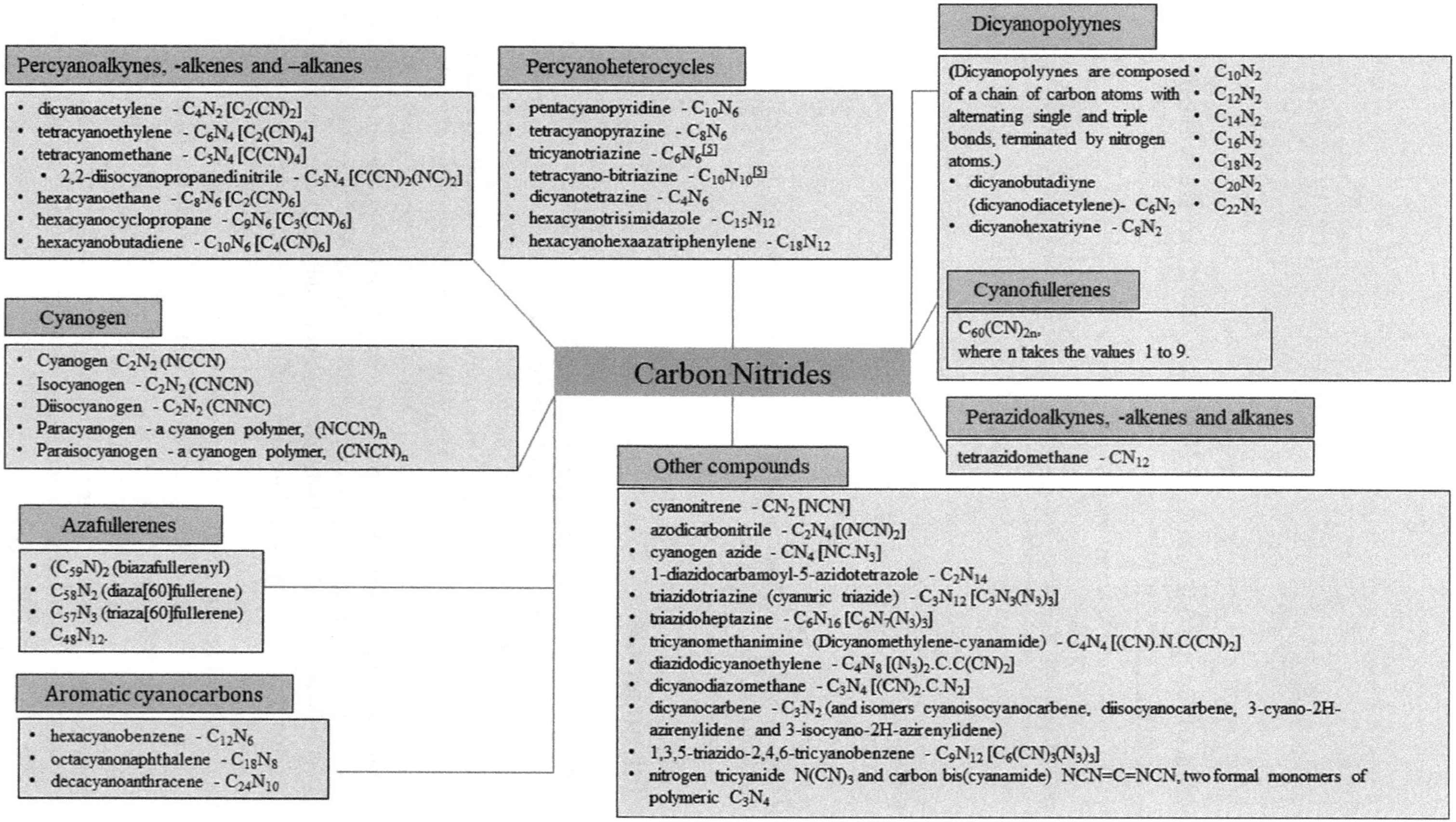

Figure 10.1 Types of carbon nitrides.

important factor is size, which ranges from 1 to 10 μm. This larger size limits its luminescent properties and water solubility [7].

On the other hand, zero-dimensional particles such as carbon quantum dots (CQDs), graphene quantum dots (GQDs), fullerenes, magnetic nanoparticles (MgNPs), inorganic quantum dots, noble metal nanoparticles, up-conversion nanoparticles (UCNPs), and polymer dots (Pdots) possess properties such as biocompatibility, ion detection, biomolecular recognition, pathogen detection, and other notable chemical and physical properties. One important phenomenon to be noted in zero-dimensional particles is the quantum confinement effect, which arises due to their ultra-small size, which in turn is responsible for the properties mentioned [8]. Although the invention of these zero-dimensional particles has played a major role in the betterment of society, their possible toxicity is still a threat. CQDs have been shown to be the least toxic of the zero-dimensional particles and have a wide range of applications due to their remarkable properties. CQDs are simple to functionalise, chemically inert, low-cost while being highly biocompatible, and can accept and donate electrons. Their properties make them stand out from other toxic zero-dimensional particles [9].

As discussed earlier, there is a wide range of applications for CQDs, but they cannot be generalised as the properties and applications vary for carbon dots synthesised via different methods and from different precursor molecules [10]. Hence, it is necessary to select the appropriate precursor and method of synthesis to produce CQDs, as the quantum yield, characteristics, properties, and applications depend on this. CQDs can be synthesised from various sources, such as organic compounds, inorganic compounds, and polymers. There are hundreds of articles reporting the synthesis of biocompatible CQDs obtained from natural products, mostly through hydrothermal synthesis [11]. However, there is a certain drawback that turns the table upside-down. Although the duration of synthesis depends on the method of synthesis, generally the duration may be comparatively longer in the case of biosynthesis. Additional separation steps might be required for complete separation of CQDs from the precursors. A specific size and shape are difficult to obtain, and a deep understanding of metal salt reduction and the chemical configuration of the biological capping has not yet been obtained, as numerous phytochemicals are present in these natural products, which makes it difficult to identify the specific phytochemical responsible for the process. These are a few demerits that should be considered in the case of biosynthesis of CQDs [12].

As noted previously, g-C_3N_4 contains a significant amount of carbon that has extensive applications, making it a viable candidate for use as a precursor in the synthesis of CQDs. Difficulties such as large size, luminescent properties, and water solubility, on the other hand, can be addressed by doping g-C_3N_4 with carbon-based nanomaterials such as graphene, carbon nanotubes, and CQDs, which improve the g-C_3N_4's photo-electrochemical activity [13]. g-C_3N_4/CQD production is widely discussed in this chapter, as are the various methods of synthesising it and its applications.

10.2 Graphitic Carbon Nitride

g-C_3N_4 was originally discovered in 1834 [14], although due to a lack of knowledge in this particular area, nothing much was achieved. But during the 1980s, it came back into fashion as researchers found it a promising two-dimensional (2D), non-metallic, π-conjugated polymeric material that had various applications [15]. In 2012, the properties of g-C_3N_4 were reported such as high intrinsic photo-absorption and photo-responsiveness, semiconductive properties, high stability under physiological conditions, and good biocompatibility. Since then it has caught the attention of scientists and has been one of the top areas of research [16].

Polymerisation of precursors with a C–N core structure or thermal polycondensation can both be used to create carbon nitride materials. Urea, thiourea, melamine, dicyandiamide, cyanamide, guanidine hydrochloride, guanidine thiocyanate, and thiourea oxide are a few of the other compounds that can be produced at between 400 and 600 °C [15, 17]. High surface regions, outstanding stability in chemistry and physics, excellent electronic band structures, and outstanding electrical, thermal, optical, and mechanical capabilities are just a few of the many benefits of this material's constitution. It was shown to be responsible for g-C_3N_4's unique sensing capacity [17]. The degree of polymerisation and the condensation process determine the characteristics and reactivity of g-C_3N_4. This material has a bandgap of between 2.4 and 2.7 eV, which makes it visibly active [15]. Moreover, the efficiency of g-C_3N_4 in the visible spectrum is lower when compared to other semiconductor materials with lower bandgaps. As a result of g-C_3N_4's bandgap, low specific surface, and crystallisation phase, it has a high number of lattice defects, which leads to frequent photogenerated species recombination and hence inhibits g-C_3N_4's photochemical ability [18]. The mechanism based on g-C_3N_4 for electron transfer and redox reactions has not been fully elucidated [19]. This is where g-C_3N_4's unusual 2D layered structure, which encourages hybridisation with other components, comes into play. As a result, researchers began doping g-C_3N_4 with a variety of different functional groups, including metal oxides, noble gases, metal-free composites, and zero-dimensional particles. CQDs are being studied in an attempt to improve their photocatalytic capabilities. g-C_3N_4 is visible light active and extensively used as a photocatalyst [16, 20].

g-C_3N_4 is the most durable of the numerous allotropic forms of carbon nitride. The carbon and nitrogen atoms in this polyconjugated semiconductor give it a graphitic structure. g-C_3N_4 has been extensively explored as a catalyst, but its structure has not been determined. As shown in Figure 10.2, a triazine-based 2D structure and a tri-s-triazine-based 2D structure have been proposed so far [21]. The most recent work on the three-dimensional (3D) structure of g-C_3N_4 employed X-ray diffraction modelling to answer a question about the structure of g-C_3N_4. However, the lack of long-term resources has resulted in an inappropriate refinement of the structure, and so the structure is still not formally defined [22].

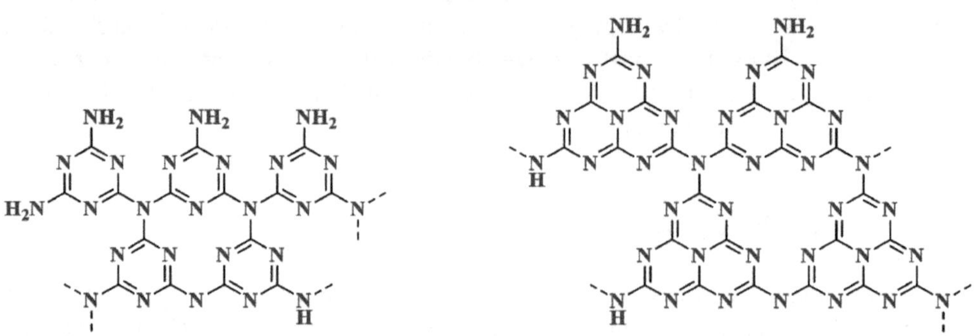

Figure 10.2 Triazine-based and tri-s-triazine-based graphitic carbon nitride structures.

10.3 Quantum Dots

Fluorescent nanoparticles were accidentally obtained as a by-product, while the purification of single-walled carbon nanotubes was investigated in 2004. These luminescent carbon nanomaterials were found to be zero-dimensional and were named carbon dots, carbon quantum dots, or carbon nanodots [23]. Carbon dots have emerged as one of the most promising materials for use as an effective catalyst over the last decade. Because they have distinct photophysical and chemical features, including light-harvesting, it is feasible to derive a variety of photovoltaic chemical reactions. Photosensitisers, bivalent redox character, chemical inertness, low toxicity, remarkable biocompatibility, and good water solubility are some of the properties of optional photoluminescence. Carbon dots are more environmentally friendly than other quantum dots because of their chemical inertness and low toxicity. They are nanoparticles with a quasi-spherical shape and a diameter of less than 5 nm. Depending on the origin of the CQDs, their size and shape may change, allowing them to be used in a wide range of configurations [24].

There are two main classifications of the synthesis of CQDs, the top-down approach and the bottom-up approach, as shown in Figure 10.3. Chemical oxidation, discharge, electrochemical oxidation, and ultrasonic techniques are all examples of the top-down approach to carbon decomposition. This method is more expensive and time-consuming than the bottom-up technique, in which tiny carbon structures are converted into larger carbon dots. Thermal degradation, pyrolysis, carbonisation, microwave synthesis, and

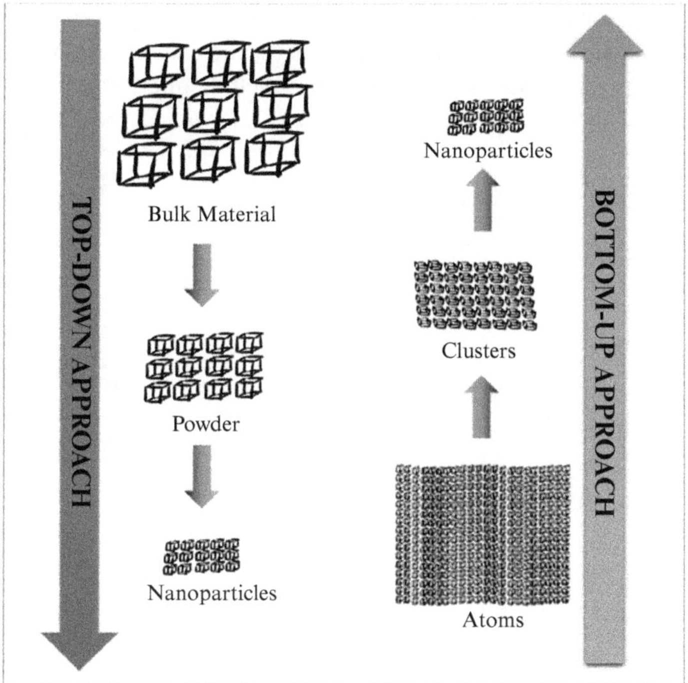

Figure 10.3 The manufacture of carbon quantum dots combines top-down and bottom-up strategies.

solvothermal procedures are all examples of bottom-up treatment approaches [25]. The synthesis procedure is solely dependent on the precursor material. Furthermore, it has been found that the addition of heteroatoms to CQDs improves their quality. It is preferable to dope N rather than other heteroatoms due to their similar size and shape. N's strong electronegativity and five-valence electrons, including two lone pairs, facilitate bonding with electro-positive ions, particularly trivalent and divalent types [24].

Precursor selection is critical since it determines the size, shape, and characteristics of the CQDs produced. As in the case of atoms, strong emission peaks are feasible. The variation in size is due to the changes in the surface-to-volume ratio with size and quantum confinement effects, which depend on the precursor. As the size changes, the photoluminescence emission colour of the CQD also changes. CQDs are commonly found between atoms and molecules. Quantum confinement effects can occur due to the size of CQDs and can occur if the energy level spacing of a nanocrystal surpasses kT when the nanocrystal becomes a nanoparticle [26]. Hundreds of suitable precursors have been identified over the course of decades of research, each with a unique set of uses. However, quantum dots derived from g-C_3N_4 capture attention due to their important features and applications. There are several methods for obtaining g-C_3N_4 quantum dots.

10.4 Methods of Synthesis of Graphitic Carbon Nitride Quantum Dots and Their Applications

g-C_3N_4 quantum dots can be synthesised using either top-down or bottom-up approaches (Figure 10.4). Electrochemical oxidation, hydrothermal treatment, and chemical oxidation are examples of top-down approaches. Bottom-up approaches include microwave, solid-phase, hydrothermal, and microwave-assisted thermal methods [27].

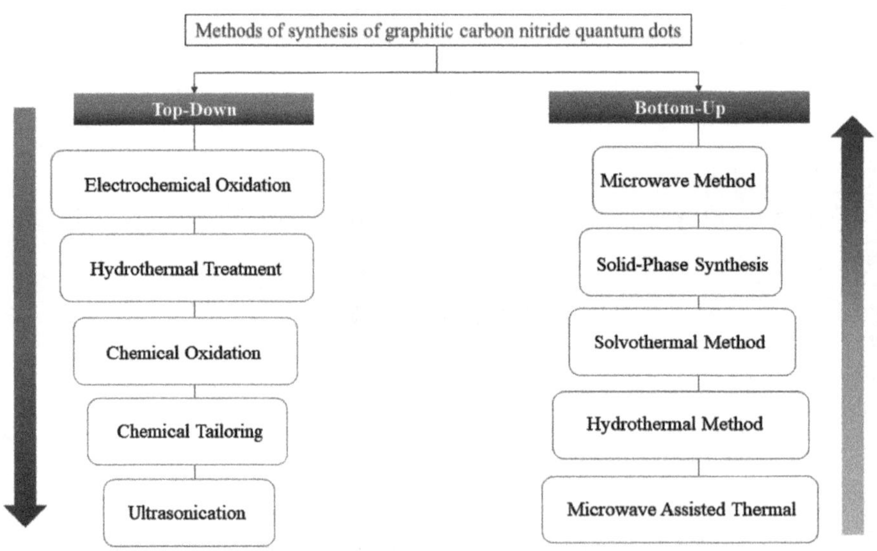

Figure 10.4 Various methods of synthesis of graphitic carbon nitride quantum dots.

Table 10.1 Bulk graphitic carbon nitride (g-C_3N_4) quantum dot production methods utilising top-down methods.

Method	Starting material	Type of photoluminescence (365 nm)	Light absorption, nm	Light excitation, nm	Light emission, nm	Average electron distribution, nm	Quantum efficiency (%)	References
Chemical oxidation	Bulk g-C_3N_4	Blue	245	220–280	367	1–5	–	[29–31]
			228	190–270	368	1–5	8.96	
Ultrasonication			350	365	406	2–6	–	[32–36]
Chemical tailoring			243	230–310	367	2–4	46	[39]
Hydrothermal treatment			400	300–400	437	5–20	16.9	[40–42]
Electrochemical oxidation			268	260–420	450	5–8	–	[45]

This chapter exclusively covers the synthesis of g-C_3N_4 quantum dots and their uses when g-C_3N_4 is used as an initial precursor. As a general rule, g-C_3N_4-based quantum dots are synthesised using the top-down technique (Table 10.1), but we will also talk about other ways to make g-C_3N_4 quantum dots.

10.4.1 Top-Down Approaches

10.4.1.1 Chemical Oxidation

Employing chemical oxidation to produce stable carbon-based nanomaterials such as CQDs is a dependable method since it is quantitative, suggesting that the amount of oxidation depends on the amount of acid used [28]. Adding a strong acid to bulk g-C_3N_4 has been shown to cause simultaneous protonation and exfoliation of the g-C_3N_4 in mass, resulting in the production of hydrophilic g-C_3N_4 quantum dots. Many researchers, including Song and his colleagues as well as Li and his co-workers, have successfully produced stable g-C_3N_4 quantum dots using chemical oxidation. Following HNO_3 oxidation, hydrothermal treatment, and ultrasonication, Song et al. exfoliated bulk g-C_3N_4 via ultrasonic treatment. The generated g-C_3N_4 quantum dots had diameters ranging from 1 to 5 nm and surfaces with hydroxyl, carboxylic acid, and amine groups, making them very dispersible in water [29]. Li et al. synthesised g-C_3N_4 quantum dots from melamine-derived bulky g-C_3N_4 using an acidic chemical oxidation technique and a liquid exfoliation procedure. It was found that the resulting g-C_3N_4 quantum dots were highly crystalline and negatively charged, and they were also water dispersible. When bulk g-C_3N_4 oxidises, the instability of hydrogen bonds in the facilities of tri-s-triazine increases, resulting in attachment and exfoliation [30]. g-C_3N_4 quantum dots were synthesised in o-dichlorobenzene by chemically oxidising bulk g-C_3N_4 and then hydrothermally treating the solution. At a 2 vol% concentration of quantum dots, polymer solar cell systems demonstrated a 40% boost in energy conversion efficiency. This highlights the photovoltaic enhancer properties of the g-C_3N_4 quantum dots generated [31]. As a result, this approach is suitable for large-scale manufacturing if certain considerations are met, such as the demand for further exfoliation treatments and the removal of excess oxidants from the reaction environment.

10.4.1.2 Ultrasonication

There is simultaneous formation and dissolution of bubbles during ultrasonication. It is through this process that the material's bonds are broken because the bubble bursts and releases its stored energy. There are two types of bonds in C_3N_4. When the 0.1316 nm link in the rings of the melon unit and the 0.1442 nm bond that connects them are disturbed, the rings are subjected to weak van der Waals forces, and robust C–N interactions are both present in the C_3N_4 layers under 180 W [32]. The bonds are broken because of the cavitation process; that is, the energy liberated from the broken bubbles is utilised to break the bonds. Because the C–N linkage establishing a connection between the melon components provides poor binding strength, strong ultrasonic energy might disrupt its C–N interconnection, resulting in reactive radicals like C and N. However, their activity and the ability to rapidly rearrange make those radicals invaluable. Wang et al. devised a solution using ethylene glycol as the solvent. Ethylene glycol is a radical scavenger with good reducibility, which aids in the rapid acceptance of active radicals. Because of this radical limitation [33], the reformation of bulk C_3N_4 is limited, resulting in C_3N_4 quantum dots (Figure 10.5). Furthermore, because of the proper viscosity of ethylene glycol, the use of ethylene glycol as the solvent has other advantages, such as the wide dispersion of quantum dots and the limitation of quantum dot collisions. Water can be used as a solvent, but the quantum dots obtained are larger, and more complex steps might be required in the case of separation [34]. There have been reports with regard to the creation of g-C_3N_4 quantum dots utilising water solvent via ultrasonication of g-C_3N_4 [35, 36]. Employing CCRF-CEM cells, autosensing investigations were performed on the synthesised g-C_3N_4 quantum dots, and the

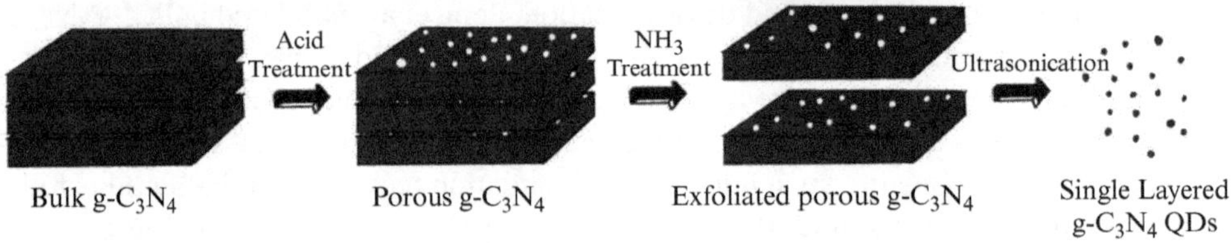

Figure 10.5 Strategy for the preparation of graphitic carbon nitride quantum dots through ultrasonication.

results demonstrated that these dots have outstanding sensing capabilities [36]. As already discussed, exfoliated porous nanosheets were obtained through the chemical oxidation method after treatment with acid. That is where ultrasonication comes into play. Only through ultrasound were single-layered g-C_3N_4 quantum dots obtained [29, 37].

10.4.1.3 Chemical Tailoring

In chemical tailoring, which is also known as chemical cleavage, specific impacts on particular chemical bonds are used to perform precise molecular cutting [38]. Large molecules are broken down into smaller, pre-determined pieces. QDs are created from g-C_3N_4 and nanowires. Zhang et al. employed larger stacked amounts of polymeric carbon nitride as a starting material. g-C_3N_4 quantum dots were created by partially hydrolysing bulk C_3N_4 in H_2SO_4, with water acting as a protic solvent to disrupt the hydrogen bonds. Hydrogen atoms were dissolved in H_2O solvent bonds while partially hydrolysing bulk C_3N_4 in H_2SO_4 [39]. The g-C_3N_4 quantum dots had a unique electronic structure and modified surface properties that allowed them to detect Fe^{3+} ions while being used as light-emitting diodes (LEDs).

10.4.1.4 Hydrothermal Treatment

Hydrothermal treatment is the most cost-efficient and greener method of all the top-down methods of synthesis of g-C_3N_4 quantum dots. When Zhang et al. reported on hydrothermal treatment, the mass g-C_3N_4 was employed in a novel way, especially as an inducer. Water-soluble, blue-coloured typical g-C_3N_4 quantum dots have an average diameter of about 10 nm and were obtained after 10 hours of heating at 180 °C. A 16.9% greater quantum yield was achieved from quantum dots, and they are excellent fluorescent probes for metal ion detection [40]. Another interesting method of g-C_3N_4 synthesis was carried out by Yu and colleagues. Although g-C_3N_4 nanosheets were obtained from bulk g-C_3N_4 by heat etching, the nanosheets were subjected to acidic cutting, resulting in nanoribbons. Finally, after the nanoribbons underwent hydrothermal cutting at 200° C for 10 hours, g-C_3N_4 quantum dots were obtained. These g-C_3N_4 quantum dots were approximately 7 nm in size, had blue emissions with tunable photoluminescence (PL), and had the possibility to employ the Vis-NIR (near-infrared) spectrum of sunlight via photocatalysis [41]. Due to the high temperature and pressure during hydrothermal treatment, a shear force is applied to the system under investigation, and 3D g-C_3N_4 is exfoliated into zero-dimensional (0D) quantum dots. According to Zhan and colleagues, quantum dots can be made in a single step by heating the autoclave holding bulk g-C_3N_4 in a mixture of concentrated potassium hydroxyl (KOH) and ethanol solution at 180 °C for 16 hours. Adding KOH to g-C_3N_4 sheets not only helps g-C_3N_4 be broken down in the process of exfoliation sheets caused by the intercalation of potassium and hydroxyl into layers, it also assists in oxidising the margins of the g-C_3N_4 sheets, as shown in Figure 10.6 [42].

10.4.1.5 Electrochemical Oxidation

The phenomenon by which the oxidation state of an ion or molecule is altered by the transfer of electrons from or to the molecule of an ion when an external current of

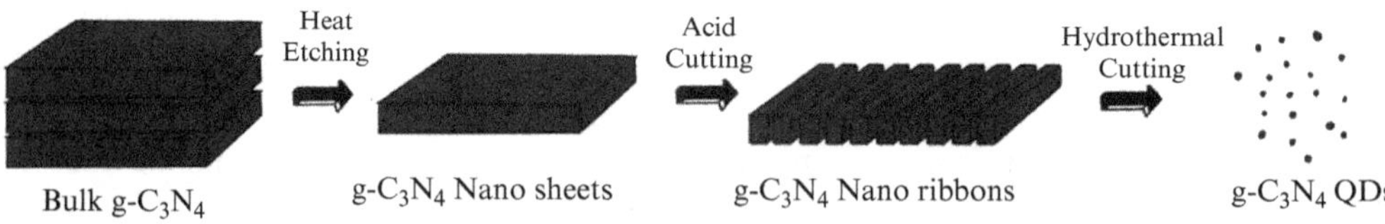

Figure 10.6 Synthesis of graphitic carbon nitride quantum dots through hydrothermal treatment.

chemical energy is applied is called electrochemical oxidation [43]. Quantum dots obtained through electrochemical oxidation show high stability. The synthesis of quantum dots by electrochemical oxidation has been reported in two ways. In one instance, the carbon–carbon bonds of the precursor are actively broken by the oxidation process. Quantum dots can be oxidatively cleaved by the formation of a hydroxyl free radical (·OH) or an oxygen free radical (·O) [44]. The electrolyte was a combination of 100 mg large bulk g-C_3N_4, 50 mg NaOH, as well as 10 mL water mixed together. The positive and negative electrodes were platinum sheets. The solution was electrolysed and diluted (Mw 1000) with H_2O for 48 hours after being exposed to 10 V (DC) for three hours and centrifuged at 10,000 rpm for 15 minutes to separate the g-C_3N_4 quantum dots. The synthesised quantum dots were extremely water stable, had high fluorescence (FL), and could be reduced at around 60 °C by Ag+ transforming them into Ag nanoparticles [45]. Although the process produced stable quantum dots, the pre-treatment of raw materials and purification of quantum dot products took longer than expected [46].

10.4.2 Other Methods of Synthesis

There are numerous works reporting the synthesis of g-C_3N_4 quantum dots through different methods of synthesis other than those methods discussed here. A few of those methods and the characteristics of the synthesised quantum dots are given in Table 10.2.

10.5 Conclusion

The methods for g-C_3N_4 quantum dot synthesis from bulk g-C_3N_4 were the focus of this chapter. Using g-C_3N_4 as a starting material for the synthesis of carbon dots is a straightforward and efficient method. Despite the fact that there are numerous methods available, the chapter focuses on the synthesis of quantum dots with bulk g-C_3N_4. Serving as a major contributor, and numerous top-down methods are being employed. The photon emission efficiency of the type of methods that have been performed can be seen clearly in their quantum yields. Even though it has proven to be extremely useful, there are still a number of application fields that need to be explored (Figure 10.7) where there is scope for improvement.

Table 10.2 Bottom-up techniques for making graphitic carbon nitride (g-C_3N_4) quantum dots from other factors.

Methods	Starting materials	Types of photolumine-scence (365 nm)	Light absorption, nm	Light excitation, nm	Light emission, nm	Average electron distribution, nm	Quantum efficiency (%)	References
Hydrothermal process	$C_3H_6N_6$ and $C_5H_8O_2$	blue	282	360	440	3–8	31	[46]
	$C_6H_8O_7$ and CH_4N_2S		338	369	444	2.78	14.5	[45, 47]
	[Bmim]BF_4 and water		240	355–385	458	2.2–6.1	8.34	[48]
Solvothermal method	CCl_4 and EN		250	360	440	1–5	11	[49]
	Citric acid monohydrate, urea, and oleic acid		268, 335, and 400	360–420	450–540	1–5	27.1	[7]
Microwave method	Guanidine hydrochloride and EDTA		260	360	453	3.2–6.5	35	[50]
	Citric acid, urea, and oleic acid		325	425	531	<10	-	[51]
	DMF and chlorosulfonic acid		266	360	443	1–6	9	[52]
	Dimethylamine and H_2SO_4		262	380	454	2–8	8.9	[53]
	Formamide		260–340	340	405	2–15	29	[54]

(Continued)

Table 10.2 (Continued)

Methods	Starting materials	Types of photolumine-scence (365 nm)	Light absorption, nm	Light excitation, nm	Light emission, nm	Average electron distribution, nm	Quantum efficiency (%)	References
Microwave-assisted thermal	Thymine, DAMN, and NaOH		271	350	445	3–8	46	[55]
Solid-phase synthesis	Urea and sodium citrate		344	360	467	2.6–5.5	42	[34]
	Melamine and EDTA		200–500	360	440	3–8	34	[56]
	EDTA.2Na and thiourea		263–358	360	433	3–13	13.4	[57]

[Bmim]BF_4, 1-butyl-3-methylimidazolium tetrafluoroborate; CCl_4, carbon tetrachloride; $C_3H_6N_6$, melamine; $C_5H_8O_2$, acetylacetone; $C_6H_8O_7$, citric acid; CH_4N_2S, thiourea; DAMN, diaminomaleonitrile; DMF, dimethylformamide; EDTA, ethylenediamine tetraacetic acid; EN, ethylenediamine.

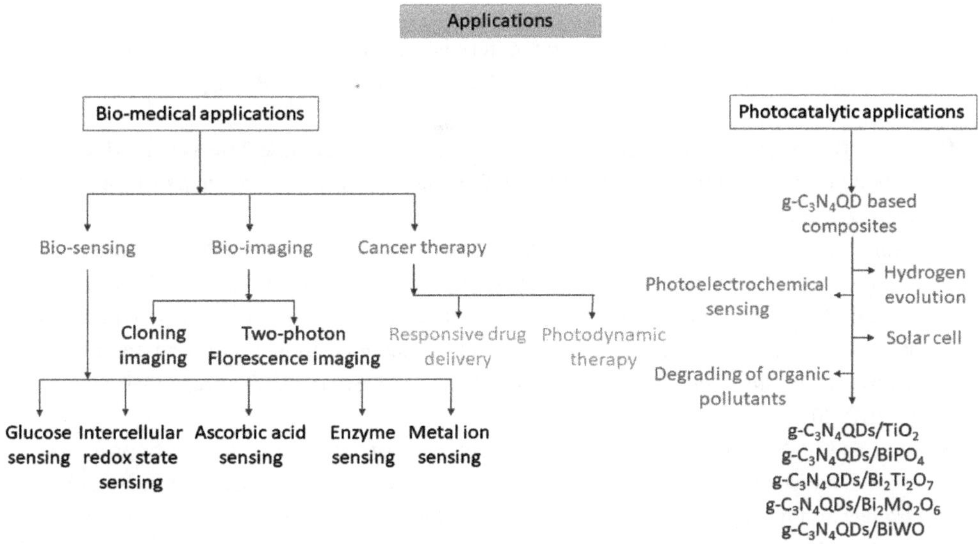

Figure 10.7 Other notable applications of graphitic carbon nitride quantum dots.

References

1 Hummelen, J.C., Knight, B., Pavlovich, J. et al. (1995). Isolation of the heterofullerene $C_{59}N$ as its dimer ($C_{59}N$) 2. *Science* 269: 1554–1556. https://doi.org/10.1126/science.269.5230.1554.

2 Webster, O.W. (1964). Hexacyanobutadiene. *Journal of the American Chemical Society* 86: 2898–2902. https://doi.org/10.1021/ja01068a026.

3 Del Sesto, R.E., Arif, A.M., Novoa, J.J. et al. (2003). Chemical reduction of 2,4,6-tricyano-1,3,5-triazine and 1,3,5-tricyanobenzene. formation of novel 4,4',6,6'-tetracyano-2,2'-bitriazine and its radical anion. *Journal of Organic Chemistry* 68: 3367–3379. https://doi.org/10.1021/jo025833h.

4 Miller, T.S., Jorge, A.B., Suter, T.M. et al. (2017). Carbon nitrides: synthesis and characterization of a new class of functional materials. *Physical Chemistry Chemical Physics* 19: 15613–15638. https://doi.org/10.1039/C7CP02711G.

5 Fang, L., Ohfuji, H., Shinmei, T., and Irifune, T. (2011). Experimental study on the stability of graphitic C_3N_4 under high pressure and high temperature. *Diamond and Related Materials* 20: 819–825. https://doi.org/10.1016/j.diamond.2011.03.034.

6 Zhu, J., Xiao, P., Li, H., and Carabineiro, S.A.C. (2014). Graphitic carbon nitride: synthesis, properties, and applications in catalysis. *ACS Applied Materials and Interfaces* 6: 16449–16465. https://doi.org/10.1021/am502925j.

7 Cao, X., Ma, J., Lin, Y. et al. (2015). A facile microwave-assisted fabrication of fluorescent carbon nitride quantum dots and their application in the detection of mercury ions. *Spectrochimica Acta Part A: Molecular and Biomolecular Spectroscopy* 151: 875–880. https://doi.org/10.1016/j.saa.2015.07.034.

8 Wang, Z., Hu, T., Liang, R., and Wei, M. (2020). Application of zero-dimensional nanomaterials in biosensing. *Frontiers in Chemistry* 8: 320. https://doi.org/10.3389/fchem.2020.00320.

9 Mallick, A., Patil, P.D., Tiwari, M.S. et al. (2021). Green and sustainable methods for dye degradation employing photocatalytic materials. In: *Photocatalytic Degradation of Dyes* (eds. M. Shah, S. Dave, and J. Das), 345–376. Amsterdam: Elsevier. https://doi.org/10.1016/B978-0-12-823876-9.00010-X.

10 Frank, B.P., Sigmon, L.R., Deline, A.R. et al. (2020). Photochemical transformations of carbon dots in aqueous environments. *Environmental Science & Technology* 54: 4160–4170. https://doi.org/10.1021/acs.est.9b07437.

11 Kang, C., Huang, Y., Yang, H. et al. (2020). A review of carbon dots produced from biomass wastes. *Nanomaterials* 10: 2316. https://doi.org/10.3390/nano10112316.

12 Omran, B.A., Whitehead, K.A., and Baek, K.-H. (2021). One-pot bioinspired synthesis of fluorescent metal chalcogenide and carbon quantum dots: applications and potential biotoxicity. *Colloids Surfaces B Biointerfaces* 200: 111578. https://doi.org/10.1016/j.colsurfb.2021.111578.

13 Jian, X., Liu, X., Yang, H. et al. (2016). Construction of carbon quantum dots/proton-functionalized graphitic carbon nitride nanocomposite via electrostatic self-assembly strategy and its application. *Applications of Surface Science* 370: 514–521. https://doi.org/10.1016/j.apsusc.2016.02.119.

14 Liebig, J. (1834). Uber einige Stickstoff – Verbindungen. *Ann der Pharm* 10: 1–47. https://doi.org/10.1002/jlac.18340100102.

15 Ghalkhani, M., Khaneghah, M.H., and Sohouli, E. (2021). Graphitic carbon nitride: synthesis and characterization. In: *Handbook of Carbon-Based Nanomaterials* (eds. S. Thomas, C. Sarathchandran, S.A. Ilangovan, and J.C. Moreno-Piraján), 573–590. Amsterdam: Elsevier. https://doi.org/10.1016/B978-0-12-821996-6.00014-2.

16 Wang, J., and Yang, M. (2019). Two-dimensional nanomaterials in cancer theranostics. In: *Theranostic Bionanomaterials* (eds. W. Cui, and X. Zhao), 263–288. Amsterdam: Elsevier. https://doi.org/10.1016/B978-0-12-815341-3.00011-0.

17 Balakumar, V., and Manivannan, R. (2021). Metal oxide-graphitic carbon nitride nanocomposite-modified electrochemical sensors for toxic chemicals. In: *Metal Oxides in Nanocomposite-Based Electrochemical Sensors for Toxic Chemicals* (eds. Pandikumar, A., and Rameshkumar, P.), 263–292. Amsterdam: Elsevier. https://doi.org/10.1016/B978-0-12-820727-7.00005-7.

18 Ansari, S.P., Fawad, A., Khan, A., and Dzudzevic-Cancar, H. (2021). Carbon polymer hybrid supported nanomaterials for hydrogen production and storage application. In: *Nanomaterials for Hydrogen Storage Applications* (eds. Sen, F., Khan, A., and Asiri, A.M.), 133–152. Amsterdam: Elsevier. https://doi.org/10.1016/B978-0-12-819476-8.00012-8.

19 Tahir, N., Zahid, M., Bhatti, I.A. et al. (2021). Metal oxide-based ternary nanocomposites for wastewater treatment. In: *Aquananotechnology* (eds. Abd-Elsalam, K., and Zahid, M.), 135–158. Amsterdam: Elsevier. https://doi.org/10.1016/B978-0-12-821141-0.00022-7.

20 Lakshmana Reddy, N., Kumbhar, V.S., Lee, K., and Shankar, M.V. (2020). Graphitic carbon nitride–based nanocomposite materials for photocatalytic hydrogen generation. In: *Nanostructured, Functional, and Flexible Materials for Energy Conversion and Storage Systems* (eds. Pandikumar, A., and Rameshkumar, P.), 293–324. Amsterdam: Elsevier. https://doi.org/10.1016/B978-0-12-819552-9.00009-9.

21 Fina, F., Callear, S.K., Carins, G.M., and Irvine, J.T.S. (2015). Structural investigation of graphitic carbon nitride via XRD and neutron diffraction. *Chemistry of Materials* 27: 2612–2618. https://doi.org/10.1021/acs.chemmater.5b00411.

22 Tyborski, T., Merschjann, C., Orthmann, S. et al. (2013). Crystal structure of polymeric carbon nitride and the determination of its process-temperature-induced modifications. *Journal of Physics Condensed Matter* 25: 395402. https://doi.org/10.1088/0953-8984/25/39/395402.

23 Ding, H., Cheng, L.-W., Ma, -Y.-Y. et al. (2013). Luminescent carbon quantum dots and their application in cell imaging. *New Journal of Chemistry* 37: 2515. https://doi.org/10.1039/c3nj00366c.

24 Pankaj, A., Tewari, K., Singh, S., and Singh, S.P. (2018). Waste candle soot derived nitrogen doped carbon dots based fluorescent sensor probe: an efficient and inexpensive route to determine Hg(II) and Fe(III) from water. *Journal of Environmental Chemical Engineering* 6: 5561–5569. https://doi.org/10.1016/j.jece.2018.08.059.

25 Sharma, A., and Das, J. (2019). Small molecules derived carbon dots: synthesis and applications in sensing, catalysis, imaging, and biomedicine. *Journal of Nanobiotechnology* 17: 92. https://doi.org/10.1186/s12951-019-0525-8.

26 Bera, D., Qian, L., Tseng, T.-K., and Holloway, P.H. (2010). Quantum dots and their multimodal applications: a review. *Materials (Basel)* 3: 2260–2345. https://doi.org/10.3390/ma3042260.

27 Liu, H., Wang, X., Wang, H., and Nie, R. (2019). Synthesis and biomedical applications of graphitic carbon nitride quantum dots. *Journal of Materials Chemistry B* 7: 5432–5448. https://doi.org/10.1039/C9TB01410A.

28 Štengl, V., Bakardjieva, S., Henych, J. et al. (2013). Blue and green luminescence of reduced graphene oxide quantum dots. *Carbon* 63: 537–546. https://doi.org/10.1016/j.carbon.2013.07.031.

29 Song, Z., Lin, T., Lin, L. et al. (2016). Invisible security ink based on water-soluble graphitic carbon nitride quantum dots. *Angewandte Chemie* 128: 2823–2827. https://doi.org/10.1002/ange.201510945.

30 Li, Y., Cai, J., Liu, F. et al. (2018). Highly crystalline graphitic carbon nitride quantum dots as a fluorescent probe for detection of Fe(III) via an inner filter effect. *Microchimica Acta* 185: 134. https://doi.org/10.1007/s00604-017-2655-8.

31 Pareek, S., Waheed, S., Rana, A. et al. (2020). Graphitic carbon nitride quantum dots (g-C_3N_4) to improve photovoltaic performance of polymer solar cell by combining Förster resonance energy transfer (FRET) and morphological effects. *Nano Express* 1: 010057. https://doi.org/10.1088/2632-959X/ab9b2f.

32 Molina, B., and Sansores, L.E. (1999). Electronic structure of six phases of C_3N_4: a theoretical approach. *Modern Physics Letters B* 13: 193–201. https://doi.org/10.1142/S0217984999000269.

33 Wang, N., Fan, H., Sun, J. et al. (2016). Fluorine-doped carbon nitride quantum dots: ethylene glycol-assisted synthesis, fluorescent properties, and their application for bacterial imaging. *Carbon* 109: 141–148. https://doi.org/10.1016/j.carbon.2016.08.004.

34 Zhou, J., Yang, Y., and Zhang, C. (2013). A low-temperature solid-phase method to synthesize highly fluorescent carbon nitride dots with tunable emission. *Chemical Communications* 49: 8605. https://doi.org/10.1039/c3cc42266f.

35 Pang, X., Pan, J., Gao, P. et al. (2015). A visible light induced photoelectrochemical aptsensor constructed by aligned ZnO@CdTe core shell nanocable arrays/carboxylated g-C_3N_4 for the detection of proprotein convertase subtilisin/kexin type 6 gene. *Biosensors and Bioelectronics* 74: 49–58. https://doi.org/10.1016/j.bios.2015.06.030.

36 Pang, X., Cui, C., Su, M. et al. (2018). Construction of self-powered cytosensing device based on ZnO nanodisks@g-C_3N_4 quantum dots and application in the detection of CCRF-CEM cells. *Nano Energy* 46: 101–109. https://doi.org/10.1016/j.nanoen.2018.01.018.

37 Wang, T., Nie, C., Ao, Z. et al. (2020). Recent progress in g-C_3N_4 quantum dots: synthesis, properties and applications in photocatalytic degradation of organic pollutants. *Journal of Materials Chemistry A* 8: 485–502. https://doi.org/10.1039/C9TA11368A.

38 Gao, P., Xie, Y., Chen, Y. et al. (2005). Large-area synthesis of single-crystal boehmite nanobelts with high luminescent properties. *Journal of Crystal Growth* 285: 555–560. https://doi.org/10.1016/j.jcrysgro.2005.09.034.

39 Zhou, Z., Shen, Y., Li, Y. et al. (2015). Chemical cleavage of layered carbon nitride with enhanced photoluminescent performances and photoconduction. *ACS Nano* 9: 12480–12487. https://doi.org/10.1021/acsnano.5b05924.

40 Zhang, S., Li, J., Zeng, M. et al. (2014). Polymer nanodots of graphitic carbon nitride as effective fluorescent probes for the detection of Fe^{3+} and Cu^{2+} ions. *Nanoscale* 6: 4157. https://doi.org/10.1039/c3nr06744k.

41 Wang, W., Yu, J.C., Shen, Z. et al. (2014). g-C_3N_4 quantum dots: direct synthesis, upconversion properties and photocatalytic application. *Chemical Communications* 50: 10148–10150. https://doi.org/10.1039/C4CC02543A.

42 Zhan, Y., Liu, Z., Liu, Q. et al. (2017). A facile and one-pot synthesis of fluorescent graphitic carbon nitride quantum dots for bio-imaging applications. *New Journal of Chemistry* 41: 3930–3938. https://doi.org/10.1039/C7NJ00058H.

43 Pimentel, M., Oturan, N., Dezotti, M., and Oturan, M.A. (2008). Phenol degradation by advanced electrochemical oxidation process electro-Fenton using a carbon felt cathode. *Applied Catalysis, B: Environmental* 83: 140–149. https://doi.org/10.1016/j.apcatb.2008.02.011.

44 Chen, W., Lv, G., Hu, W. et al. (2018). Synthesis and applications of graphene quantum dots: a review. *Nanotechnology Reviews* 7: 157–185. https://doi.org/10.1515/ntrev-2017-0199.

45 Lu, Q., Wang, H., Liu, Y. et al. (2017). Graphitic carbon nitride nanodots: as reductant for the synthesis of silver nanoparticles and its biothiols biosensing application. *Biosensors and Bioelectronics* 89: 411–416. https://doi.org/10.1016/j.bios.2016.05.064.

46 Shen, J., Li, Y., Su, Y. et al. (2015). Photoluminescent carbon–nitrogen quantum dots as efficient electrocatalysts for oxygen reduction. *Nanoscale* 7: 2003–2008. https://doi.org/10.1039/C4NR06484D.

47 Lu, Y.-C., Chen, J., Wang, A.-J. et al. (2015). Facile synthesis of oxygen and sulfur co-doped graphitic carbon nitride fluorescent quantum dots and their application for mercury(II) detection and bioimaging. *Journal of Materials Chemistry C* 3: 73–78. https://doi.org/10.1039/C4TC02111H.

48 Xiao, D., Li, S., Liu, S. et al. (2016). One-step hydrothermal synthesis of photoluminescent carbon nitride dots derived from ionic liquids. *New Journal of Chemistry* 40: 320–324. https://doi.org/10.1039/C5NJ01717C.

49 Liu, S., Tian, J., Wang, L. et al. (2011). Preparation of photoluminescent carbon nitride dots from CCl_4 and 1,2-ethylenediamine: a heat-treatment-based strategy. *Journal of Materials Chemistry* 21: 11726. https://doi.org/10.1039/c1jm12149a.

50 Tang, Y., Su, Y., Yang, N. et al. (2014). Carbon nitride quantum dots: a novel chemiluminescence system for selective detection of free chlorine in water. *Analytical Chemistry* 86: 4528–4535. https://doi.org/10.1021/ac5005162.

51 Shorie, M., Kaur, H., Chadha, G. et al. (2019). Graphitic carbon nitride QDs impregnated biocompatible agarose cartridge for removal of heavy metals from contaminated water samples. *Journal of Hazardous Materials* 367: 629–638. https://doi.org/10.1016/j.jhazmat.2018.12.115.

52 Liu, S., Wang, L., Tian, J. et al. (2011). Acid-driven, microwave-assisted production of photoluminescent carbon nitride dots from N,N-dimethylformamide. *RSC Advances* 1: 951. https://doi.org/10.1039/c1ra00249j.

53 Liu, S., Tian, J., Wang, L. et al. (2012). A general strategy for the production of photoluminescent carbon nitride dots from organic amines and their application as novel peroxidase-like catalysts for colorimetric detection of H_2O_2 and glucose. *RSC Advances* 2: 411–413. https://doi.org/10.1039/C1RA00709B.

54 Barman, S., and Sadhukhan, M. (2012). Facile bulk production of highly blue fluorescent graphitic carbon nitride quantum dots and their application as highly selective and sensitive sensors for the detection of mercuric and iodide ions in aqueous media. *Journal of Materials Chemistry* 22: 21832. https://doi.org/10.1039/c2jm35501a.

55 Achadu, O.J., and Revaprasadu, N. (2018). Microwave-assisted synthesis of thymine-functionalized graphitic carbon nitride quantum dots as a fluorescent nanoprobe for mercury(II). *Microchimica Acta* 185: 461. https://doi.org/10.1007/s00604-018-3004-2.

56 Fan, X., Feng, Y., Su, Y. et al. (2015). A green solid-phase method for preparation of carbon nitride quantum dots and their applications in chemiluminescent dopamine sensing. *RSC Advances* 5: 55158–55164. https://doi.org/10.1039/C5RA05397H.

57 Patir, K., and Gogoi, S.K. (2018). Facile synthesis of photoluminescent graphitic carbon nitride quantum dots for Hg^{2+} detection and room temperature phosphorescence. *ACS Sustainable Chemistry & Engineering* 6: 1732–1743. https://doi.org/10.1021/acssuschemeng.7b03008.

11

Mechanochemistry for Sustainable Drug Design and Active Pharmaceutical Ingredient Synthesis

Pedro Brandão[1] and Marta Pineiro[2]

[1] *Egas Moniz Center for Interdisciplinary Research (CiiEM); Egas Moniz School of Health & Science, Caparica, Portugal*
[2] *Coimbra Chemistry Centre (CQC)–Institute of Molecular Sciences (IMS), Department of Chemistry, University of Coimbra, Coimbra, Portugal*

CONTENTS

11.1 Introduction

Sustainability, meeting the needs of the present without compromising the ability of future generations to meet their own needs [1], is a broad concept that encompasses all aspects of life, namely sustainable economy, sustainable energy, sustainable agriculture, sustainable tourism, and, of course, sustainable chemistry.

Sustainability has taken centre stage of our everyday life and is now a cornerstone for scientific and technological development. Academia, industry, and regulatory authorities are turning their attention to the increasing demand for sustainable manufacturing processes with lower environmental demands and impact [2].

The crucial importance of sustainable chemistry for sustainable development was highlighted in the *Green and Sustainable Chemistry: Framework Manual* published by the United Nations (UN) Environment programme in 2020 [3]. Sustainable chemistry is related, among other things, to water purification, alternative energies, chemical policies, and also green chemistry and it is in line with the objectives of the UN for sustainable development. Using the words of I.T. Horváth, 'resources, including energy, should be used at a rate at which they can be replaced naturally, and the generation of wastes cannot be faster than the rate of their remediation' [4]. The green chemistry concept, elaborated through the well-known 12 principles, is focused on the design, development, and

Sustainable Approaches in Pharmaceutical Sciences, First Edition. Edited by Kamal Shah, Durgesh Nandini Chauhan, and Nagendra Singh Chauhan.

implementation of chemical products and processes and is also in line with sustainable development. Green chemistry looks to reduce pollution at its origin by minimising or eliminating the hazards of chemical feedstocks, reagents, solvents, and products by looking at the solvent applied in the process, exploring the potential use of catalysts, seeking the inclusion of renewable feedstocks, reducing energy utilisation, and identifying materials that do not persist or bioaccumulate. These goals are summarised in the 12 principles of green chemistry [2] and are depicted in Figure 11.1.

Several strategies have been implemented to accomplish green chemistry goals, including bottom-up strategies to develop new materials, synthetic strategies and processes in academic and industrial innovation and development (I&D) labs to develop sustainable process at an industrial level, and implementation of international regulation of chemicals use and chemical processes, which forces the chemical industry to change and move to sustainable chemistry.

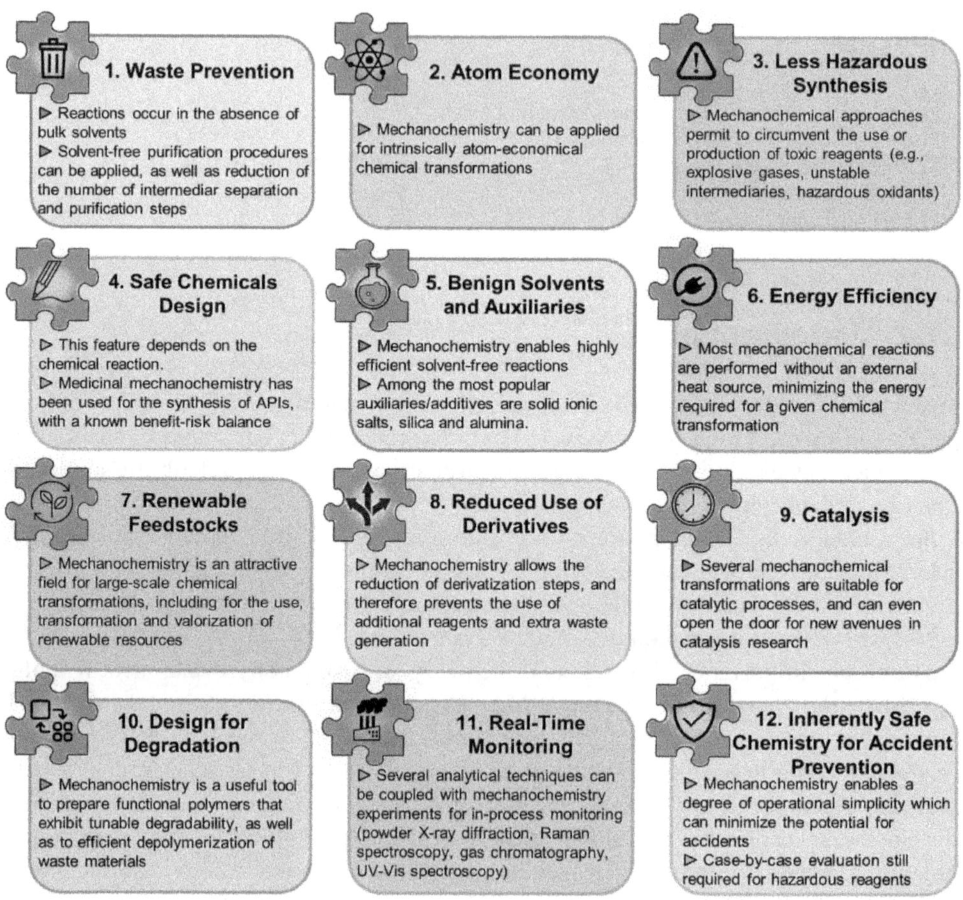

Figure 11.1 Mechanochemistry compliance with green chemistry principles.

The pharmaceutical industry is devoted to discovering, developing, producing, and commercialising drugs, in order to increase the life expectancy and life quality of patients. These advances are largely responsible for the increase, almost doubling, of life expectancy from 1900 to 2000. In contrast, the fine chemicals industry is one of the sectors that produce large amounts of chemical waste, potentially decreasing the health of the planet. To be able to increase life expectancy and the quality of populations while increasing the quality of life, the pharmaceutical industry was one of the sectors that first embraced the field of green chemistry [5]. The pharmaceutical industry offers some commonly used examples of reduced manufacturing costs of active pharmaceutical ingredients (APIs), including many award-winning green chemistry technologies, such as the eight Presidential Green Chemistry Challenge programme awards that were attributed to companies working in this sector [6]. In 2005, the ACS Green Chemistry Institute® and several worldwide pharmaceutical companies founded the ACS GCI Pharmaceutical Roundtable, currently composed of 22 pharmaceutical companies and 19 associate and affiliate companies, to promote innovation while encouraging the assimilation of green chemistry and green engineering in the production of medicines. These industry competitors collaborate to find alternatives and solutions to the environmental impact of the pharmaceutical industry [7].

To address the goals of green chemistry, several approaches can be used and combined. From the reactivity point of view, one-pot, domino, or multicomponent reactions are desirable, as well as regio- and stereoselective synthetic procedures. Catalysis (acid–base and transition metals catalysis) and biocatalysis have an important impact in the increase of sustainability. Synthesis under non-classical conditions such as using supercritical fluids and alternative solvents, namely water and ionic liquids, and of course alternative activation methods are required.

One of the major causes of chemical waste in a chemical transformation is the use of solvent, identified as responsible for more than 80% of the waste produced in a chemical transformation [8]. Once the major cause of waste had been acknowledged, the solution to the waste problem was clear – remove the reaction solvent – but it did not seem to be an easy solution to implement, since the phrase attributed to Aristotle, ‘corpora non agunt nisi fluida seu solute’ (compounds do not react unless fluid or if dissolved), was a general belief among chemists [2, 9].

Mechanochemistry is a branch of chemistry that comprises the chemical and physicochemical transformations of substances in all states of aggregation, produced by the effect of mechanical energy [10]. Solvent-free reactions may efficiently evolve in homogeneous conditions, that is as solid–gas or solid–liquid mixtures. However, heterogeneous systems pose more challenges in order to develop efficient chemical reactions. To carry out reactions in solid–solid state without solvents, it is required to provide the necessary energy to the reactants, which could be achieved in the high-pressure conditions produced by mechanical action.

A mechanochemical reaction was defined in the Gold Book of the International Union of Pure and Applied Chemistry (IUPAC) as “a chemical reaction that is induced by the direct absorption of mechanical energy” [11]. Although mechanochemical reactions have been around for many centuries, namely for inorganic reactions, their application in organic chemical transformations is rather recent.

11.2 Mechanochemistry for Sustainable Processes

For the chemical industry, and for sustainable API production, green chemistry and its 12 principles emerged as guidelines for the design and construction of new synthetic routes [12, 13]. The recent focus by synthetic organic chemists on mechanochemistry is highly driven by this demand for the development of green synthetic alternatives.

The first obvious advantage is intertwined with green chemistry's first principle, waste prevention, as mechanochemical approaches allow reactions of different substances under solvent-free conditions, or by applying small amounts of liquid reaction media (liquid-assisted grinding, LAG), as will be addressed later in this chapter. Solvents are a major contribution to waste production in conventional chemical transformations (reaction, separation, and purification steps all often require considerable amounts of solvents). Mechanochemical transformations are feasible to generate chemical reactivity in the absence of bulk solvents. However, they might still require considerable amounts of solvents for work-up procedures [14]. To circumvent this requirement, researchers have already described the possibility of coupling solvent-free mechanochemical protocols with purification procedures that do not require solvents, such as sublimation [15, 16], or other less energy-consuming purification techniques such as filtration, requiring minimal amounts of water or organic solvents [17, 18]. The use of mechanochemistry to perform multicomponent reactions [19, 20] or multistep synthesis also reduces waste production [21, 22] by decreasing the number of intermediary separation and purification steps.

The second green chemistry principle is atom economy. With the incorporation of all of the reactant atoms in a single final product, atom economy is a concept at the centre of green chemical transformations [23]. More than the activation technique used, a good atom economy is intrinsically related to the chemical transformation being studied. Nevertheless, mechanochemistry has been successfully employed in several of these transformations (e.g. cycloadditions, isomerisations, molecular rearrangements) and has proved to be a suitable alternative for metal-organic framework synthesis, with a better atom economy index than well-established protocols [24, 25].

Less hazardous chemical synthesis is the third green chemistry principle, and it is intrinsically related to the properties of the starting materials and products (and by-products) of a given chemical transformation. However, several examples showcase how mechanochemistry can avoid the usage or production of toxic substances, such as explosive gases, by applying safer reagents than conventional chemical transformations [14].

The fourth principle, designing safer chemicals, is quite dependent on the final product to be obtained. If we consider APIs as compounds with a well-established benefit–risk assessment and balance, thorough knowledge of potential by-products of their synthesis, and overall safety in terms of human and environmental health should be known. It is noteworthy that mechanochemical approaches have been successfully applied to the synthesis of APIs [26, 27], as will be detailed later in this chapter. Mechanochemistry, in particular ball milling, can also be used for studies on drugs' stability under mechanical stress [28].

Safer or benign solvents and auxiliaries, the fifth principle of green chemistry, can be easily attained using mechanochemistry approaches, for the reasons already described. By removing or decreasing to a minimal level the solvent requirements for a chemical transformation, mechanochemistry can enable highly efficient solvent-free reactions and therefore meet this principle. Furthermore, exploring solvent-free protocols under mechanochemistry allowed the synthesis of products that were difficult to access using conventional methodologies [14]. In the case of LAG, the use of catalytic volumes of solvents can operate in multiple ways, whereas it can help to mimic the potential of a bulk solvent to accelerate or steer chemical transformations, or even to discover and tune chemical reactivity [29, 30]. It is important to understand that in LAG, the solvent is placed in the reaction vessel not to operate strictly as a reaction medium, but to work as a catalytic additive. From the sustainability point of view, the small quantities employed make their use acceptable, regardless of their safety profile. In what concerns solid auxiliaries, ionic salts (such as sodium chloride), silica, and alumina are among the most used in mechanochemistry. Larger amounts are required when compared to LAG, because their role is to dilute the reaction mixture or to disperse catalysts. They can also absorb reactants, making the mixtures physically more suitable for the milling process. These additives will necessarily cause more waste, and therefore their application should be critically evaluated for the desired transformation [31, 32].

As far as energy efficiency is concerned, mechanochemistry can also make a strong contribution to meeting this green chemistry principle. Most mechanochemical transformations occur without external heating, minimising the energy required for a given chemical process, especially when compared to their solvothermal counterparts. Despite the high value of achieving chemical transformations without external heating from the energy and process safety points of view, temperature control in mechanochemical transformations can be a suitable option to increase the efficiency, reproducibility, and robustness of this kind of process [14, 33–35].

The use of renewable feedstocks, the seventh principle of green chemistry, also caught the attention of researchers working in the field of mechanochemistry. Easy-to-perform protocols allow the polymerisation, modification, and/or depolymerisation of relevant biopolymers, such as chitin [36, 37], cellulose [38, 39], lignin [40, 41], among others. The use of biomass as starting point to achieve high-value products, including materials, has also been reported [42, 43].

Reducing the use of chemical derivatives, corresponding to the eighth principle of green chemistry, can be achieved in mechanochemistry by reducing derivatisation steps, simplifying the synthetic route, and preventing the use of additional reagents and generation of extra waste. One good example of the suitability of mechanochemistry to avoid over-processing of raw materials is the use of mineral ores as catalysts directly in mechanochemical transformations, without their use to refine the material to a pure inorganic metal catalyst, or even as a replacement for classical bases [14, 44–46].

Concerning catalysis, the ninth green chemistry principle, mechanochemistry has opened the door to new endeavours in the field of catalysis research. For example, the surface itself of the milling medium/container/balls can operate as a catalyst for a given chemical transformation [47, 48]. Mechanochemistry apparatus has also proven to be suitable for a wide range of metal catalysts [49], organocatalysts [50, 51], and biocatalysts [52].

The design for degradation principle is highly oriented to material synthesis in the mechanochemistry context. Several efforts have been developed to generate mechanochemical protocols to prepare functional polymers with tunable degradability [14].

Over the past few years, considerable efforts have been dedicated to real-time monitoring of mechanochemical reactions, increasing the compliance with principle eleven of green chemistry. To achieve this goal, several analytical techniques were successfully coupled with mechanochemistry equipment, including synchrotron powder X-ray diffraction [53],

Raman spectroscopy [54], real-time thermal sensors [55], real-time manometric monitoring [56], gas chromatography [57], non-dispersive infrared spectroscopy [58], X-ray absorption spectroscopy [59], X-ray diffraction [59], solid state nuclear magnetic resonance (NMR) [60], real-time UV-Vis spectroscopy [61], and so on. The implementation of in-process control systems in the field of mechanochemistry allows the elucidation of reaction mechanisms, as well as investigation of the correlation between mechanochemical parameters and the course of the chemical reaction.

The development of inherently safe chemistry for accident prevention, the twelfth principle of green chemistry, is driven, in the case of mechanochemistry, by the level of operational simplicity required, which can help to reduce risks and accident potential. Nevertheless, transformations requiring contact-unstable or explosive reactants need to have their risk potential assessed for each case, especially when scaling-up procedures are considered [62, 63]. The previously described real-time monitoring, as well as the development of low-temperature mechanochemical protocols, can also be suitable options to perform chemical transformations under safe conditions, namely exothermic reactions [33].

Figure 11.1 illustrates the main features of mechanochemical transformations, supporting their application under the 12 principles of green chemistry. It becomes clear that the use of mechanochemistry can provide green synthetic protocols for well-established reactions, as well as to discover new chemical reactivity and synthetic routes, and to prepare elusive products under mild conditions that could not be prepared under conventional conditions.

11.3 Mechanochemistry Apparatus

The birth of mechanochemistry applied to organic chemistry is credited to the preparation of quinhydrone derivatives [64]. Following a slow start, mechanochemistry is one of the most recent techniques in organic synthesis and has great potential for the development of faster and cleaner solvent-free synthetic methodologies for pharmaceuticals [65]. This development goes hand in hand with the development of equipment to perform mechanochemistry at the lab scale.

Manual grinding, performed using a mortar and a pestle, was the first approach used to perform mechanochemical transformations in the lab [66] and was extended to all types of laboratories, including industry, academia, and secondary schools. However, the high reliance on the operator and consequent lack of reproducibility led to the search for the development of alternatives. Nowadays there are several types of grinding and milling apparatus of diverse brands commercially available, including automatic mortars. Among them can be highlighted ball milling instruments that include planetary ball mills and vibrational ball mills, and extruders. These ball milling systems are an automated apparatus that enables the control of energy input by adjusting the milling frequency, allowing an increase in reproducibility and performing reactions with longer reaction times [67]. The main difference between them is the type of movement to promote mechanical energy input: planetary ball mills involve rotation, and mixer milling systems are based on back-and-forth swinging. These laboratory-scale systems were designed for batch production and could suffer from some reactor cleaning issues, especially when the final reaction crude is not a free-flowing powder and the goal is to keep the entire process solvent free [68].

In addition, mechanochemical reactions can also be performed via flow extrusion techniques, where the mixing of solid materials is promoted by forcing them through constrained spaces. This is an alternative mechanochemical process with great interest for the pharmaceutical industry, but with limitations for the laboratory-scale development phase of drugs, which requires the synthesis of a large number of molecules [69]. Depending on the device used, the mechanical energy could be afforded via impact, compression, shear, or friction, as depicted in Figure 11.2.

Several processes occur during mechanical grinding of solids, such as generation of new surfaces, formation of dislocations and point defects in the crystalline structure, as well as decrease of the particle size and phase transformations. The occurrence of chemical reactions, which has been associated with the heat generated in the milling process and favoured by phase transformations and the large area of contact between the solids, has been explained using different models, namely the hot-spot theory [70–72], the magma-plasma model [73], the hierarchical model [74, 75], or the theory of short-lived active centres [76].

The limitations and capabilities of mechanochemistry to scale up depend on the type of equipment and technology used [77]. Ball mills, mixer mills, or planetary mills are batch-mode systems, and their scaling up and applicability in the chemical industry, and particularly in the pharmaceutical industry, have some limitations mainly due to safety issues, as well as to localised hot spots and temperature control. However, extrusion (twin and single-screw extruders) works in flow mode and has been used in the transformation industry. Extrusion, along with flow chemistry in solution, was identified by IUPAC as one of the top ten most relevant chemical innovations that could change the world [78]. These techniques can provide a scalable continuous solution and, when fully developed, lead to the full implementation of mechanochemistry in industry.

11.4 Selected Examples of Active Pharmaceutical Ingredient Production Using Mechanochemistry

A wide range of equipment can be used to carry out API synthesis under mechanochemical conditions. From the examples reported in the literature, ball milling is by far the method most commonly used by researchers.

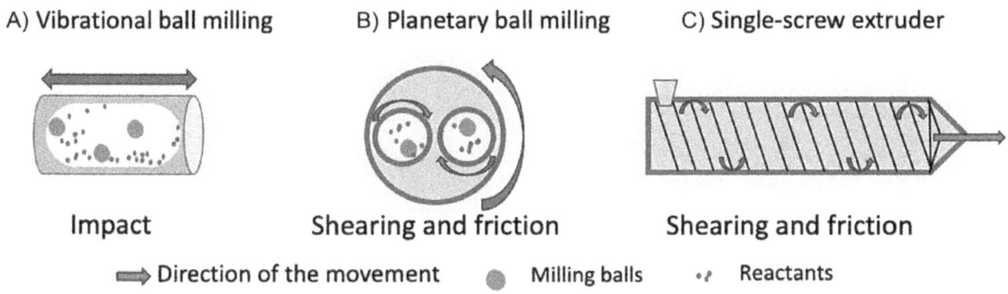

Figure 11.2 Schematic representation of (A) vibrational ball milling; (B) planetary ball milling; and (C) single-screw extruder.

Portada et al. explored the catalytic transfer hydrogenation of aromatic nitro derivatives under mechanochemical conditions, and applied it successfully to two well-established APIs [79], the analgesic and antipyretic paracetamol (or acetaminophen) [80] and the anti-arrhythmic procainamide [81]. Paracetamol was obtained by solvent-free sequential mechanochemical hydrogenation of *p*-nitrophenol and acetylation of the newly formed amino group (Figure 11.3A). Silica was used as a solid grinding auxiliary in both steps. In the case of procainamide, a two-step procedure was also designed and optimised, with the first step consisting of the amide coupling of 4-nitrobenzoylchloride and *N,N*-diethylenediamine promoted by potassium carbonate to afford a 4-nitrobenzoyldiethylenediamine precursor, which after chromatography-free purification (88% yield) was subjected to catalytic transfer hydrogenation under LAG conditions (methanol was used as auxiliary) to provide the desired API quantitatively (Figure 11.3B) [79].

Sulfonylureas, widely used in clinical practice in treatment of type 2 diabetes [82], are a class of drugs that has been widely studied in synthetic approaches using mechanochemistry. Friščić and co-workers [83] reported the synthesis of first-generation sulfonylureas tolbutamide and chlorpropamide using ball milling under LAG reaction conditions. The synthetic protocol consisted in promoting the copper(I)-catalysed coupling reaction between sulfonamides and isocyanates. Among the different catalysts screened, copper(I) chloride proved to be suitable to promote the synthesis of tolbutamide at high yield (91%) even in the absence of LAG. However, thorough screening of different grinding liquids showed that nitromethane enabled the reaction to occur with a similar yield (90%), but with a considerable decrease in the catalyst load required (from 20 mol% to 5 mol%), improving the overall sustainability of the synthetic protocol (Figure 11.4A). With the best conditions in hand, the researchers proved the protocol to be suitable for the synthesis of chlorpropamide (92% yield) (Figure 11.4B) and could also be adapted to a two-step mechanochemical protocol for the synthesis of second-generation glibenclamide (92% yield) (Figure 11.4C) [83]. Later on, the same group explored the synthesis of tolbutamide using the same

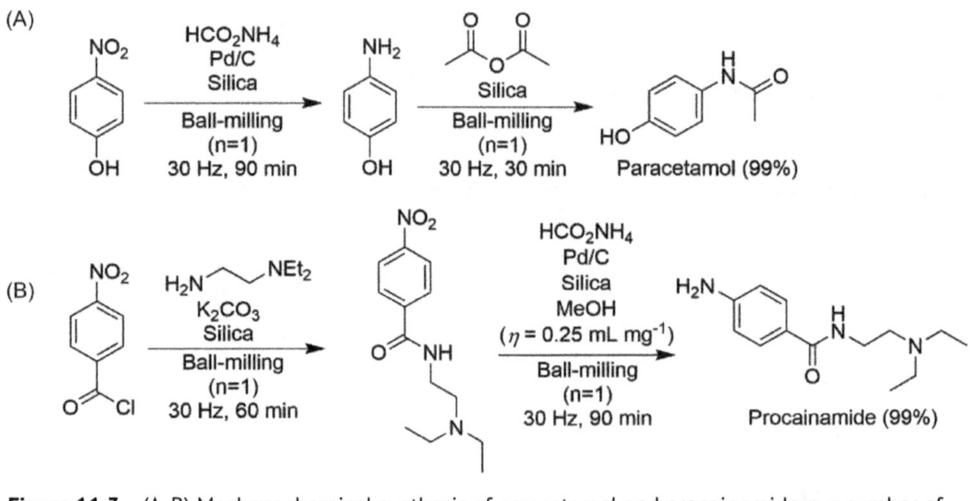

Figure 11.3 (A, B) Mechanochemical synthesis of paracetamol and procainamide. n = number of balls placed in the ball mill.

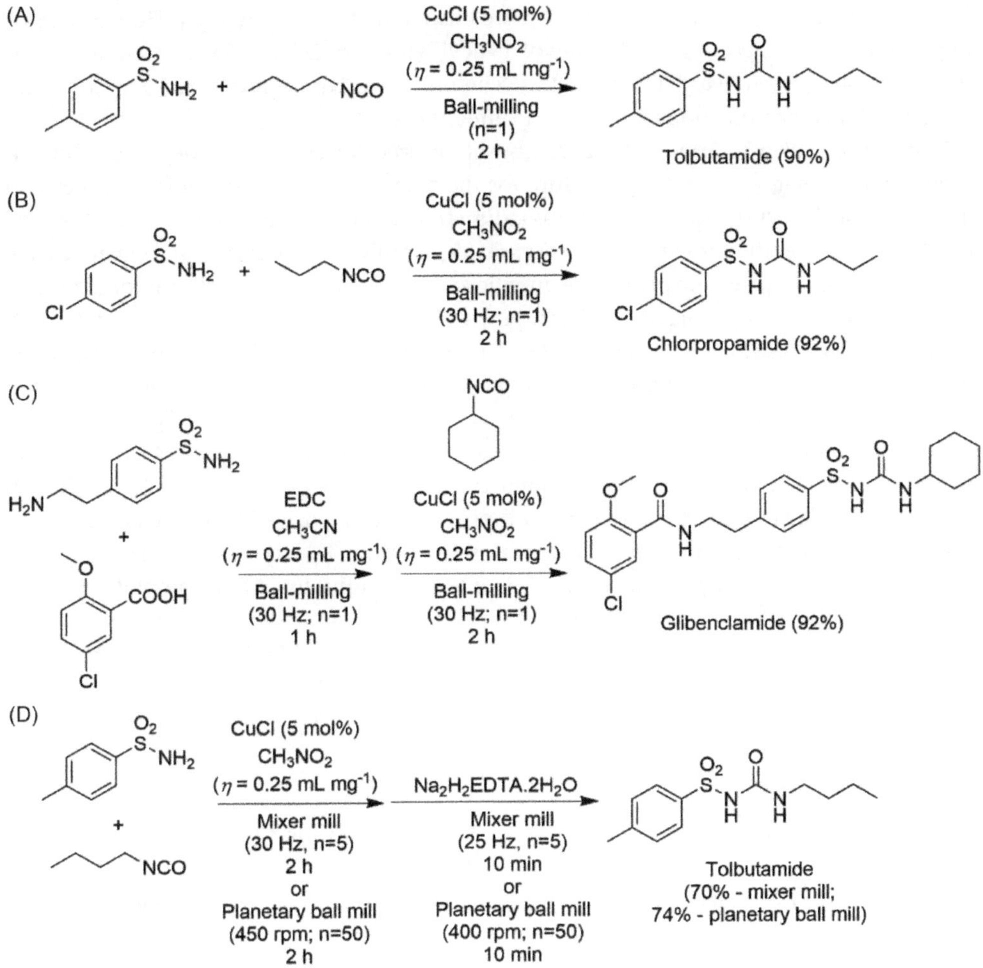

Figure 11.4 (A–D) Mechanochemical synthesis of sulfonylureas. n = number of balls placed in the ball mill; EDC, *N*-ethyl-*N'*-(3-dimethylaminopropyl)carbodiimide.

protocol, but this time assessing the suitability of this process for being performed in a mixer mill and in a planetary ball mill [84]. The synthetic process included a work-up step, performed under milling conditions, consisting of the addition of disodium dihydrogen ethylenediaminetetraacetate dihydrate ($Na_2H_2EDTA.2H_2O$) and water directly to the jar, for removal of the copper catalyst through a complexation reaction (Figure 11.4D). This example was developed in order to introduce the concept of mechanochemistry to students and showcase the sustainability inherent in the application of these technologies for the synthesis of APIs [84].

The versatility of mechanochemistry can also be portrayed by the ability to couple this methodology with other sustainable approaches. Jiang et al. highlighted this versatility by using a mechanochemical system to perform an enzyme-catalysed multicomponent reaction [85]. Antihypertensive calcium channel blockers felodipine and nifedipine,

1,4-dihydropyridine derivatives, were prepared using the three-component Hantzsch reaction, promoted by Lipozyme® (triacylglycerol acylhydrolase, EC3.1.1.3), in moderate yields (69% and 54%, respectively) (Figure 11.5). The only auxiliary required was sodium chloride, which is very innocuous for the environment [85].

Enzymes can also be applied for deracemisation procedures. Pérez-Venegas and Juaristi reported a mechanoenzymatic procedure for the resolution of racemic chiral amines and applied it for the synthesis of API (*R*)-rasagiline [86], a monoamine oxidase inhibitor used as a therapeutic option for Parkinson's disease [87]. Briefly, immobilised *Candida antarctica* Lipase B (CALB) enzyme promotes the enantioselective acylation of (*R*)-1-aminoindan with ethyl acetate as the acylating agent. Next, propargyl mesylate was added, affording the (*S*)-enantiomer of rasagiline. The acylated (*R*)-1-aminoindan is then deprotected in the presence of an acid, and the resulting enantiomeric pure (*R*)-1-aminoindan was milled with propargyl mesylate to achieve the final (*R*)-rasagiline in enantiopure form (Figure 11.6) [86].

Teriflunomide, a drug approved for the treatment of multiple sclerosis [88], was synthesised using planetary ball milling through the use of *N,N'*-carbonyldiimidazole (CDI)-promoted amide bond formation. After milling 5-methyl-4-isoxazolecarboxylic acid in the presence of CDI for 20 minutes, 4-(trifluoromethyl)aniline hydrochloride was added, and the reaction allowed to proceed under solvent-free conditions. After completion of the

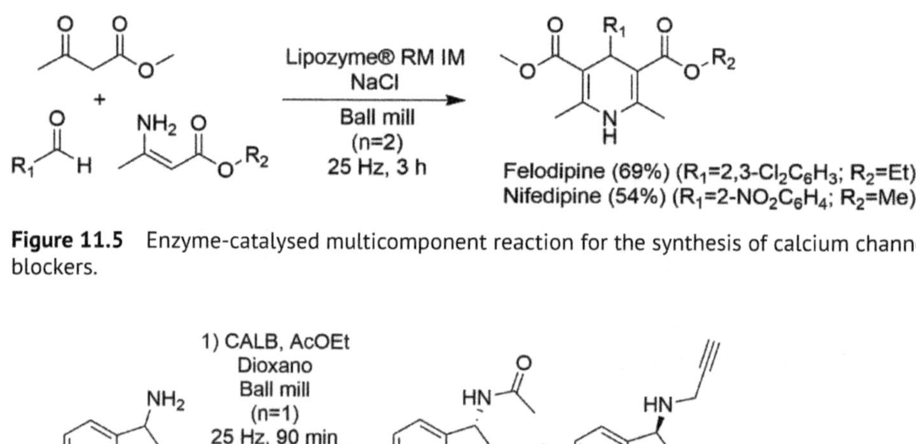

Figure 11.5 Enzyme-catalysed multicomponent reaction for the synthesis of calcium channel blockers.

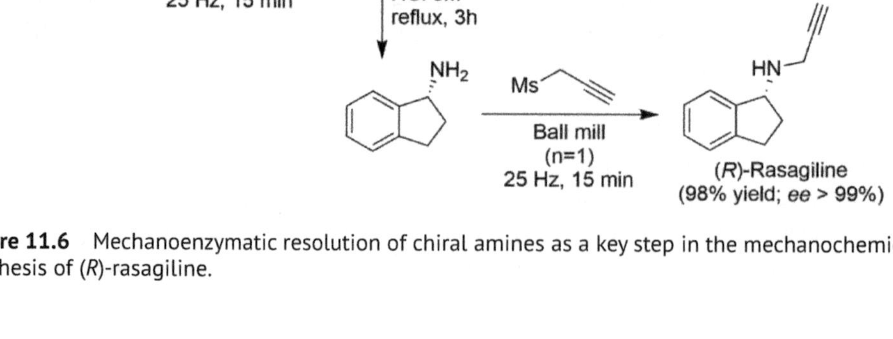

Figure 11.6 Mechanoenzymatic resolution of chiral amines as a key step in the mechanochemical synthesis of (*R*)-rasagiline.

reaction, water was added and milled with the crude reaction, in order to optimise the transfer to a round-bottomed flask, to promote the isoxazole ring opening in acidic conditions (Figure 11.7) [89].

Yu and co-workers recently reported the use of a planetary ball mill to attain the API axitinib [90], a drug used in clinical practice for the treatment of renal cell carcinoma [91]. A total of five reaction steps were performed under mechanochemical conditions, including palladium-catalysed Heck-Migita coupling (Figure 11.8). This is a clear example of the application of mechanochemistry for multistep synthesis, where fine tuning of the reaction conditions can lead to satisfactory yields and great environmental gains [90].

Another example of API synthesis using a planetary ball mill was reported by Colacino and co-workers [92]. In this case, phenytoin, used as an antiseizure drug in the treatment of epilepsy [93], was successfully prepared using a water-assisted mechanochemical protocol. Briefly, using 5,5-diphenylglycine methyl ester hydrochloride as a starting material, in the

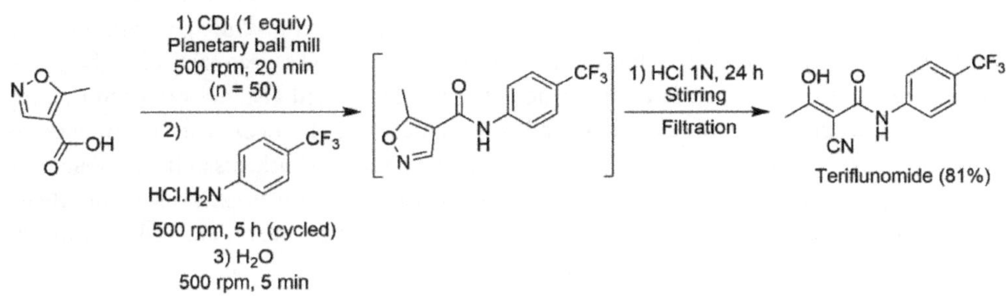

Figure 11.7 Mechanochemical synthesis of teriflunomide.

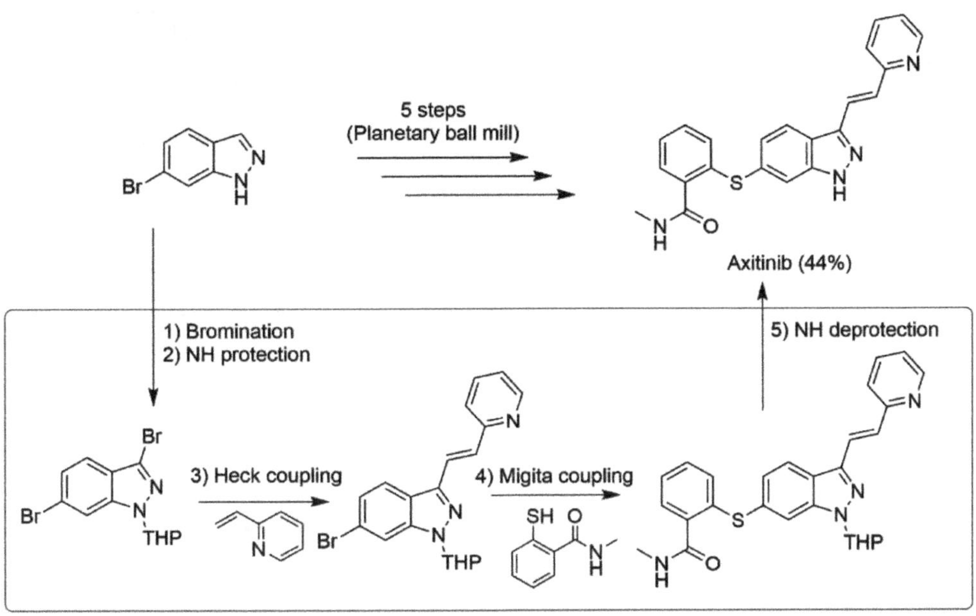

Figure 11.8 Multistep mechanochemical synthesis of axitinib.

presence of an excess of trimethylsilyl isocyanate (TMS-NCO) and water, leads to in situ formation of the base hexamethyldisilazane (HMDS), crucial for the formation of the amino nucleophile, after hydrolysis of the *N*-protected trimethylsilyl group. In a second step, caesium carbonate is added and ground with the mixture, to afford the final phenytoin at a very good yield (84%), without the requirement of a chromatography work-up procedure, which contributes to the overall sustainability of this synthetic process (Figure 11.9).

Another hydantoin derivative, the muscle relaxant dantrolene used in the treatment of malignant hyperthermia [94], was also synthesised using a mechanochemical approach. The main novelty featured in this synthetic protocol is the ability to monitor the reaction by in situ Raman spectroscopy, enabled by the use of translucid poly(methyl methacrylate) (PMMA) plastic ball mills (Figure 11.10A). This approach was also carried out using a LAG procedure with acetonitrile [95].

In the same year, the same research group used this API as a model to explore another mechanochemistry apparatus, the twin-screw extrusion. As previously referred to, apart from the difference in the type of mechanical forces, the twin-screw extrusion system allows continuous manufacturing and easy scale-up of the API, while ball mill systems only enable batch production. The synthetic protocol, using the same reaction as the previous example, does not require the presence of any solvent, and also does not require any work-up procedure, supporting the overall compliance of this process with green chemistry principles. This mechanochemical apparatus also enabled synthesis of the antibacterial drug nitrofurantoin (Figure 11.10B) [96]. Twin-screw extrusion presents several advantages, since it can be easily fine-tuned, subjected to high temperatures, and when properly optimised can drastically reduce reaction time [35].

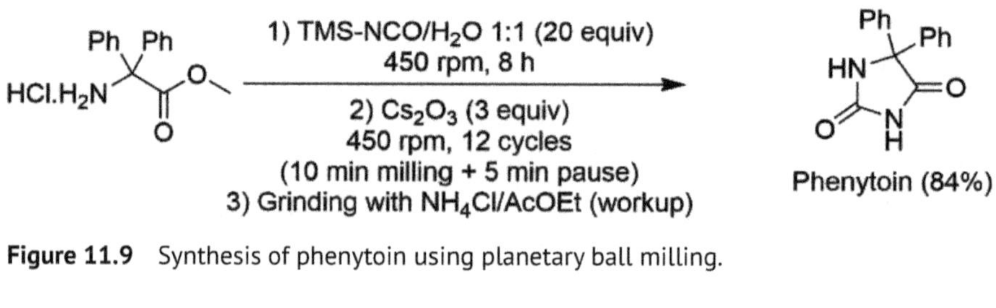

Figure 11.9 Synthesis of phenytoin using planetary ball milling.

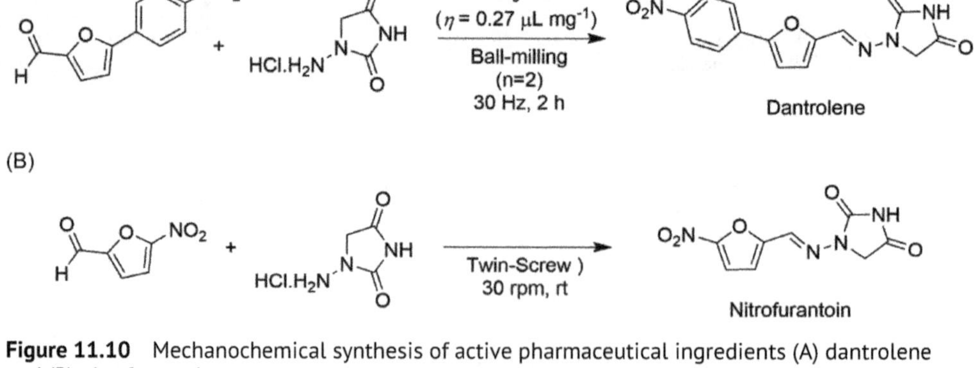

Figure 11.10 Mechanochemical synthesis of active pharmaceutical ingredients (A) dantrolene and (B) nitrofurantoin.

11.5 Conclusion

Mechanochemical approaches display several advantages for API synthesis, from the access to unexplored reactivity to the high compliance with sustainability parameters and green chemistry principles. The wide variety of apparatus, the number of variables to optimise, and safety concerns regarding scale-up procedures remain some of the most relevant challenges in years to come in the field of mechanochemistry. The still fairly unexplored field of continuous manufacturing under mechanochemical conditions might open the door to new, safer, and cleaner API synthesis protocols, easily applied in the industrial setting.

Acknowledgement

Authors thanks CQC supported by the Portuguese Agency for Scientific Research, "Fundação para a Ciência e a Tecnologia" (FCT) through projects UIDB/00313/2020 and UIDP/00313/2020, cofounded by COMPETE2020-UC and project CENTRO-45-2021-30 - Sistema de Apoio à Investigação Científica e Tecnológica (SAICT) - 01/SAICT/2021 - Projetos de Prova de Conceito (PdC); Project nº 180078. This work is financed by national funds through the FCT - Foundation for Science and Technology, I.P., under the project UIDB/04585/2020 (PB).

References

1 Brundtland, G.H. (1987). *Report of the World Commission on Environment and Development: Our Common Future*. Geneva: United Nations.
2 James, S.L., Adams, C.J., Bolm, C. et al. (2012). Mechanochemistry: opportunities for new and cleaner synthesis. *Chemical Society Reviews* 41: 413–447.
3 Halpaap, A. (2020). *Green and Sustainable Chemistry: Framework Manual*. Geneva: United Nations Environment Programme.
4 Horváth, I.T. (2018). Introduction: sustainable chemistry. *Chemical Reviews* 118 (2): 369–371.
5 Sheldon, R. (2010). Introduction to green chemistry, organic synthesis and pharmaceuticals. In: *Green Chemistry in the Pharmaceutical Industry* (eds. Dunn, P.J., Wells, A.S., and Williams, M.T.), ch. 1. Weinheim: Wiley.
6 Arnaut, L.G., Caldwell, R.A., Elbert, J.E., and Melton, L.A. (1992). Recent advances in photoacoustic calorimetry: theoretical basis and improvements in experimental design. *Review of Scientific Instruments* 63: 5381–5389.
7 ACS Green Chemistry Institute Pharmaceutical Roundtable. (2005). www.acsgcipr.org.
8 Curzons, A.D., Jiménez-González, C., Duncan, A.L., Constable, D.J.C., and Cunningham, V.L. (2007). Fast life cycle assessment of synthetic chemistry (FLASC™) tool. *International Journal of Life Cycle Assessment* 12: 272–280.
9 Tanaka, K., and Toda, F. (2000). Solvent-free organic synthesis. *Chemical Reviews* 100: 1025–1074.

10 Kajdas, C. (2013). General approach to mechanochemistry and its relation to tribochemistry. In: (ed. Pihtili, H.), *Tribology in Engineering*, ch. 11. Rijeka: InTech.

11 McNaught, A.D., and Wilkinson, A. (eds.) (1997). *IUPAC Compendium of Chemical Terminology*. Oxford: Blackwell Scientific Publications.

12 Anastas, P.T., and Warner, J.C. (1998). *Green Chemistry: Theory and Practice*. Oxford: Oxford University Press.

13 Anastas, P., and Eghbali, N. (2010). Green chemistry: principles and practice. *Chemical Society Reviews* 39: 301–312.

14 Ardila-Fierro, K.J., and Hernández, J.G. (2021). Sustainability assessment of mechanochemistry by using the twelve principles of green chemistry. *ChemSusChem* 14 (10): 2145–2162.

15 Huskić, I., Halasz, I., Friščić, T., and Vančik, H. (2012). Mechanosynthesis of nitrosobenzenes: a proof-of-principle study in combining solvent-free synthesis with solvent-free separations. *Green Chemistry* 14: 1597.

16 Qareaghaj, O.H., Mashkouri, S., Naimi-Jamal, M.R., and Kaupp, G. (2014). Ball milling for the quantitative and specific solvent-free Knoevenagel condensation + Michael addition cascade in the synthesis of various 2-amino-4-aryl-3-cyano-4H-chromenes without heating. *RSC Advances* 4: 48191–48201.

17 Ding, W., Wang, C., Tan, J.R. et al. (2020). Site-selective aromatic C–H λ3-iodanation with a cyclic iodine(iii) electrophile in solution and solid phases. *Chemical Science* 11: 7356–7361.

18 Métro, T.-X., Bonnamour, J., Reidon, T. et al. (2015). Comprehensive study of the organic-solvent-free CDI-mediated acylation of various nucleophiles by mechanochemistry. *Chemistry Europe* 21 (36): 12787–12796.

19 Leonardi, M., Villacampa, M., and Menéndez, J.C. (2018). Multicomponent mechanochemical synthesis. *Chemical Science* 9: 2042–2064.

20 Polindara-García, L.A., and Juaristi, E. (2016). Synthesis of Ugi 4-CR and Passerini 3-CR adducts under mechanochemical activation. *European Journal of Organic Chemistry* 6: 1095–1102.

21 Ferguson, M., Giri, N., Huang, X., Apperley, D., and James, S.L. (2014). One-pot two-step mechanochemical synthesis: ligand and complex preparation without isolating intermediates. *Green Chemistry* 16: 1374–1382.

22 Zhao, Y., Rocha, S.V., and Swager, T.M. (2016). Mechanochemical synthesis of extended iptycenes. *Journal of the American Chemical Society* 138 (42): 13834–13837.

23 Trost, B.M. (1991). The atom economy – a search for synthetic efficiency. *Science* 254 (5037): 1471–1477.

24 Mottillo, C., and Friščić, T. (2017). Advances in solid-state transformations of coordination bonds: from the ball mill to the aging chamber. *Molecules* 22 (1): 144.

25 Stolar, T., and Užarević, K. (2020). Mechanochemistry: an efficient and versatile toolbox for synthesis, transformation, and functionalization of porous metal–organic frameworks. *CrystEngComm* 22: 4511–4525.

26 Pérez-Venegas, M., and Juaristi, E. (2020). Mechanochemical and mechanoenzymatic synthesis of pharmacologically active compounds: a green perspective. *ACS Sustainable Chemistry & Engineering* 8 (24): 8881–8893.

27 Ying, P., Yu, J., and Su, W. (2021). Liquid-assisted grinding mechanochemistry in the synthesis of pharmaceuticals. *Advanced Synthesis & Catalysis* 363 (5): 1246–1271.

28 Urlaub, J., Kaiser, R.P., Scherf-Clavel, O., Bolm, C., and Holzgrabe, U. (2021). Investigation of isomerization of dexibuprofen in a ball mill using chiral capillary electrophoresis. *Electrophoresis* 42 (17–18): 1790-1799.

29 Howard, J.L., Sagatov, Y., Repusseau, L., Schotten, C., and Browne, D.L. (2017). Controlling reactivity through liquid assisted grinding: the curious case of mechanochemical fluorination. *Green Chemistry* 19: 2798–2802.

30 Howard, J.L., Brand, M.C., and Browne, D.L. (2018). Switching chemoselectivity: using mechanochemistry to alter reaction kinetics. *Angewandte Chemie International Edition* 57 (49): 16104–16108.

31 Shao, Q.-L., Jiang, Z.-J., and Su, W.-K. (2018). Solvent-free mechanochemical Buchwald-Hartwig amination of aryl chlorides without inert gas protection. *Tetrahedron Letters* 59 (23): 2277–2280.

32 Szuppa, T., Stolle, A., Ondruschka, B., and Hopfe, W. (2010). An alternative solvent-free synthesis of nopinone under ball-milling conditions: investigation of reaction parameters. *ChemSusChem* 3: 1181–1191.

33 Andersen, J., and Mack, J. (2018). Insights into mechanochemical reactions at targetable and stable, sub-ambient temperatures. *Angewandte Chemie International Edition* 57 (40): 13062–13065.

34 Andersen, J., Brunemann, J., and Mack, J. (2019). Exploring stable, sub-ambient temperatures in mechanochemistry via a diverse set of enantioselective reactions. *Reaction Chemistry & Engineering* 4: 1229–1236.

35 Crawford, D.E. (2017). Extrusion – back to the future: using an established technique to reform automated chemical synthesis. *Beilstein Journal of Organic Chemistry* 13: 65–75.

36 Di Nardo, T., and Moores, A. (2019). Mechanochemical amorphization of chitin: impact of apparatus material on performance and contamination. *Beilstein Journal of Organic Chemistry* 15: 1217–1225.

37 Margoutidis, G., Parsons, V.H., Bottaro, C.S., Yan, N., and Kerton, F.M. (2018). Mechanochemical amorphization of α-chitin and conversion into oligomers of N-acetyl-D-glucosamine. *ACS Sustainable Chemistry & Engineering* 6 (2): 1662–1669.

38 Kaufman Rechulski, M.D., Käldström, M., Richter, U., Schüth, F., and Rinaldi, R. (2015). Mechanocatalytic depolymerization of lignocellulose performed on hectogram and kilogram scales. *Industrial & Engineering Chemistry Research* 54 (16): 4581–4592.

39 Shrotri, A., Lambert, L.K., Tanksale, A., and Beltramini, J. (2013). Mechanical depolymerisation of acidulated cellulose: understanding the solubility of high molecular weight oligomers. *Green Chemistry* 15 (10): 2761.

40 Kleine, T., Buendia, J., and Bolm, C. (2013). Mechanochemical degradation of lignin and wood by solvent-free grinding in a reactive medium. *Green Chemistry* 15 (1): 160–166.

41 Sun, C., Zheng, L., Xu, W., Dushkin, A.V., and Su, W. (2020). Mechanochemical cleavage of lignin models and lignin via oxidation and a subsequent base-catalyzed strategy. *Green Chemistry* 22 (11): 3489–3494.

42 Cova, C.M., and Luque, R. (2019). Advances in mechanochemical processes for biomass valorization. *BMC Chemical Engineering* 1: 16.

43 Muñoz-Batista, M.J., Rodriguez-Padron, D., Puente-Santiago, A.R., and Luque, R. (2018). Mechanochemistry: toward sustainable design of advanced nanomaterials for electrochemical energy storage and catalytic applications. *ACS Sustainable Chemistry & Engineering* 6 (8): 9530–9544.

44 Anselmi, M., Stavole, P., Boanini, E. et al. (2020). Green synthesis of bioactive oligopeptides promoted by recyclable nanocrystalline hydroxyapatite. *Future Medicinal Chemistry* 12 (6): 479–491.

45 Landeros, J.M., and Juaristi, E. (2017). Mechanochemical synthesis of dipeptides using Mg-Al hydrotalcite as activating agent under solvent-free reaction conditions. European Journal of Organic Chemistry 2017 (3): 687–694.

46 Puccetti, F., Schumacher, C., Wotruba, H., Hernández, J.G., and Bolm, C. (2020). The use of copper and vanadium mineral ores in catalyzed mechanochemical carbon–carbon bond formations. *ACS Sustainable Chemistry & Engineering* 8 (19): 7262–7266.

47 Haley, R.A., Mack, J., and Guan, H. (2017). 2-in-1: catalyst and reaction medium. *Inorganic Chemistry Frontiers* 4 (1): 52–55.

48 Pickhardt, W., Grätz, S., and Borchardt, L. (2020). Direct mechanocatalysis: using milling balls as catalysts. *Chemistry Europe* 26 (57): 12903–12911.

49 Porcheddu, A., Colacino, E., De Luca, L., and Delogu, F. (2020). Metal-mediated and metal-catalyzed reactions under mechanochemical conditions. *ACS Catalysis* 10 (15): 8344–8394.

50 Chauhan, P., and Chimni, S.S. (2012). Mechanochemistry assisted asymmetric organocatalysis: a sustainable approach. *Beilstein Journal of Organic Chemistry* 8: 2132–2141.

51 Williams, M.T.J., Morrill, L.C., and Browne, D.L. (2022). Mechanochemical organocatalysis: do high enantioselectivities contradict what we might expect? *ChemSusChem* 15 (2): e202102157.

52 Pérez-Venegas, M., and Juaristi, E. (2021). Mechanoenzymology: state of the art and challenges towards highly sustainable biocatalysis. *ChemSusChem* 14 (3): 2682–2688.

53 Friščić, T., Halasz, I., Beldon, P.J. et al. (2013). Real-time and in situ monitoring of mechanochemical milling reactions. *Nature Chemistry* 5: 66–73.

54 Gracin, D., Štrukil, V., Friščić, T., Halasz, I., and Užarević, K. (2014). Laboratory real-time and in situ monitoring of mechanochemical milling reactions by raman spectroscopy. *Angewandte Chemie International Edition* 53 (24): 6193–6197.

55 Užarević, K., Ferdelji, N., Mrla, T. et al. (2018). Enthalpy vs. friction: heat flow modelling of unexpected temperature profiles in mechanochemistry of metal–organic frameworks. *Chemical Science* 9 (9): 2525–2532.

56 Brekalo, I., Yuan, W., Mottillo, C. et al. (2020). Manometric real-time studies of the mechanochemical synthesis of zeolitic imidazolate frameworks. *Chemical Science* 11 (8): 2141–2147.

57 Temnikov, M.N., Anisimov, A.A., Zhemchugov, P.V. et al. (2018). Mechanochemistry – a new powerful green approach to the direct synthesis of alkoxysilanes. *Green Chemistry* 20 (9): 1962–1969.

58 Eckert, R., Felderhoff, M., and Schüth, F. (2017). Preferential carbon monoxide oxidation over copper-based catalysts under in situ ball milling. *Angewandte Chemie International Edition* 56 (9): 2445–2448.

59 De Oliveira, P.F.M., Michalchuk, A.A.L., Buzanich, A.G. et al. (2020). Tandem X-ray absorption spectroscopy and scattering for in situ time-resolved monitoring of gold nanoparticle mechanosynthesis. *Chemical Communications* 56 (71): 10329–10332.

60 Schiffmann, J.G., Emmerling, F., Martins, I.C.B., and Van Wüllen, L. (2020). In-situ reaction monitoring of a mechanochemical ball mill reaction with solid state NMR. *Solid State Nuclear Magnetic Resonance* 109: 101687.

61 May, P.A., Munaretto, N.F., Hamoy, M.B., Robb, M.J., and Moore, J.S. (2016). Is molecular weight or degree of polymerization a better descriptor of ultrasound-induced mechanochemical transduction? *ACS Macro Letters* 5 (2): 177–180.

62 Achar, T.K., Maiti, S., and Mal, P. (2014). IBX works efficiently under solvent free conditions in ball milling. *RSC Advances* 4 (25): 12834–12839.

63 Alam, M.T., Maiti, S., and Mal, P. (2018). The mechanochemical synthesis of quinazolin-4(3H)-ones by controlling the reactivity of IBX. *Beilstein Journal of Organic Chemistry* 14: 2396–2403.

64 Ling, A.R., and Baker, J.L. (1893). XCVI.—Halogen derivatives of quinone. Part III. Derivatives of quinhydrone. *Journal of the Chemical Society, Transactions* 63: 1314–1327.

65 Tan, D., Loots, L., and Friščić, T. (2016). Towards medicinal mechanochemistry: evolution of milling from pharmaceutical solid form screening to the synthesis of active pharmaceutical ingredients (APIs). *Chemical Communications* 52 (50): 7760–7781.

66 Takacs, L. (2013). The historical development of mechanochemistry. *Chemical Society Reviews* 42 (18): 7649.

67 Stolle, A., Szuppa, T., Leonhardt, S.E.S., and Ondruschka, B. (2011). Ball milling in organic synthesis: solutions and challenges. *Chemical Society Reviews* 40: 2317–2329.

68 Beyer, M.K., and Clausen-Schaumann, H. (2005). Mechanochemistry: the mechanical activation of covalent bonds. *Chemical Reviews* 105 (8): 2921–2948.

69 Thiry, J., Krier, F., and Evrard, B. (2015). A review of pharmaceutical extrusion: critical process parameters and scaling-up. *International Journal of Pharmaceutics* 479 (1): 227–240.

70 Bowden, F.P., and Yoffe, A.D. (1985). *Initiation and Growth of Explosion in Liquids and Solids*. Cambridge: Cambridge University Press.

71 Boldyrev, V.V. (1990). Mechanochemistry and mechanical activation of solids. *Bulletin of the Academy of Sciences of the USSR Division of Chemical Science* 39: 2029–2044.

72 Urakaev, F.K., and Boldyrev, V.V. (2000). Mechanism and kinetics of mechanochemical processes in comminuting devices: 2. Applications of the theory. Experiment. *Powder Technology* 107: 197–206.

73 Thiessen, P.A., Meyer, K., and Heinicke, G. (1967). *Grundlagen der Tribochemie*. Berlin: Akademie.

74 Balaz, P. (2008). *Mechanochemistry in Nanoscience and Minerals Engineering*. Berlin: Springer.

75 Heegn, H. (1988). Change in the properties of solids during mechanical activation and fine comminution. *Siberian Chemistry Journal* 2 (1): 3–9.

76 Streletskii, A.N., and Butyagin, P.Y. (1973). Nature of luminescence observed during deformation, breaking and friction of polymers. *Vysokomolekulyarnye Soedineniya Seriya A* 15: 654–661.

77 Bolt, R.R.A., Leitch, J.A., Jones, A.C., Nicholson, W.I., and Browne, D.L. (2022). Continuous flow mechanochemistry: reactive extrusion as an enabling technology in organic synthesis. *Chemical Society Reviews* 51 (11): 4243–4260.

78 Gomollón-Bel, F. (2020). Ten chemical innovations that will change our world. The developing science that will fight the pandemic and reshape the chemical landscape. *Chemistry International* 42 (4): 3–9.

79 Portada, T., Margetić, D., and Štrukil, V. (2018). Mechanochemical catalytic transfer hydrogenation of aromatic nitro derivatives. *Molecules* 23 (12): 3163.

80 Prescott, L.F. (2000). Paracetamol: past, present, and future. *American Journal of Therapeutics* 7 (2): 143–147.

81 Trujillo, T.C., and Nolan, P.E. (2000). Antiarrhythmic agents. *Drug Safety* 23 (6): 509–532.

82 Sola, D., Rossi, L., Schianca, G.P.C. et al. (2015). Sulfonylureas and their use in clinical practice. *Archives of Medical Science* 11 (4): 840–848.

83 Tan, D., Štrukil, V., Mottillo, C., and Friščić, T. (2014). Mechanosynthesis of pharmaceutically relevant sulfonyl-(thio)ureas. *Chemical Communications* 50 (40): 5248–5250.

84 Colacino, E., Dayaker, G., Morère, A., and Friščić, T. (2019). Introducing students to mechanochemistry via environmentally friendly organic synthesis using a solvent-free mechanochemical preparation of the antidiabetic drug tolbutamide. *Journal of Chemical Education* 96: 766–771.

85 Jiang, L., Ye, L.-D., Gu, J.-L., Su, W.-K., and Ye, W.-T. (2019). Mechanochemical enzymatic synthesis of 1,4-dihydropyridine calcium antagonists and derivatives. *Journal of Chemical Technology & Biotechnology* 94 (8): 2555–2560.

86 Pérez-Venegas, M., and Juaristi, E. (2018). Mechanoenzymatic resolution of racemic chiral amines, a green technique for the synthesis of pharmaceutical building blocks. *Tetrahedron* 74 (44): 6453–6458.

87 Chang, Y., Wang, L.-B., Li, D., Lei, K., and Liu, S.-Y. (2017). Efficacy of rasagiline for the treatment of Parkinson's disease: an updated meta-analysis. *Annals of Medicine* 49 (5): 421–434.

88 Miller, A.E. (2021). An updated review of teriflunomide's use in multiple sclerosis. *Neurodegenerative Disease Management* 11 (5): 387–409.

89 Métro, T.-X., Bonnamour, J., Reidon, T. et al. (2012). Mechanosynthesis of amides in the total absence of organic solvent from reaction to product recovery. *Chemical Communications* 48 (96): 11781.

90 Yu, J., Hong, Z., Yang, X. et al. (2018). Bromide-assisted chemoselective Heck reaction of 3-bromoindazoles under high-speed ball-milling conditions: synthesis of axitinib. *Beilstein Journal of Organic Chemistry* 14: 786–795.

91 Keating, G.M. (2015). Axitinib: a review in advanced renal cell carcinoma. *Drugs* 75 (16): 1903–1913.

92 Konnert, L., Reneaud, B., De Figueiredo, R.M. et al. (2014). Mechanochemical preparation of hydantoins from amino esters: application to the synthesis of the antiepileptic drug phenytoin. *Journal of Organic Chemistry* 79 (21): 10132–10142.

93 Patocka, J., Wu, Q., Nepovimova, E., and Kuca, K. (2020). Phenytoin – an anti-seizure drug: overview of its chemistry, pharmacology and toxicology. *Food and Chemical Toxicology* 142: 111393.

94 Krause, T., Gerbershagen, M.U., Fiege, M., Weißhorn, R., and Wappler, F. (2004). Dantrolene – a review of its pharmacology, therapeutic use and new developments. *Anaesthesia* 59 (4): 364–373.

95 Sović, I., Lukin, S., Meštrović, E. et al. (2020). Mechanochemical preparation of active pharmaceutical ingredients monitored by in situ raman spectroscopy. *ACS Omega* 5 (44): 28663–28672.

96 Crawford, D.E., Porcheddu, A., McCalmont, A.S. et al. (2020). Solvent-free, continuous synthesis of hydrazone-based active pharmaceutical ingredients by twin-screw extrusion. *ACS Sustainable Chemistry & Engineering* 8 (32): 12230–12238.

Index

Sustainable Approaches in Pharmaceutical Sciences, First Edition. Edited by Kamal Shah, Durgesh Nandini Chauhan, and Nagendra Singh Chauhan.

l

m

n

o

p

q

r

s